Medical-Surgical
Nursing
at a Glance

This title is also available as an e-book.
For more details, please see
www.wiley.com/buy/9781118902752
or scan this QR code:

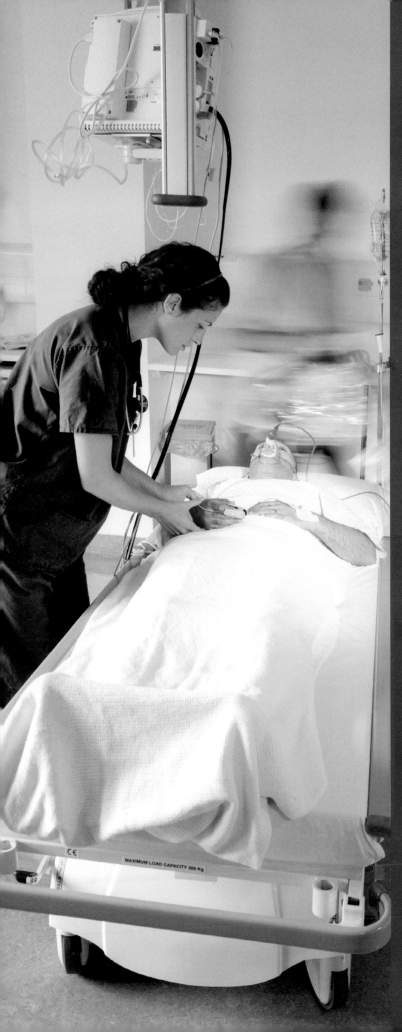

Medical-Surgical Nursing
at a Glance

Ian Peate

Professor of Nursing
Head of School
School of Health Studies
Gibraltar

Series editor: Ian Peate

WILEY Blackwell

This edition first published 2016 © 2016 by John Wiley & Sons Ltd.

Registered office: John Wiley & Sons, Ltd, The Atrium, Southern Gate, Chichester,
                     West Sussex, PO19 8SQ, UK

Editorial offices: 9600 Garsington Road, Oxford, OX4 2DQ, UK
                     The Atrium, Southern Gate, Chichester, West Sussex, PO19 8SQ, UK
                     350 Main Street, Malden, MA 02148-5020, USA

For details of our global editorial offices, for customer services and for information about how to apply for permission to reuse the copyright material in this book please see our website at www.wiley.com/wiley-blackwell

Library of Congress Cataloging-in-Publication Data
Peate, Ian, author.
  Medical-surgical nursing at a glance / Ian Peate.
    p. ; cm. -- (At a glance series)
  Includes bibliographical references and index.
  ISBN 978-1-118-90275-2 (pbk.)
  I. Title.   II. Series: At a glance series (Oxford, England)
  [DNLM: 1. Perioperative Nursing. 2. Nursing Care. 3. Nursing Process. WY 161]
  RT41
  610.73--dc23
                                                    2015024293

A catalogue record for this book is available from the British Library.

Wiley also publishes its books in a variety of electronic formats. Some content that appears in print may not be available in electronic books.

Cover image: © Getty Images/David Leahy

Set in 9.5/11.5pt Minion Pro by Aptara Inc., New Delhi, India
Printed and bound in Singapore by Markono Print Media Pte Ltd

1   2016

Contents

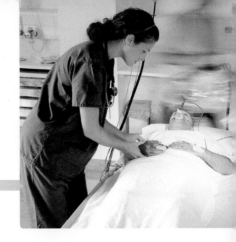

Part 4 Surgical nursing 103

Preface

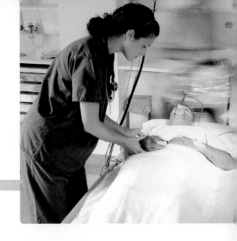

Medical-Surgical Nursing at a Glance is the ideal revision and consolidation book for undergraduate nurses and other healthcare workers. The text breaks down complex aspects of medical and surgical care in an accessible and inviting way against the backdrop of continually changing surroundings.

There have and there will continue to be many changes that will have an impact on the care that nurses offer patients in medical and surgical care settings. Key trends that may emerge over the next ten years or so are related to the socioeconomic and political environments, the health and care sectors, regulation concerning health and social care, the nursing and midwifery sectors as well as education and training provision for nurses and healthcare assistants. These changes will affect the ways in which nurses deliver care in the various health and social care settings. Rapid technological progress has the potential to alter the dynamic between the nurse and the patient. Telehealth is being increasingly used in providing healthcare along with the implementation of the electronic patient record.

Despite these changes, caring, kindness and compassion remain central to the role of the medical or surgical nurse. The use of an evidence base to offer care that is safe and effective is now a prerequirement of any healthcare provision.

This is a user-friendly, accessible aid for study and revision for preregistration nursing students. There are 77 chapters with 4 parts divided into medical and surgical nursing. The text adopts a concise and simple approach and is accompanied by detailed illustrations. The chapters are presented in bite sizes, in a double-page spread with colour diagrams, tables and line drawings. It is a practical text that addresses issues from a number of perspectives including anatomy and physiology, where relevant, and associated pathophysiology.

This book has been written to meet the needs of those working in the dynamic and ever-changing medical and surgical setting. The key aim of the book is to orientate and guide readers through the important and salient issues that they may face when providing safe and effective medical and surgical care. This text is offered at an introductory level, capturing all that the healthcare practitioner needs to know during their initial education and beyond. The approach used provides a better understanding of the issues related to medical and surgical nursing, walking the reader through the key issues and the significant points. The text reminds readers that there are physical and psychological issues that must be given careful consideration as well as recognising patient safety and the legal and ethical issues that must be taken into account when providing contemporary and up-to-date care.

The text builds on the strengths of existing 'At a Glance' titles already published; it is more accessible and less intimidating than other revision aids related to medical and surgical nursing. The At a Glance approach incorporates images and text, appealing to a number of learning styles.

I have enjoyed writing this text and I hope that you enjoy reading it.

Ian Peate

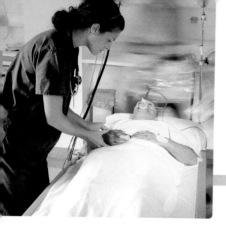

Acknowledgements

I would like to thank my partner Jussi Lahtinen for his enduring encouragement and Mrs Frances Cohen for her ongoing support. I acknowledge the help given to me by the library staff at St Bernard's Hospital, Gibraltar. Finally, I am indebted to my talented brother Anthony Peate who contributed to the illustrations.

Ian Peate

We acknowledge with thanks the use of material from other John Wiley & Sons publications:

Davey, P. (ed.) (2014) *Medicine at a Glance*, 4th edn.
Nair, M. and Peate, I. (2013) *Fundamentals of Applied Pathophysiology*, 2nd edn.
Nair, M. and Peate, I. (2015) *Pathophysiology for Nurses at a Glance*.
Peate, I. and Glencross, W. (2015) *Wound Care at a Glance*.
Peate, I., Wild, K. and Nair, M. (eds) (2014) *Nursing Practice*.
Wicker, P. (2015) *Perioperative Practice at a Glance*.

About the companion website

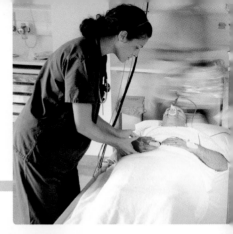

Don't forget to visit the companion website for this book:

www.ataglanceseries.com/nursing/medsurg

There you will find valuable material designed to enhance your learning, including interactive multiple choice questions.

Scan this QR code to visit the companion website.

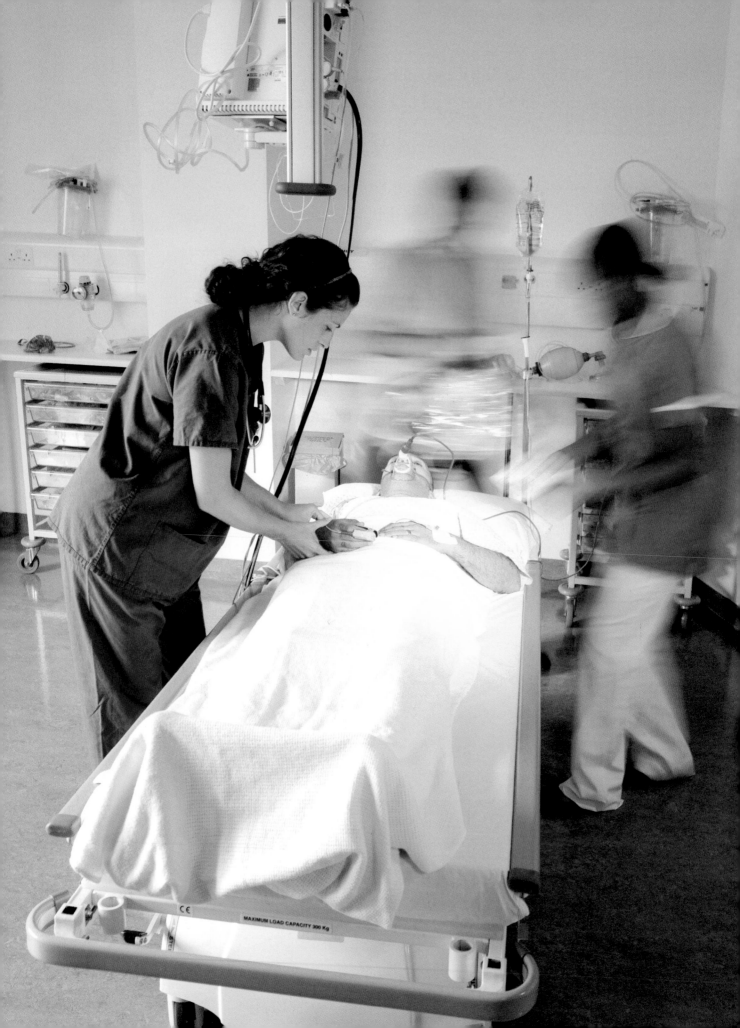

Nursing practice

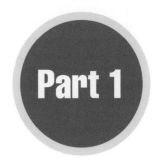

Part 1

Chapters

1 What is Nursing?

Figure 1.1 Three definitions of nursing

International Council of Nursing

Nursing encompasses autonomous and collaborative care of individuals of all ages, families, groups and communities, sick or well and in all settings. Nursing includes the promotion of health, prevention of illness, and the care of ill, disabled and dying people. Advocacy, promotion of a safe environment, research, participation in shaping health policy and in patient and health systems management, and education are also key nursing roles

The American Nurses Association

Nursing is the protection, promotion, and optimization of health and abilities, prevention of illness and injury, alleviation of suffering through the diagnosis and treatment of human response, and advocacy in the care of individuals, families, communities, and populations

Royal College of Nursing

The use of clinical judgment in the provision of care to enable people to improve, maintain, or recover health, to cope with health problems, and to achieve the best possible quality of life, whatever their disease or disability, until death

Figure 1.2 Some elements associated with the role of the nurse

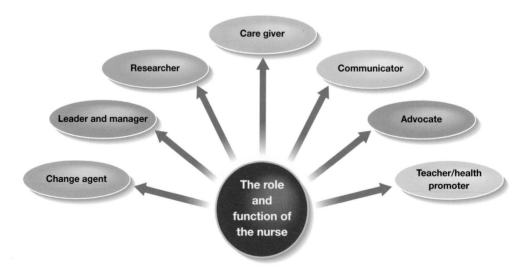

Medical-Surgical Nursing at a Glance, First Edition. Ian Peate. © John Wiley & Sons, Ltd. Published 2016 by John Wiley & Sons, Ltd.
Companion website: www.ataglanceseries.com/nursing/medsurg

To care safely and effectively for a person, the nurse must understand what nursing is, the role of the nurse and the function of the nurse. Attempting to do this, however, brings with it challenges.

Defining nursing

The International Council of Nursing suggests that nursing encompasses the autonomous and collaborative care of people of all ages, families, groups and communities, be these sick or well and in all settings. Nurses in undertaking their work promote health, prevent illness and care for those who are ill or disabled and people who are dying. Central to the nurse's role is advocacy, the promotion of a safe environment, research, participating in shaping health policy in patient and health systems management and education.

The American Nurses Association explains that nursing is concerned with the protection, promotion and optimisation of health and ability, preventing illness and injury, and relief from suffering. Nurses do this through diagnosis and treatment of the human response; nurses also act as advocates caring for individuals, families, communities and populations.

The Royal College of Nursing (2003: www.rcn.org.uk/__data/assets/pdf_file/0003/604038/Defining_Nursing_Web.pdf) professes that nursing can be described as the provision of care that is underpinned by clinical judgement, enabling individuals to improve or maintain health or recover from illness. Nurses assist people to cope with health problems; they contribute to enhancing the quality of life regardless of the person's disease or disability until their death.

Figure 1.1 provides an overview of three definitions of nursing.

The fact that there are so many definitions of nursing (not to mention what it is that nurses do) would suggest that the term is elusive and is difficult if not impossible to define. When working in a variety of contexts, for example, a hospital ward, person's own home or general practice, the role and function of the nurse will change in response to the context in which care is being offered. However, there are still central components of the nurse's role that will never change, for example, offering support, providing information and making decisions that are in the best interests of the person. What must be remembered, however, is that different kinds of definitions are needed for different purposes.

Nursing is a dynamic activity and as such it is constantly developing to meet the needs of people. Nursing and what nurses do take account of new knowledge from a variety of disciplines, for example, the social (psychology, social anthropology, sociology) and physical (chemistry, biology, physics) sciences. No one definition of nursing will ever suffice due to the complex nature of the human being. Trying to define nursing could be too limiting but without a definition, it would be difficult to formulate policy, specify services and develop educational curricula and therefore some specification is required.

The function of the nurse

Just as it is a challenge to attempt to define nursing, it is also a challenge to describe the role and function of the nurse. Figure 1.2 provides some elements that are associated with the role of the nurse.

Care giver

This aspect of the role has traditionally included those activities that assist the person from a physical and psychological perspective while preserving the person's dignity, providing comfort and respecting the person. The notion of care giving embodies physical, psychosocial, developmental, cultural and spiritual aspects; this is often referred to as a holistic approach.

Communicator

The most important aspect of the role of the nurse concerns communication which is central to all nursing roles. The nurse communicates with the person, the person's family (as well as those who support the person), a variety of health professionals and others in the community. Communication takes many forms, non-verbal (i.e. body language, the ability to actively listen, and written communication) and verbal. The quality of a nurse's communication (efficacy) is an important element in nursing care.

Advocate

The role of an advocate is to protect the person; when required, the nurse represents the needs of the person, assisting the person in exercising their rights and helping them speak up for themselves.

Teacher/health promoter

The nurse as teacher/health promoter helps people to learn about their health and what they need to do to restore or maintain their health. Assessing the person's learning needs and readiness to learn, the nurse working with the person sets learning goals, performing teaching strategies and measuring learning.

Change agent

The nurse acts as a change agent when assisting others, helping them to make modifications in their own behaviour. Nurses also work with others to make changes in the healthcare system.

Leader and manager

The nurse as leader influences others to work together to accomplish specific goals. This is often carried out at different levels: individual person, family, groups of people, colleagues or the community. The nurse manages the nursing care of individuals, families and communities, appropriately delegating activities to others, supervising and evaluating their performance.

Researcher

Nurses use and conduct research to enhance care. As researchers and consumers of research, they must be aware of the process and language of research.

The changing role of the nurse

As the role of the nurse continues to expand, there are a number of new aspects developing alongside the function of the nurse.

Consultant nurses and clinical nurse specialists have usually completed a doctorate or Master's degree in a specialty and have a considerable range of clinical expertise in that specialty. These nurses provide expert care to individuals, participate in educating healthcare professionals and undertake research.

The nurse practitioner is skilled at making nursing assessments, performing examinations, counselling, teaching and treating minor and self-limiting illness.

A nurse educator teaches in clinical and educational settings, teaches theoretical knowledge and clinical skills and conducts research.

2 The 6 Cs

Figure 2.1   The 6Cs of nursing

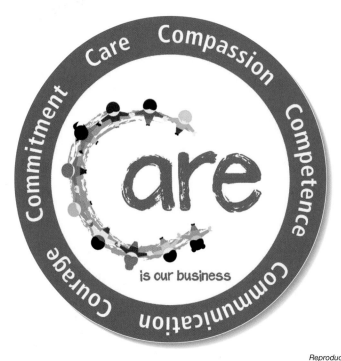

Reproduced with permission of NHS England

Medical-Surgical Nursing at a Glance, First Edition. Ian Peate. © John Wiley & Sons, Ltd. Published 2016 by John Wiley & Sons, Ltd.
Companion website: www.ataglanceseries.com/nursing/medsurg

Compassion in practice

Care is at the centre of all that nurses do. Being a nurse brings with it a number of privileges; it is an extraordinary role. What the nurse does every day can have a tremendous impact on the health and well-being of the people we are privileged to provide care for. Nurses are central in helping people keep themselves independent, healthy and well for longer. Helping people to recover from illness and supporting them in living with illness from a medical and surgical perspective is a part of this.

The provision of care and comfort when a person's life comes to an end, the compassion and humanity that nurses show are the hallmarks of our care and support system. Nurses provide care for everyone, regardless of their background, their gender or their age, from the beginning of a new life to the end of a life. This care is provided to people in their own homes, in their local general practice, in the community, in residential and care homes, in hospices and in hospitals. Nurses support people and their families often when they may be at their most vulnerable.

The Chief Nursing Officer for England and the Director of Nursing at the Department of Health have drawn up a 3-year vision and strategy for nursing, midwifery and care staff – Compassion in Practice – introduced in December 2012. The vision is underpinned by six fundamental values: care, compassion, competence, communication, courage and commitment (Figure 2.1).

The 6 Cs

The Chief Nursing Officer's vision acknowledges that the context for healthcare and support is changing and always in a state of flux. In particular, people are living longer, there are a greater number of older patients and people who require and will continue to require support, there are a growing number of people with multiple and complex needs as well as people with higher expectations of what healthcare and support can and should provide. Offering people health and care support and services requires the nurse to work with people in a new partnership, engaging with people when they make choices about their health and care.

No one of the 6 Cs is more important than the other five; each one (the values and behaviours) carries equal weight. The 6 Cs instinctively focus on ensuring that the person being cared for is at the heart of the care they receive.

Care

Care is central to the work of our core business and that of our organisations and the care that nurses deliver can help the individual person and improve the health of the whole community. Caring defines nurses and nursing. Those who receive care should be able to expect it to be right for them, always, throughout every stage of their life.

Compassion

This concept concerns how care is given through relationships that are rooted in empathy, respect and dignity. Compassion can also be seen as intelligent kindness and is crucial to how people perceive the care they receive.

Competence

All those who provide care must have the capability and capacity to understand a person's heath and social needs along with the expertise, clinical and technical understanding to deliver care that is effective and treatment that is safe and based on research and evidence.

Communication

Nurses are at the heart of the communication process, ensuring that care and support planning is in place based on the identified needs of the person being cared for.

This concept is key to effective caring relationships and successful team work. In order for 'no decision about me without me' to become a reality, listening is just as important as what we say and do. Communication is the key to a good workplace with benefits for those in our care and staff alike.

Courage

Being courageous empowers the nurse to do the right thing for the people we offer care to, to make it known when we have concerns and to mobilise our personal strength and imagination to innovate and welcome new ways of working.

Commitment

Commitment is a cornerstone of what nurses do and what people expect. Nurses are committed to improving the care and experience of the people they care for, in order to meet the health, care and support challenges that will lie ahead.

Areas of action

Along with the 6 Cs go six areas of action.

1 Helping people to stay independent, maximising well-being and improving health.
2 Working with people to provide a positive experience of care.
3 Delivering high-quality care.
4 Measuring its impact.
5 Building and strengthening leadership.
6 Ensuring we have the right staff, with the right skills in the right place

Person-centred care in the NHS requires the nurse and other healthcare workers to look at all the elements of care a person experiences – from the clinical care they receive to how the person is greeted by a cleaner or receptionist, or how easy it is to find their way round a hospital or health centre. Often, it is the little things that make a big difference to how people feel about the way their care needs are met. Together with the 6 Cs and the six areas of action, nurses can work towards the ultimate aim of ensuring that the patient is truly at the heart of all that is done.

3 Accountability and Responsibility

Table 3.1 The purpose of the Code

- Inform the profession of the standard of professional conduct that is demanded of them in the exercise of their professional accountability and practice

- Inform the public, other professions and employers of the standard of professional conduct that they can expect of a registered nurse

Table 3.2 The key facets of the Code

Make the care of people your first concern, treating them as individuals and respecting their dignity

- Treat people as individuals, holistically
- Maintain people's confidentiality
- Cooperate with those in your care
- Ensure consent is gained
- Uphold clear professional boundaries

Work with others to protect and promote the health and wellbeing of those in your care, their families and carers, and the wider community

- Communicate information with colleagues
- Work effectively as part of a team
- Delegate effectively
- Manage risk

Provide a high standard of practice and care at all times

- Utilise the best available evidence
- Keep your skills and knowledge up to date
- Keep clear and accurate records

Be open and honest, act with integrity and uphold the reputation of your profession

- Act with honesty
- Deal with problems
- Be unbiased
- Uphold the standing of the profession

Figure 3.1 Four spheres of accountability

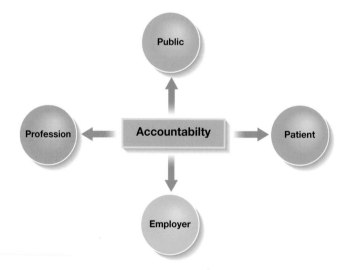

The role of the nurse is complex and is in a constant state of flux and because of this the nurse must be acutely aware of responsibility and accountability. The two concepts of responsibility and accountability are often discussed together but at other times they are seen as two very distinct entities.

Statutory regulation

Some healthcare professions that involve the potential risk of serious harm to people are statutorily regulated; the law requires this regulation. This regulation is carried out by regulatory bodies with legal responsibility for ensuring that registers of people entitled to practise in the United Kingdom are kept. They also set appropriate standards and take action when these standards have not been met.

The regulatory body for nurses and midwives is the Nursing and Midwifery Council (NMC). There are nine health and care professional regulatory bodies in the UK. Other regulatory bodies regulate other professions; for example, the Health and Care Professions Council (HCPC) is responsible for regulation of 17 health and care professional groups. Doctors are regulated by the General Medical Council (GMC) and the General Dental Council (GDC) regulates seven dental professional groups (dental nurses are included here).

The various health and care regulators have been set up with one overriding aim and that is to protect the public. The Professional Standards Authority (PSA) has responsibility for overseeing the UK's nine health and care professional regulatory bodies. It has oversight and scrutiny of the regulators, which is important in order to protect users of health and social care services and the public.

Nursing and Midwifery Council

There are around 676,547 nurses and midwives on the professional register. In the UK, the NMC is the regulatory body that sets the standards for nurses and midwives to meet in their working lives.

Nurses have a code of conduct that they must adhere to. This states how they must work and behave without exception, regardless of whether the nurse is involved in hands-on practice or is a manager, an academic or researcher.

The NMC also sets and monitors the national education and training requirements needed to qualify as a nurse. The standards make sure that nurses have the right skills and qualities when they start work. Standards are also set for education throughout nurses' careers, after they initially register with the NMC. Nurses are required to continually take part in learning activities to demonstrate that their skills and knowledge are up to date.

By maintaining a register of all nurses in the UK, the NMC decides who is able to call themselves a registered nurse. It is illegal to work as a nurse without being on the NMC register. In order to be on the register, nurses must pay a yearly fee and provide evidence that they fulfil requirements for keeping their skills and knowledge up to date.

The NMC sets requirements for nurses and midwives to help them to provide safe and appropriate care, taking firm but fair action where those obligations have not been met. If an allegation is made about a nurse or midwife that they do not meet the standards for skills, education and behaviour, or that there is a problem with their work, the NMC will investigate, calling the nurse to account and, if necessary, removing a nurse from the register permanently or for a set period of time. They may also place restrictions on the nurse's right to practise in the UK.

The Code of Professional Conduct

Codes of professional conduct, also known as codes of ethics, are regularly updated and renewed (an ethical code for nurses in the UK dates back to 1983). *The Code: Standards of Conduct, Performance and Ethics for Nurses and Midwives* (the Code) guides nurses with regard to their professional behaviour, helping to ensure that nurses work within ethical and moral frameworks.

The Code is not law; it is a guide informing the general public and other professionals of the standard of conduct that should be expected from a registered nurse. Codes of conduct do not solve problems; they reflect professional morality, operating to remind the nurse of the standards required by the profession. An overview of the purpose of the Code can be found in Table 3.1.

There are a number of key facets incorporated within Code – see Table 3.2.

Accountability

Being accountable for actions and omissions is a central tenet of the Code. All healthcare professionals in carrying out their duties have the potential to do good as well as to harm the people they offer care to. To be accountable, the nurse needs to be in possession of up-to-date knowledge and to have the appropriate nursing skills.

Professional accountability is constant; the nurse is accountable at all times for their actions or omissions and the first section of the Code makes this clear. The nurse is personally accountable for their own practice and may be called to account for actions and omissions. There are four spheres associated with accountability (Figure 3.1).

Public accountability

This occurs through the criminal courts as defined by criminal law. Where accountability is in question, the police are likely to investigate and a decision may be made to prosecute the nurse for a criminal offence. Public accountability is generally associated with a social contract between the public and the profession.

Accountability to the patient

The injured party may seek a civil remedy via the criminal law in the courts. The person making the complaint or bringing the action for negligence may also sue the NHS for the nurse's negligence (indirect liability).

Employer accountability

The nurse is accountable through the contract of employment. In some cases, the nurse may be in breach of contract if they have not acted with due care and skill and disciplinary action may ensue.

Accountability to the profession

The nurse is accountable to the NMC through its Conduct and Competence Committee. The NMC determines if a nurse is deemed incompetent through their actions or omissions.

4 Risk and Safety

Table 4.1 Resources available to help nurses manage risk and enhance patient safety

Preventing falls	**Clinical Practice Guideline for the Assessment and Prevention of Falls In Older People** – *National Institute for Health and Care Excellence*
	The 'How to' Guide for Reducing Harm from Falls – *Patient Safety First*
	Up and About: Pathways for The Prevention and Management of Falls and Fragility Fractures – *NHS Quality Improvement Scotland*

Nutrition and hydration	**Food, Fluid and Nutritional Care in Hospitals** – *NHS Quality Improvement Scotland*
	Hospital Hydration Best Practice Toolkit – *Royal College of Nursing, National Patient Safety Agency*
	Nutritional Factsheets *National Patient Safety Agency*
	Nutrition Now – *Royal College of Nursing*
	Observation Prompts and Guidance for Monitoring Compliance: Guidance for CQC Inspectors. Outcome 5: Meeting Nutritional Needs – *Care Quality Commission and Royal College of Nursing*

Prevention of pressure ulcers	**The Management of Pressure Ulcers in Primary and Secondary Care: A Clinical Practice Guideline** – *Royal College of Nursing*
	Pressure Ulcer Treatment: Quick Reference Guide – *European Pressure Ulcer Advisory Panel and National Pressure Ulcer Advisory Panel*
	Best Practice Statement. Prevention and Management of Pressure Ulcers – *NHS Quality Improvement Scotland, Tissue Viability*

Infection prevention and control	**Infection Control: Prevention of Healthcare-Associated Infection in Primary and Community Care** – *National Institute for Health and Care Excellence*
	Standards: Healthcare Associated Infection – *NHS Quality Improvement Scotland*
	Infection Prevention and Control: Minimum Standards – *Royal College of Nursing*

Table 4.2 An example of a Modified Early Warning System (there are various systems available)

A score of **0, 1, 2,** or **3** is allocated to a vital sign, as follows:

Heart rate:	Score of **0** (50 to 100 beats per minute), **1** (41 to 50 or 101 to 110), **2** (40 or fewer or 111 to 129), or **3** (130 or greater)
Systolic blood pressure:	Score of **0** (101 to 199 mm Hg), **1** (81 to 100), **2** (71 to 80 or 200 or greater), or **3** (70 or lower)
Respiratory rate:	Score of **0** (9 to 14 breaths per minute), **1** (15 to 20), **2** (8 or fewer or 21 to 29), or **3** (30 or more)
Temperature:	Score of **0** (36.1–38 degrees centigrade), **2** (more than 39.1) or **3** (if lower than 35)
Level of consciousness:	Score of **0** (alert), **1** (responds to voice), **2** (responds to pain), or **3** (unresponsive)

Medical-Surgical Nursing at a Glance, First Edition. Ian Peate. © John Wiley & Sons, Ltd. Published 2016 by John Wiley & Sons, Ltd.
Companion website: www.ataglanceseries.com/nursing/medsurg

In all aspects of health and social care there will always be elements of care that are associated with risk and issues concerning safety. We can never guarantee that patients will never be harmed by the system that is meant to look after them. Issues concerning risk and safety may be associated with people being cared for or those who are delivering care. Healthcare systems are complex so preventing adverse events and improving patient safety require a multifaceted approach. Patient safety is seen as a priority in most organisations. Nurses have a key role to play in the investigation and implementation of improvements in patient safety.

Nurses are required by law and from a professional perspective to manage risk, be aware of risk and help to ensure that everyone is kept safe in the places where they are receiving healthcare. Patient safety is a key component of high-quality healthcare; it is something that patients have a right to expect. Nurses need to know how to manage patient safety and risk in all care settings.

Risk management can be considered from many perspectives; it is not a one-off event but rather a process that can help to raise the quality and safety of services provided. It focuses on occurrences where patients may have been harmed by their treatment or where that treatment had the potential to cause them harm. It is the collective responsibility of healthcare organisations and an individual responsibility of those who work in them to manage risk and improve the safety of care. Nurses need to understand that it is not just the harm that is caused to the patient but also the knock-on effect this has on families, loved ones and friends.

In organisations as large and as complex as the NHS, things will sometimes go wrong and as such patients will suffer unintended harm. When this does happen, an opportunity to learn and not to blame should be taken.

Resources

There are several resources available to help nurses deliver high-quality, safe and effective care (Table 4.1). The pace of change in contemporary nursing practice, the introduction of policy statements and the amount of new evidence emerging have the potential to lead to frontline staff such as nurses feeling swamped.

Risk assessment tools

A variety of assessment tools are available. For example, the Waterlow score is a pressure ulcer risk assessment tool that can be used to alert staff to the need to implement certain actions to prevent a deterioration in the patient's condition. Other examples of risk assessment tools include those for malnutrition, suicide and falls.

Regardless of the risk assessment tool being used, these are only as good as the nurse undertaking the assessment. Risk assessment tools can help to predict the probable degree of risk to the patient. Risk awareness is associated with understanding risk-prone situations and having the skill to anticipate or predict hazards, risks and incidents and reduce the ensuing personal and organisational risk.

Early warning systems

Early warning scoring systems proactively help nurses and other staff to identify those patients at risk of deterioration. Using these systems has the potential to lead to fewer cardiopulmonary emergencies and deaths.

The Modified Early Warning System is a simple scoring system that routinely measures patients' physiological vital signs to identify those who are likely to deteriorate. It prompts nurses to notify medical staff and other care givers when appropriate and take other essential steps in order to prevent further decline in condition. A score is allocated to each vital sign and these scores are combined to provide the patient's overall score. Table 4.2 identifies some of the components of a Modified Early Warning System.

Surgical safety checklist

A surgical safety checklist has been devised by the World Health Organization (WHO) with the intention of reducing the number of surgical deaths across the world. The checklist addresses important safety issues, including inadequate anaesthetic safety practices, avoidable surgical infection and poor communication among team members. These factors have proved to be common, deadly and preventable problems.

The checklist is not a regulatory device nor is it a component of official policy; it is intended to be used by nurses and others interested in improving the safety of surgical procedures and reducing unnecessary surgical deaths and associated complications. There are three areas that the checklist addresses; these can be modified to meet local needs.

1 *Before the induction of anaesthesia*: patient confirmation, site marked (if appropriate), anaesthesia safety check completed, pulse oximeter on the patient and working, any known allergies, airway risk, risk of blood loss.

2 *Before skin incision*: team introductions, patient verbally confirmed, site and procedure, anticipated critical events, surgeon review, anaesthetist team review, nursing team review, need for antibiotic prophylaxis, essential imaging displayed.

3 *Before the patient leaves the operating room*: the nurse verbally confirms with the team the name of the procedure recorded, instrument, sponge and needle counts are correct, how specimens were labelled (including patient's name), if there are any equipment problems to be addressed, surgeon, anaesthesia professional and nurse review the key concerns for recovery and management of the patient.

Improving the safety of patient care is a weighty challenge for the NHS; patient safety is at the heart of the healthcare agenda. The provision of healthcare relies on a range of complex interactions between people, skills, technologies and drugs. Sometimes things can and do go wrong. Adverse events that do occur can be avoided, if lessons from previous incidents are learned.

5 Patient-Centred Care

Figure 5.1 Some components of patient-centred care

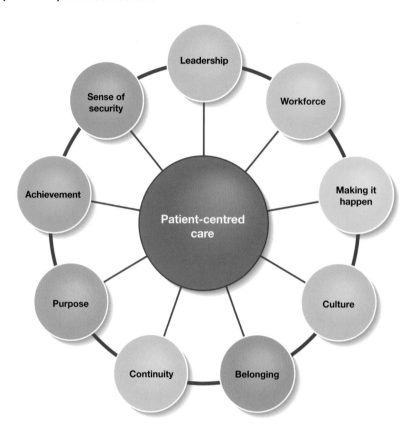

Table 5.1 Types of patient-centred care

Type of care	Description
Person-centred care	An approach used in practice that seeks to establish, form and foster therapeutic relationships between all care providers, patients and others who are significant to them. Central to this concept are the values of respect for persons, individual right to self-determination, reciprocal respect and understanding
Patient-centred care	All those involved in caring (the person, family carers and paid or voluntary carers) should experience relationships that promote a sense of security, belonging, continuity, purpose, achievement and significance
Family-centred care	This is a way of caring for people as well as their families within health services, ensuring that care is planned around the whole family, not just the person and in which all the family members are recognised as care recipients (if appropriate)
Relationship-centred care	Having an understanding of the personal meaning of the illness for the patient by finding out what their concerns are, what ideas they have, their expectations, their needs and how they feel and how they function. Promoting the understanding of the patient within their individual psychosocial context; sharing power and responsibility, and developing therapeutic goals that resonate with the patient's values

Medical-Surgical Nursing at a Glance, First Edition. Ian Peate. © John Wiley & Sons, Ltd. Published 2016 by John Wiley & Sons, Ltd.
Companion website: www.ataglanceseries.com/nursing/medsurg

Patient-centredness

Person-centred care is a term being used with increasing frequency within health and social care; indeed, it is the focus of many government initiatives, with the patient at the heart of all we do. The patient is at the centre of care delivery. Person-centredness is recognised as a multidimensional concept (Figure 5.1).

Patient-centred care is healthcare that is respectful of, and responsive to, the preferences, needs and values of individual patients. The key principles of patient-centred approaches include:

- treating patients, consumers, carers and families with dignity and respect
- encouraging and supporting participation in decision making by patients, consumers, carers and families
- communicating and sharing information with patients, consumers, carers and families
- promoting collaboration with patients, consumers, carers, families and health professionals in programmes and policy development and in health service design, delivery and evaluation.

Patient-centred care is seen as an important feature of high-quality healthcare in its own right and there is evidence that a patient-centred focus has the potential to lead to improvements in healthcare quality and outcomes by enhancing safety, cost-effectiveness and patient, family and staff satisfaction.

Partnership working

There are a number of strategies that can be used to promote patient-centred care and partnerships with patients and their families (see Table 5.1). Considering service provision from a patient's perspective can be a powerful motivator to provide care that is patient and not organisation centred.

Most nurses work to the highest standards to deliver safe and high-quality care for patients. The nursing profession needs to demonstrate the need for a continuous duty to deliver high-quality, safe and effective patient care combined with a determination to uphold high standards and to make known concerns and to challenge those who are responsible for poor practice. The provision of high-quality, safe patient care relies not only on the clinical skills of those who are treating and caring for patients. It also involves teamwork, communication, leadership and a culture where nurses and others can discuss patient safety openly with peers, senior clinicians and healthcare managers as well as with patients themselves. Those who face illness or disability, loss or bereavement may need the support of those who understand what they are going through, who can offer empathy and demonstrate humanity. These are central features that are essential to good nursing.

Fundamental needs

Nurses who put the patient at the centre of all they do will take into account the needs of each patient as an individual, ensuring that the person's dignity is maintained throughout their treatment and care. This takes into account their needs for:

- food and drink and help to eat and drink
- personal care
- relief from pain and other distressing symptoms.

These are basic and fundamental needs and ensuring they have been met is a key concern for the nurse.

People first

As well as demonstrating that they have the requisite knowledge and skills, the nurse must also demonstrate that they have compassion and are kind. Nurses have a duty at all times to ensure that they put the people they care for first and as soon as they believe that patients are at risk, they must make this known, raising their concerns.

Nurses are ideally placed to encourage partnership working, working across professional boundaries, with the aim of focusing on delivering positive, effective and compassionate care for patients. These professional values are laid out in the NMC's Code of Conduct where nurses are required to treat people as individuals, respect their dignity, take immediate action if they think that they, someone they work with or the location in which they are delivering care is or is potentially putting someone at risk. It is an expectation that nurses will be kind and considerate when they provide care to the patient, their carers and families.

Working with others

Working constructively with colleagues, listening to and working in partnership with them, can demonstrate patient-centred care, acknowledging that multidisciplinary teamwork, fostering constructive debate from all team members, adopting a safety-focused leadership approach and a culture based on openness and learning when things do not go as well as expected are central to accomplishing high-quality care.

Nurses of today face very different challenges from those faced by their predecessors; regardless of this, those human values are crucial to the role of the nurse and remain steadfast, underpinning the trust which lies at the heart of the therapeutic nurse–patient relationship.

6 Team Working

Table 6.1 Features of a team

- Team members have shared objectives in relation to their work

- Team members interact with each other to achieve these shared objectives

- Team members have well-defined roles, some of which are differentiated from each other

- Teams have an organisational identity – they have a defined organisational function and are recognised as a team by others outside the team

- The tasks the team perform have consequences that affect others inside or outside the organisation

Figure 6.1 Characteristics of an effective team

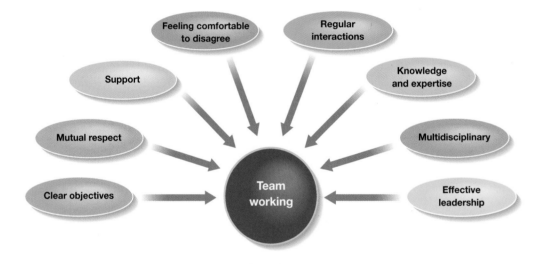

Medical-Surgical Nursing at a Glance, First Edition. Ian Peate. © John Wiley & Sons, Ltd. Published 2016 by John Wiley & Sons, Ltd.
Companion website: www.ataglanceseries.com/nursing/medsurg

Team working has an important if not essential contribution to make to the effective delivery of healthcare. If teams are to be effective, then they need to be given the support of team leaders and to be located in organisations that actively support team working. The Nursing and Midwifery Council demands that nurses work effectively as part of a team. They must work in a co-operative manner within teams, respecting the skills, expertise and contributions of other colleagues. Nurses have to be willing to share their skills and experience to help and assist colleagues.

Principles underpinning team work

Every healthcare team is unique and has its own purpose, size, setting and set of core members as well as methods of communication. Regardless of these differences, there are core principles that exemplify 'teamness'. There are a number of key principles related to team work, including shared goals, clear roles, reciprocal trust, effective communication and measurable processes and outcomes. These principles are not to be seen in isolation, rather they are interlaced and each one is reliant on the other. The most important organisational factor required for effective team-based healthcare is institutional leadership that fully and explicitly embraces and supports these principles in words and what they do.

Characteristics of teams

Those teams that work well together have certain characteristics (Table 6.1).

Team members have joint objectives with respect to their work and each member of the team has a well-defined role along with a clear understanding of how they can contribute to achieving these objectives. Members of the team interact regularly with each other so as to achieve the team's shared objectives and are able to offer their knowledge and expertise to decision making in the team. Team members have a shared responsibility to accomplish excellence and a focus on quality. Team members support innovation by providing each other with practical and social support as innovation is introduced. An effective team will regularly reflect on how the members work together.

Effective teams are multidisciplinary in nature. Those with a varied range of professional groups are likely to produce higher levels of innovation in patient care. Good-quality, focused meetings, communication and integration of processes in healthcare teams enhance new and improved ways of delivering patient care. Teams with clear leadership have more efficient team processes, provide better quality patient care and are more innovative. Overall, teams that display these characteristics (Figure 6.1) will produce better quality patient care and better team member well-being.

Team values

While teams are groups, it must be remembered that they are also made up of individuals. As well as the particular characteristics that facilitate the function of the team, there are also certain personal values required for individuals to function effectively within the team. These personal values typify the most effective members of high-functioning teams in healthcare.

Honesty

Team members value effective communication within the team, including transparency about aims, decisions, uncertainty and mistakes. Key to continued improvement and for preserving the mutual trust required for a high-functioning team is honesty.

Discipline

Members of the team perform their roles and responsibilities with discipline, even when it seems difficult. Concurrently, team members are disciplined in seeking out and sharing new information to advance individual and team functioning, even though at times this may be uncomfortable. Such discipline enables team members to develop and maintain their standards and protocols even when they are seeking new ways to improve.

Creativity

Team members are motivated by the chance of tackling new or emerging problems creatively. They consider errors and unanticipated bad outcomes as possible opportunities to learn and improve.

Humility

Team members understand differences in training but do not think that one type of training or viewpoint is superior to the training that others have received. They are also aware that they are human and that mistakes will be made. Therefore a key value of working in a team is that team members can rely on each other to help recognise and prevent failures, wherever they are in the hierarchy.

Curiosity

Team members are committed to reflecting upon lessons learned in the course of their daily activities and using those insights for continuous improvement of their own work and team functioning.

Barriers to effective team working

It has been demonstrated that there are substantial benefits to patient care and team members that can be gained from the development of team work. Despite this, in practice, team working has proved difficult to achieve. Some of the barriers to effective team working include the following.

- Differences in status and gender.
- Division between professional groups.
- Different professional groups with different agendas.
- Team members have different terms and conditions of employment.
- Difficulties with communication.
- Lack of awareness of each other's roles and responsibilities.
- Lack of support and help with developing team working.

Conflict

When there is unresolved conflict within a team, this has the potential to interfere with the achievement of successful clinical outcomes, as well as with personal and professional satisfaction (individual or collective). The aim of conflict resolution is to avoid deadlock and blame and to restore stability and to engender healthy and functional communication within the team.

Resolving conflict in the workplace necessitates intentionality and active approaches that support workplace goals. Effective conflict resolution means that a deliberate decision to actively address workplace issues is required, as well as considering the emotional concerns of colleagues. A positive approach to conflict resolution can benefit patients and staff and support the effective functioning of the team.

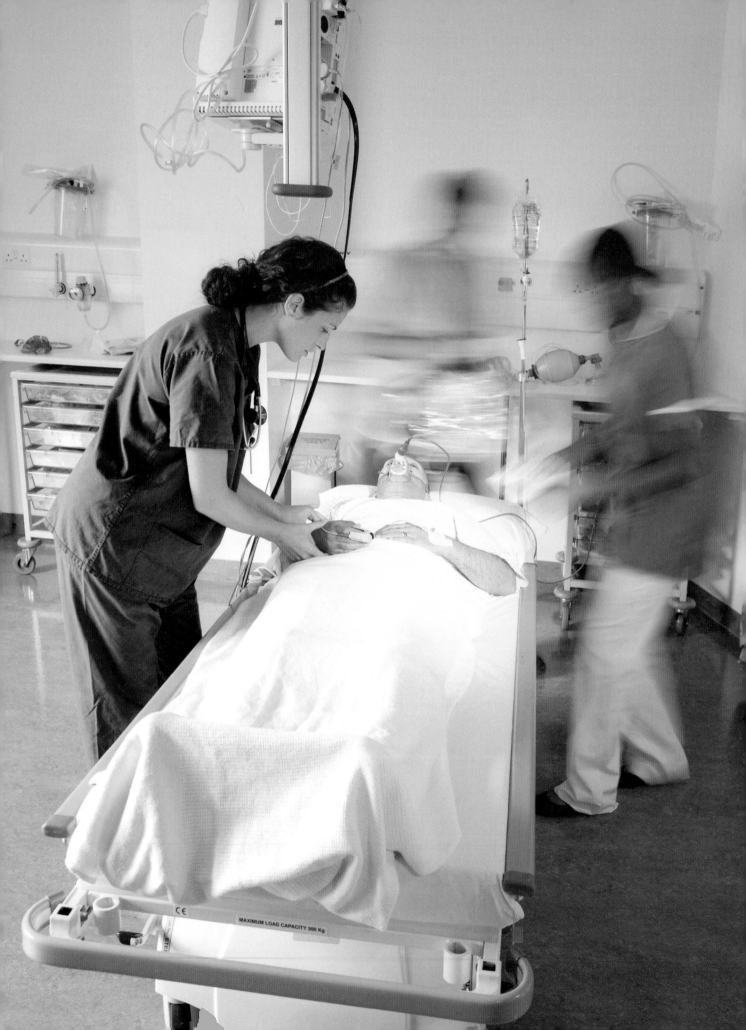

General care

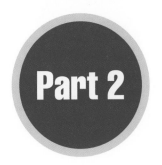

Part 2

Chapters

7 Health Assessment

Figure 7.1 The nursing process

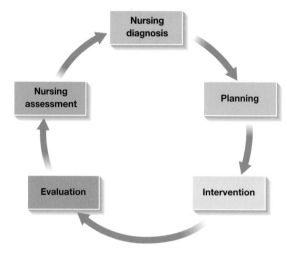

Nursing diagnosis → Planning → Intervention → Evaluation → Nursing assessment → (cycle back to Nursing diagnosis)

Table 7.1 Some assessment techniques

Communication	Without effective communication other assessment techniques will fail
Inspection	This is the most frequently used assessment technique. Inspection is important as it usually leads to further investigation of findings. The nurse looks for conditions that can be observed with your eyes, ears, or nose. When inspecting the skin, for example, observe for colour, location of lesions, bruises or rash, symmetry, size of body parts and abnormal findings and odours
Auscultation	Usually undertaken after inspection. When auscultating, ensure the room in which the assessment is taking place is quiet, auscultate over bare skin, never over clothing or a gown
Palpation	This technique requires the nurse to touch the patient with different parts of the hand
Percussion	Percussion requires skill and practice. Used to elicit tenderness or sounds that could provide clues to any underlying problems. The nurse should monitor the patient for signs of discomfort

Figure 7.2 Abdominal palpation

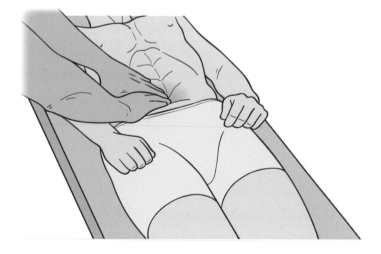

Table 7.2 The SMART approach to goal setting

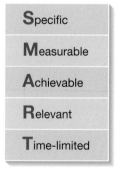

Specific
Measurable
Achievable
Relevant
Time-limited

Medical-Surgical Nursing at a Glance, First Edition. Ian Peate. © John Wiley & Sons, Ltd. Published 2016 by John Wiley & Sons, Ltd.
Companion website: www.ataglanceseries.com/nursing/medsurg

Health

Defining health is complex, if not impossible, as health means different things to different people at different times in their lives and in different contexts. In 1948, the World Health Organization provided a definition of health, describing it as a state of complete physical, mental and social well-being and not merely the absence of disease or infirmity. When this definition was devised, it was radical because of its breadth and ambition. This definition did not have negative connotations, health was seen as an absence of disease and it included the physical, mental and social spheres. As populations age and the pattern of illnesses changes, this definition may hinder as opposed to help. The current WHO definition has limitations and this should be taken into account when choosing to use it.

Assessing needs

Assessing a person's health is one part of the role and function of the nurse. Assessment of patient needs varies depending on the nurse's role and the setting. A cardiac care nurse, for example, will be more familiar with cardiac issues whereas a nurse working with people with gastrointestinal problems will be more familiar with more complex gastrointestinal conditions and the associated investigations and examinations. Throughout all aspects of the care experience, the nurse must give consideration to the person's privacy and develop open, honest two-way communication.

Health history

Obtaining a health history serves a number of purposes. It provides the nurse with a description of the person's symptoms and how they developed. It provides information about the person's physical status, as well as their spiritual needs, cultural requirements and functional living status. During the history taking, communication must respect the person as an individual and physical examination must be performed in a respectful and culturally sensitive manner. Privacy is essential and the nurse must be aware of their own body language and tone of voice whilst interviewing the person.

A systematic approach to care: the nursing process

The nursing process is a cyclical approach with five aspects (Figure 7.1). It provides a systematic approach to planning and delivering nursing care. The nurse uses a problem-solving cycle, taking into account the unique individual needs of the patient, working in partnership with the patient and their family. This approach requires the nurse to think critically about possible nursing interventions, to develop a care strategy and to evaluate the outcomes of care provision.

Assessment

During the assessment, an opportunity arises to develop a relationship with the person and their family. Interactions at this stage provide the person and family with impressions about you, other nurses and how care will be managed. Using a systematic process and acknowledging that this is a dynamic activity enables the nurse to gather and analyse data about a person, the first step in delivering nursing care. Assessment includes not only physiological data, but also psychological, sociocultural, spiritual, economic and lifestyle factors. For example, when assessing the needs of a person in pain, this will include the physical causes and manifestations of pain as well as the patient's response, an inability to mobilise, withdrawal from family members, anger directed at hospital staff, fear, or request for more pain medication.

A full, detailed and skilled assessment provides invaluable information about the patient, obtaining descriptions about their symptoms, how the symptoms developed and a process to discover any related physical findings that will assist in the development of differential diagnoses. The nurse uses both subjective and objective data. It is the patient who provides the subjective data. Objective assessment data includes data that is observable and measurable. A number of assessment tools are available to help the nurse gather information that is objective and measurable. Table 7.1 provides examples of some assessment techniques and Figure 7.2 demonstrates abdominal palpation.

Nursing diagnosis

The nursing diagnosis is the nurse's clinical judgement concerning the person's response to actual or potential health conditions or needs. The nursing diagnosis provides the basis for a range of nursing interventions that will result in positive patient outcomes for which the nurse has accountability. A nursing diagnosis can only occur once a comprehensive nursing assessment has been undertaken. The diagnosis provides the basis for the nurse's care plan.

Planning

When the assessment and diagnosis have been made, the nurse sets measurable and achievable short- and long-term goals with the patient and a plan of care is formulated.

Patient-centred goals should be clear, avoiding ambiguity. The nursing process should always be clearly linked to the person receiving care.

All outcomes must be patient orientated and communicated in the form of a statement. The goal should clearly specify what the patient would be able to do once a nursing intervention takes place. If the goal is unclear, it becomes difficult to assess patient progression or to encourage the patient towards the desired outcome. Nurses need to set goals for the short and long term. A SMART approach to goal statements is advocated (Table 7.2).

Implementation

This phase of the systematic approach to nursing care is also called the intervention stage. During this stage, nursing care is implemented according to the care plan (the plan of care was formulated during the planning stage), in order for continuity of care to occur while the person is receiving care and also in preparation for discharge. Any care that has been given (or omitted) must be documented according to local policy and procedure in the patient's record.

Evaluation

Both the patient's status and the effectiveness of the nursing care provided must be continuously evaluated; this is an ongoing process dependent upon the changing condition of the person. The care plan must be modified as needed, providing evidence that care has been adjusted to meet the needs of the person. Evaluation involves reassessment of needs.

8 **Intravenous Therapy**

Table 8.1 Types of vascular access device (VAD). These can be inserted peripherally or centrally

Peripheral lines are cannulae and midlines	• Peripheral cannulae are the most commonly used type of VAD in secondary care settings.
	• They are used for short-term (one to five days) infusions of fluids, blood products and medication, and are inserted by health-care professionals
	• A midline catheter provides venous access in a large peripheral vein but does not enter the central venous system. Midlines are often inserted into a vein situated in the antecubital fossa area of the arm, the tip extends into the vein of the upper arm up to 20 cm
Centrally inserted devices are peripherally inserted central catheters (PICCs), non-tunnelled central venous catheters (CVCs), tunnelled central venous catheters, and implantable ports	• A CVC is a device whose tip is positioned into the superior vena cava or right atrium by direct entry into the antecubital fossa, jugular or subclavian veins
	• CVCs are used to monitor central venous pressure, administer large amounts of fluid or blood products, provide long-term access for administration of vesicant drugs, such as cytotoxic and antibiotic infusions, for repeated specimen collection and total parenteral nutrition (TPN)
	• Four types are available: peripherally inserted central catheters (PICCs), centrally inserted catheters (non-tunnelled and tunnelled), and implantable ports
	• A peripherally inserted central line is a catheter that is advanced into the superior vena cava. The tip position is usually confirmed radiologically
	• Used when there is a lack of peripheral access for infusion of vesicant and irritant drugs/fluids, TPN and hyperosmolar solutions. They are also used when long-term access is required
	• Tunnelled CVCs are often referred to as Hickmann lines, used when the person requires long-term infusional therapy, such as chemotherapy, and TPN. They also provide access for blood sampling
	• This type of line is usually inserted in theatre or radiology using an image intensifier to ensure correct positioning. Patients are often lightly sedated
	• Non-tunnelled – this type of CVC is sometimes called a short-term percutaneous central venous catheter (non-tunnelled) it is the most commonly used CVC in secondary care, directly inserted into a central vein
	• Implantable ports are VADs inserted into the chest, abdomen or antecubital area for long-term intravenous therapy, bolus injections, blood sampling and TPN use
	• Ports are inserted under subcutaneous skin

Figure 8.1 Intramuscular, intravenous and subcutaneous injections

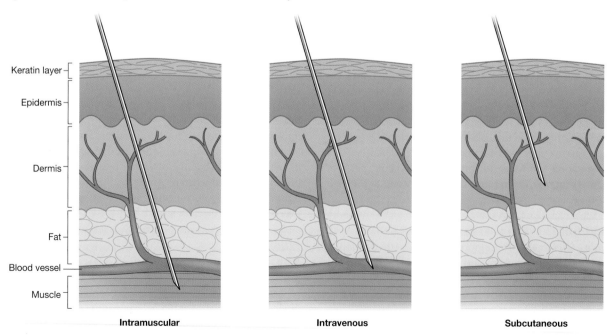

Keratin layer
Epidermis
Dermis
Fat
Blood vessel
Muscle

Intramuscular   Intravenous   Subcutaneous

Medical-Surgical Nursing at a Glance, First Edition. Ian Peate. © John Wiley & Sons, Ltd. Published 2016 by John Wiley & Sons, Ltd.
Companion website: www.ataglanceseries.com/nursing/medsurg

Most people admitted to hospital will at some stage during their stay have some type of vascular access device inserted. Infusion therapy, it must be remembered, is not confined solely to the hospital setting. The traditional perception that infusion therapy should be confined to the hospital environment is being challenged.

All nurses will come into contact with people in the medical or surgical setting who require some form of intravenous (IV) therapy, which is one of the most common forms of treatment provided in acute care. They will be responsible for the administration and management of IV therapy. Nurses working in partnership with other members of the interdisciplinary healthcare team have an important role in providing evidence-based care to people who require IV therapy.

This chapter provides a brief overview of the main types of IV fluids and routes for administration.

Vascular access devices

Vascular access devices (VADs) are a common and essential part of clinical practice for the administration of parenteral fluids, nutrients, medications and blood products. VADs also provide a method to monitor the haemodynamic status of a person. There are several types of VAD (Table 8.1). New technology and advanced new treatment regimens continue to emerge and as such, nurses are required to support best practices in order to ensure more effective vascular access care.

Administration of IV fluid is the practice of giving fluid directly into a person's vein. In effect, IV medication and all IV fluids must be prescribed; IV fluids may also contain medications.

Methods of administering IV fluid may include giving the fluid by rapid injection into the vein using a syringe, giving the fluid intermittently over a specific amount of time or giving the fluid continuously. IV fluids are usually given through a peripheral line (as opposed to a central venous catheter). At all times, the nurse must adhere to local policy and procedure concerning the administration of medications.

Prior to commencing IV therapy, nurses must consider a number of factors:

- the person
- the type of device to be used
- the reason for the IV therapy
- the duration of therapy
- the fluids to be infused.

An in-depth holistic assessment of the person is needed in order to ensure that their needs are being met.

The choice of the most appropriate VAD for an individual is not easy; there may not be one single device that will meet all requirements. Thought must be given to the reason a person requires the device, their medical history, vascular accessibility, the type of therapy to be provided as well as the length of time that the line is required.

It is essential to ensure that local protocols for care and maintenance of VADs are adhered to; these are usually based on national guidance and best available evidence.

The principles of care

There are several advantages of intravenous over intramuscular (IM) injections. There is an immediate therapeutic effect when using the IV route as well as control over the rate of administration of the fluid being infused which can lead to prolonged action (a steady amount of medication in the bloodstream). The IV route allows those people who cannot tolerate drugs or fluids orally to receive medications and to ensure hydration. The IV route permits those drugs that cannot be absorbed by any other route to be used therapeutically.

Potential complications

As well as the distinct advantages of using this route, there are also some disadvantages and complications. The speed at which the drug takes effect can be a disadvantage as there is no drug recall; the direct IV route can lead to toxicity. Mechanical/chemical irritation (phlebitis), thrombophlebitis, infiltration and extravasation can occur as well as microbial contamination and infection.

Insufficient control of administration can lead to speed shock, resulting in circulatory overload. The risk of anaphylaxis or an allergic reaction (itching, rash, shortness of breath) is heightened when medication is given via the IV route.

Adhering to aseptic technique is vital in the prevention of intravenous-related infections. Asepsis should be maintained at insertion, during clinical use and at removal of the device. Local policy and procedure should be adhered to at all times.

Avoiding complications and enhancing patient comfort are essential requirements when caring for people with IVs *in situ*, and planning care can help. The person should be given an explanation of the procedure and informed consent should be obtained. Understanding the associated risks and using aseptic non-touch technique (ANTT) at all times are prerequisites. The practitioner should be familiar with the products and infusion sets being used.

Care issues

The person receiving the infusion may be anxious so they will require explanations and reassurance. Explain to the person that they should not alter the infusion rate or tamper with the infusion set or the equipment. If the person is experiencing pain or discomfort associated with the IV infusion then this will indicate complications.

Should complications arise, the practitioner needs to know when to seek extra help and from whom. It is essential that the local drug policy is adhered to as well as any professional guidance issued by regulatory bodies such as the Nursing and Midwifery Council or the Health and Care Profession Council.

It is essential that a comprehensive record is made, including type of access device, location and condition of entry site; a visual infusion phlebitis score is also recorded. The aim is to be patient centred, ensuring patient safety and well-being.

Fluid balance

Fluid balance means maintaining the correct amount of fluid in the body. It is the continuance of the fluid input and output of the body. Fluid balance may change with disease and illness.

Patients can make a valuable contribution to their fluid balance. If a patient needs IV fluids, explain the decision and discuss the signs and symptoms they need to look out for if their fluid balance needs adjusting.

All patients receiving IV fluids need regular monitoring. Initially this should include at least daily reassessments of clinical fluid status, laboratory values (urea, creatinine and electrolytes) and fluid balance charts, along with weight measurement twice weekly.

Patients' intake and output are recorded on fluid balance charts, and accurate recording is crucial for their wellbeing. Input and output should be recorded with a clear indication of the amount of urine passed and fluid taken in – this includes IV fluids.

9 Blood Transfusion

Figure 9.1   Blood groups

Blood type	Antigen (RBC membrane)	Antibody (plasma)	Can receive blood from	Can donate blood to
A	A antigen	Anti-B antibodies	A, O	A, AB
B	B antigen	Anti-A antibodies	B, O	B, AB
AB	A antigen / B antigen	No antibodies	A, B, AB, O	AB
O	No antigen	Both anti-A and anti-B antibodies	O	O, A, B, AB

Figure 9.2   Barcodes used to reduce risk

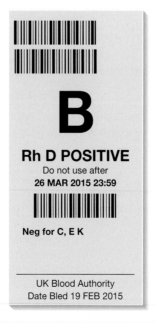

B

Rh D POSITIVE

Do not use after
26 MAR 2015 23:59

Neg for C, E K

UK Blood Authority
Date Bled 19 FEB 2015

Medical-Surgical Nursing at a Glance, First Edition. Ian Peate. © John Wiley & Sons, Ltd. Published 2016 by John Wiley & Sons, Ltd.
Companion website: www.ataglanceseries.com/nursing/medsurg

The blood

When blood is donated special equipment is used to separate the donation into various blood components.

Red blood cells transport oxygen around the body and are used to treat anaemia. Platelets help to stop bleeding, so platelet transfusions can be used to prevent excessive bleeding in some groups of people, for example, those who are having chemotherapy treatment. Plasma makes up most of the volume of blood, containing nutrients required by the body's cells, as well as proteins helping the blood to clot if there is haemorrhage. White cells are used to fight infection.

Blood types

Every person has one of the following blood types: A, B, AB or O. Also, every person's blood is either rhesus (Rh) positive or Rh negative. So, if the person has type A blood, it is either A positive or A negative.

The blood used in a transfusion must be compatible with the patient's blood type. If it is not, antibodies in the blood cause an incompatibility reaction.

For almost everyone, type O blood is safest. Approximately 40% of the population has type O blood. Those with this blood type are universal donors. Type O blood is used for emergencies when there is no time to test a person's blood type. People who have type AB blood are called universal recipients. This means they can receive any type of blood (Figure 9.1).

If the person has Rh-positive blood, they can receive Rh-positive or Rh-negative blood but if they have Rh-negative blood, they should only be given Rh-negative blood. Rh-negative blood is used for emergencies when there is no time to test a person's Rh type.

Alternatives to blood transfusion

There are alternatives to blood transfusion but there is no man-made alternative to human blood. Surgeons try to reduce the amount of blood lost during surgery so that fewer patients will need blood transfusions.

Autologous blood

This involves using the person's own blood. Preoperative donation requires that the person donate their own blood prior to surgery. The blood bank draws the blood and stores it until needed during or after surgery. This option is only for elective surgery. It has the advantage of eliminating or minimising the need for someone else's blood during and after surgery. There are some medical conditions that may prevent the preoperative donation of blood products.

Intraoperative autologous transfusion occurs when the person's blood is recycled during surgery; this blood is filtered and transfused back into the person's body. This can be done for emergency and elective surgeries but cannot be used if the person has cancer or an infection.

Postoperative autologous transfusion involves recycling blood after surgery; this blood is collected, filtered and returned to the person. This can be done in emergency and elective surgeries but cannot be used in those with cancer or infection.

Need for transfusion

Blood transfusions are very common; the procedure is used for people of all ages. Those undergoing surgery need blood transfusions due to blood loss during their operations. People who have serious injuries, for example, road traffic accidents and burns, need blood transfusions to replace blood lost.

A blood transfusion may be needed if a person has a severe infection or liver disease, preventing the body from producing blood or some parts of blood. Kidney disease or cancer may result in anaemia as well as certain medications or radiation used to treat a medical condition; blood transfusion can counteract these conditions. There are a number of types of anaemia, including aplastic, haemolytic, iron deficiency, pernicious and sickle cell anaemias and thalassaemia. A bleeding disorder, such as haemophilia or thrombocytopenia, may require transfusion. When there is loss of plasma, as in the case of burns, a transfusion of plasma may be needed.

Transfusion safety

Blood used for transfusions in the UK is very safe and normally free from disease. All donated blood is tested. It is very rare to get a disease through a blood transfusion.

The main risk in a blood transfusion is getting the wrong blood type by accident although this is rare. Transfusion with the wrong blood type can cause anaphylaxis that may be life-threatening, but this is also very rare. If a person has a blood transfusion, they are more likely to have problems from immune system reactions. A reaction happens when the body rejects the new blood. If possible, prior to a blood transfusion, blood is tested to determine blood type and the blood to be transfused is tested to ensure it matches the person's blood. A mild allergic reaction may occur even if the person gets the correct blood type. Signs of a reaction include:

- pyrexia
- tachycardia
- hives
- shortness of breath
- pain (flank, abdomen, chest)
- chills
- hypotension
- oliguria.

A mild reaction can cause anxiety but it is seldom dangerous if treated quickly.

Fluid overload

This occurs when too much fluid is transfused or too quickly, leading to pulmonary oedema and acute respiratory failure. Those at particular risk are patients with chronic anaemia who are normovolaemic or hypervolaemic and those with symptoms of cardiac failure prior to transfusion. In these patients, packed cells rather than whole blood should be given via slow transfusion, with diuretics if required.

Reducing transfusion errors

In order to reduce the possibility of transfusion risks, robust hospital transfusion protocols should be implemented. All staff involved in blood administration/taking samples for cross-matching should be trained. Improved information technology, the use of a unique barcode on the patient's wristband/blood sample and prepared blood can reduce errors (Figure 9.2).

10 Nutrition

> "Every careful observer of the sick will agree in this, that thousands of patients are starved in the midst of plenty, from want of attention to the ways which make it possible for them to take food"
>
> *(Florence Nightingale)*

Figure 10.1 Chemical degradation

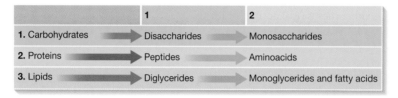

	1	**2**
1. Carbohydrates	Disaccharides	Monosaccharides
2. Proteins	Peptides	Aminoacids
3. Lipids	Diglycerides	Monoglycerides and fatty acids

Figure 10.2 The eatwell plate

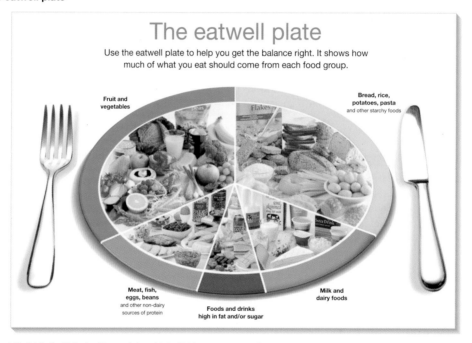

Crown copyright. Public Health England in association with the Welsh government, the Scottish government and the Food Standards Agency in Northern Ireland

Table 10.1 Basic information required to make an assessment of nutritional needs

- Height and weight
- Eating and drinking likes and dislikes
- Food allergies and medical dietary requirements (for example gluten-free diet for those with coeliac disease)
- Cultural/ethnic/religious requirements (halal for Muslims or kosher for Jews or vegan meals)
- Social/environmental mealtime needs
- Physical difficulties with eating and drinking (such as tremor)
- Need for equipment to assist with eating and drinking

Medical-Surgical Nursing at a Glance, First Edition. Ian Peate. © John Wiley & Sons, Ltd. Published 2016 by John Wiley & Sons, Ltd.
Companion website: www.ataglanceseries.com/nursing/medsurg

ursing care that promotes nutritional intake when and as appropriate has the potential to significantly aid recovery from illness and enhance a person's health and well-being.

The role of the nurse

The nurse's role with respect to the nutritional care of patients is diverse; this can range from promoting a healthy diet for a person with a brain injury to the provision of parenteral nutrition to a person who is critically ill.

Over the past few decades, the focus of nursing activities in the delivery of nutritional care has changed. The nurse is becoming more involved in aspects of nutritional care relating to health education, specifically related to the rise in the incidence of obesity as well as non-insulin-dependent diabetes mellitus. There are other areas where the role of the nurse has advanced, for example, enteral nutrition via a gastrostomy tube and parenteral nutrition. These interventions are now being used more and more in hospital and community settings.

For nurses and other healthcare professionals, nutrition is a key issue but the management of nutritional problems is often poor. For those in hospital, malnutrition is a significant risk.

Malnutrition

Malnutrition is a term used frequently in healthcare to refer to undernourished individuals who have an inadequate intake of energy in their diet. Undernutrition can occur as a result of inadequate intake as well as disorders of digestion or absorption of protein and calories. It can also refer to deficiencies in the intake of a particular vitamin or mineral.

Malnutrition related to inadequate intake, digestion or absorption of protein or calories is often referred to as 'protein-energy malnutrition' (PEM). This is common and can be associated with poor eating habits, social conditions, acute or chronic illness and disorders of the digestive tract. Acute illness made worse by PEM can lead to a risk of infection, diminished immune response, poor skin integrity, delays in wound healing, increased risk of complications and a lengthy hospital stay.

Assessment

Nutritional assessment is undertaken to assess nutritional status, identify disorders of nutrition and establish which individuals need support. Assessment should include screening for malnutrition using a validated tool. Screening must be carried out initially on all patients in order to identify those who are in need of further investigation and subsequent nutritional support.

Table 10.1 identifies some of the information that should be recorded during assessment on admission to hospital; the exact nature of the information to be collected will depend on the person's individual needs. The information suggested in Table 10.1 will help nurses to recognise and respond to some of the many issues that may be a cause of PEM in hospital patients.

Those people who are at risk of malnutrition will require more detailed questioning to evaluate the nature of their risk. Assessing the nutritional status of a patient should include a general observation of the person, observing for signs of malnutrition, for example, the appearance of hair and skin. In some people who are malnourished, the hair may appear dull, brittle and dry, and there may also be signs of hair loss. The skin can be pale, dry and rough; if the person has any wounds, these will take longer to heal. The nurse should also look for signs of weight loss such as thin appearance and a lack of subcutaneous fat and clothing that is poorly fitting.

Dietary history along with medical history can be used to create a nutritional treatment plan, while recent medical history along with a dietary history may identify illnesses or conditions that can increase the risk of malnutrition. A patient may, for example, describe loss of appetite, nausea and vomiting, change in bowel habit, weight loss or tiredness, all of which may point to an underlying condition such as cancer.

Assessment tools

There are a variety of assessment tools available, including anthropometric measurements, biochemical analyses and specific nurse-administered screening tools (such as the malnutrition universal screening tool), as well as physical assessment and dietary history taking.

Nutrients

Proteins are essential to growth and repair of muscle and other body tissues. Fats provide one source of energy and are important in relation to fat-soluble vitamins. Carbohydrates are the main source of energy. Minerals (inorganic elements) occurring in the body are critical to its normal functions. Water and fat-soluble vitamins play important roles in many chemical processes in the body. Water is essential for normal body function; it acts as a vehicle for carrying other nutrients, and 60% of the human body is water. The fibrous indigestible portion of our diet, roughage, is essential to the health of the digestive system.

Carbohydrates, proteins and lipids are absorbed in a form that cannot be taken up by the cells, so food needs to be broken into small pieces (mechanical digestion) and broken down chemically (chemical digestion) (Figure 10.1).

The eatwell plate

The eatwell plate (Figure 10.2) defines the UK government's advice on a healthy balanced diet; it is a visual representation of how different foods contribute towards such a diet. The plate model has been tested extensively with consumers and health professionals. The nurse can use it when promoting healthy eating. The size of the segments for each of the food groups is in alignment with government recommendations for a diet that would provide all the nutrients required for a healthy adult or child over the age of 5.

The eatwell plate, based on the five food groups, makes healthy eating easier to understand by giving a visual representation of the types and proportions of foods needed for a healthy balanced diet. Choosing a variety of foods from within the four main food groups will add to the range of nutrients consumed. This includes plenty of fruit and vegetables, plenty of bread, rice, potatoes, pasta and other starchy foods, some milk and dairy foods, some meat, fish, eggs, beans and other non-dairy sources of protein. Foods and drinks high in fat and/or sugar are not essential to a healthy diet and should only be consumed in small amounts.

11 Pain

Figure 11.1 Chronic pain

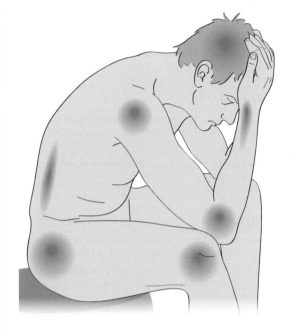

Table 11.1 Factors influencing pain

- The person's past experience
- Level of anxiety being experienced by the individual
- The person's mental health status (e.g. if the person is depressed)
- An individual's culture
- The person's gender
- Genetic make up

Table 11.2 The main changes associated with chronic pain

- Depression
- An attempt to keep pain-related behaviour to a minimum
- Sleeping disorders
- Preoccupation with the pain
- Tendency to deny pain

Figure 11.2 The analgesic ladder

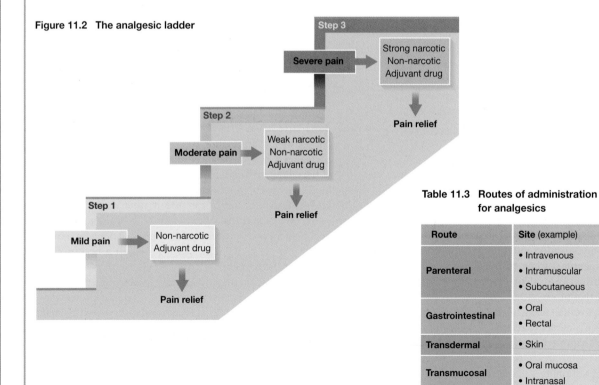

Step 3

Severe pain → Strong narcotic / Non-narcotic / Adjuvant drug → Pain relief

Step 2

Moderate pain → Weak narcotic / Non-narcotic / Adjuvant drug → Pain relief

Step 1

Mild pain → Non-narcotic / Adjuvant drug → Pain relief

Table 11.3 Routes of administration for analgesics

Route	Site (example)
Parenteral	• Intravenous • Intramuscular • Subcutaneous
Gastrointestinal	• Oral • Rectal
Transdermal	• Skin
Transmucosal	• Oral mucosa • Intranasal
Topical	• Skin
Epidural	• Epidural space
Intraspinal	• Spinal canal

Medical-Surgical Nursing at a Glance, First Edition. Ian Peate. © John Wiley & Sons, Ltd. Published 2016 by John Wiley & Sons, Ltd.
Companion website: www.ataglanceseries.com/nursing/medsurg

Many people experience pain. Acute pain can be protective as it can cause a person to move away from a dangerous situation. However, chronic pain serves no function. Pain is the most common reason for people seeking healthcare. People can have a painful diagnosed condition such as arthritis or diabetes neuropathy or they may have a painful condition that is not fully understood, for example, long-term back pain.

Because perception and tolerance of pain vary from person to person, it is difficult to define and describe. Despite this, there are several definitions of pain; it can be said to be a disagreeable sensory and emotional experience resulting in actual or potential tissue damage. Some suggest it is the fifth vital sign.

Pain receptors

Pain is sensed when specific pain receptors are activated. The description of pain is subjective and objective and is based on duration, speed of sensation and location.

Pain receptors, called nociceptors, are the primary afferent neurons with specific nerve endings that have the ability to distinguish between noxious (thermal, chemical and mechanical) and innocuous events and initially transmit this information centrally to the spinal cord. The transmission of pain is known as nociception. Chemical substances such as prostaglandins (which increase sensitivity of pain receptors), endorphins and enkephalins (which suppress pain reception) also play an important part in the perception of pain. Other chemicals that cause or worsen pain include histamine, bradykinin and serotonin.

Factors influencing pain

There are several factors that have the potential to influence pain (Table 11.1).

Types of pain

There are a number of types of pain, for example, acute pain, chronic (continuing) pain, cancer-related pain. It is also possible to classify pain according to location or aetiology.

Acute pain

Acute pain is a protective mechanism alerting the individual to a condition or experience that is immediately harmful to the body. The onset of acute pain is usually sudden and it lasts less than 6 months.

Stimulation of the autonomic nervous system can be observed during this type of pain (tachycardia, tachypnoea, sweating, vasoconstriction). There may be hypertension, pallor or flushing, hyperglycaemia, reduced acid secretion and gastric motility. Blood flow to the viscera (kidney, skin) is decreased.

Chronic pain

Chronic pain (persistent or intermittent pain) lasting longer than 6 months can severely affect a person's health and well-being. This type of pain can develop insidiously; often it is associated with a sense of hopelessness and helplessness. Intermittent pain produces a physiological response similar to acute pain. Persistent pain allows for adaptation; body functions are normal but the pain is not relieved. Persistent low back pain is the most common type of chronic pain; this type of pain can also

be associated with cancer. Chronic pain produces significant behavioural and psychological changes (Table 11.2).

Location of pain

Pain felt by a pinprick or the scraping of a knee is cutaneous pain; this is felt on the skin or subcutaneous tissue and is localised. Deep somatic pain is pain that comes from the bones, skeletal muscles or blood vessels, for example; this type of pain is slow pain and may radiate along a nerve root. Pain in the abdominal or thoracic cavity is known as visceral pain; this is often severe and localised but may be referred, for example, angina, pancreatitis. Referred pain is pain that is felt in an area other than the location of injury, making it difficult to identify the exact origin.

Assessment of pain

Assessment of the person's pain should be undertaken holistically, from a multidimensional perspective. The nurse should consider the person's goal or expectations of comfort and pain relief, what pain means for the patient, the physical and psychological behaviours associated with the pain and the physical responses being made to the pain. Characteristics of the pain such as intensity, timing, location and quality and any aggravating or alleviating factors should be noted during the assessment.

Pain scales

There are several types of pain intensity rating scales available that will enable the nurse, with the patient, to make an objective assessment of the severity of pain. These include visual analogue scales, numeric pain intensity scale, descriptive pain intensity scale and face pain scale.

Pain management

Effective pain management demands competent, consistent and compassionate care that is delivered in a timely manner. Pain management is ongoing and the outcomes of pain management strategies should be documented in the person's care plan.

Pharmacological interventions

Opioid analgesics (for example, morphine) act on the central nervous system, inhibiting activity of ascending nociceptive pathways. Non-steroidal anti-inflammatory drugs (NSAIDs) decrease pain by inhibiting cyclo-oxygenase (the enzyme involved in the production of prostaglandin). Local anaesthetics act by blocking nerve conduction when applied to the nerve fibres. The WHO suggests using a step-by-step approach to pain control – the analgesic ladder (Figure 11.2). Administration routes for analgesia can be found in Table 11.3.

Non-pharmacological interventions

Cutaneous stimulation (such as transcutaneous electrical nerve stimulation – TENS), massage and use of heat and cold may help to relieve pain. Cautious use of heat and cold changes blood flow to the area and can promote healing. Heat should not be applied to a painful area that is the site of acute, untreated infection as this could cause increased pain with increased blood flow to the site.

The use of distraction, relaxation and guided imagery may redirect attention, promote muscle relaxation and affect perception or reception of pain stimulus in the brain.

12 Infection Prevention and Control: I

Figure 12.1 The chain of infection

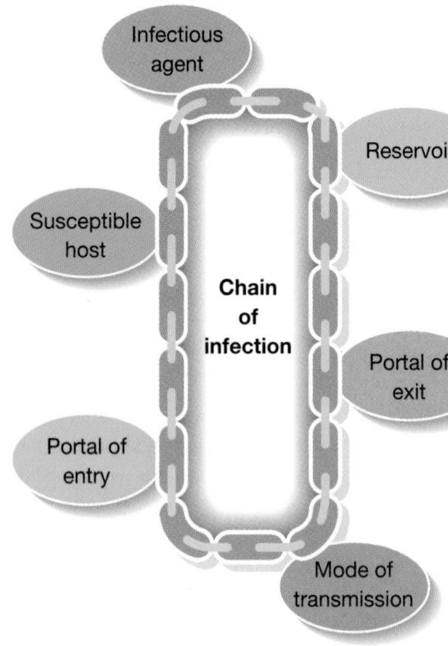

Infectious agent

Reservoir

Susceptible host

Chain of infection

Portal of exit

Portal of entry

Mode of transmission

Figure 12.2 Five moments of hand washing

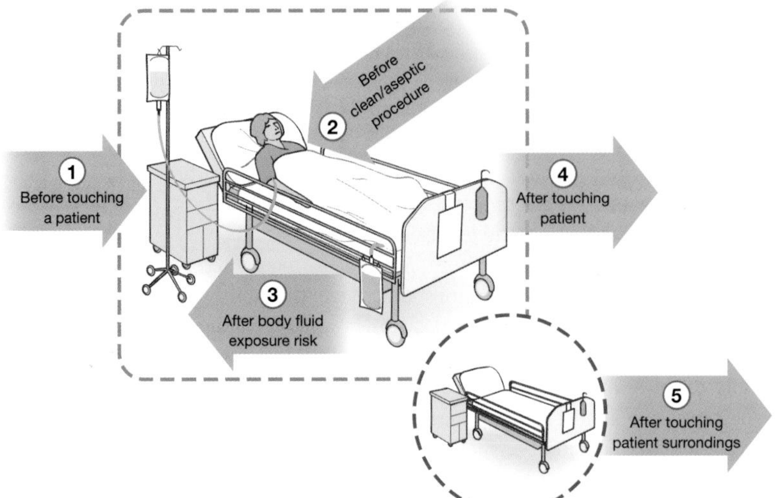

① Before touching a patient

② Before clean/aseptic procedure

③ After body fluid exposure risk

④ After touching patient

⑤ After touching patient surrondings

Source: Reproduced with permission of WHO

Figure 12.3 Hand washing technique

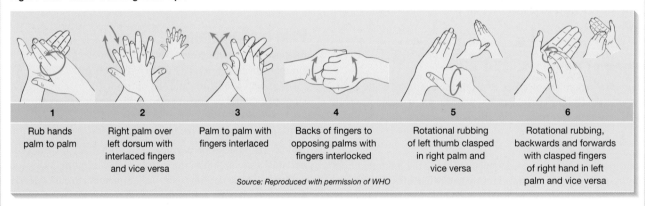

1	2	3	4	5	6
Rub hands palm to palm	Right palm over left dorsum with interlaced fingers and vice versa	Palm to palm with fingers interlaced	Backs of fingers to opposing palms with fingers interlocked	Rotational rubbing of left thumb clasped in right palm and vice versa	Rotational rubbing, backwards and forwards with clasped fingers of right hand in left palm and vice versa

Source: Reproduced with permission of WHO

Table 12.1 The modes of transmission

Contact transmission	Occurs when the transfer of microorganisms results from direct physical contact between an infected or colonised individual and a susceptible host. Indirect transmission involves the passive transfer of an infectious agent to a susceptible host via an intermediate object or fomite (instruments, bed rails, bed tables and other environmental surfaces)
Droplet transmission	Occurs when respiratory droplets via coughing, sneezing or talking contact susceptible mucosal surfaces, such as the eyes, nose or mouth. Can also occur indirectly via contact with contaminated fomites with hands and then mucosal surfaces. Respiratory droplets are large and are not able to remain suspended in the air, they are usually dispersed over short distances
Airborne transmission	Refers to infectious agents spread via droplet nuclei (residue from evaporated droplets) containing infective microorganisms. These organisms can survive outside the body, remaining suspended in the air for long periods of time. Infecting others via the upper and lower respiratory tracts

Medical-Surgical Nursing at a Glance, First Edition. Ian Peate. © John Wiley & Sons, Ltd. Published 2016 by John Wiley & Sons, Ltd.
Companion website: www.ataglanceseries.com/nursing/medsurg

Infection prevention and control are essential components of healthcare. Healthcare-associated infections (HCAIs) cost the health service millions of pounds per year as well as causing patients and their families unnecessary suffering and concern.

Healthcare-associated infections

The Health Care Act (2006) defines an HCAI as:

Any infection to which an individual may be exposed or made susceptible (or more susceptible) in circumstances where healthcare is being, or has been provided to that or any other individual, and the risk of exposure to the infection, or susceptibility (or increased susceptibility) to it, is directly or indirectly attributable to the provision of healthcare.

Healthcare-associated infections are the most common complication affecting patients in hospital. However, the problem does not just affect patients and workers in hospitals, as HCAIs can occur in any healthcare setting, including general practice settings, clinics, dental surgeries and also long-term care facilities. HCAI is a potentially preventable adverse event as opposed to an unpredictable complication. Anybody working in or entering any healthcare facility is at risk of transmitting infection or being infected. When effective infection prevention and control procedures are implemented, this can significantly reduce the rate of HCAI.

Not all infections are preventable but managing infection control and ensuring best practice can improve patient outcomes and service user safety significantly.

The transmission of infections such as meticillin-resistant *Staphylococcus aureus* (MRSA) and *Clostridium difficile* can occur through the contaminated hands of a healthcare worker, the equipment and the medical devices that they use.

Healthcare workers will come into contact with people who have infections and/or contagious diseases and they must know how to prevent or reduce the transmission of infection.

Incorporating evidence-based infection prevention and control advice into routine clinical care activities is important in reducing the incidence of preventable HCAIs. As a result of this, the National Institute for Health and Care Excellence has produced guidelines on how to prevent and control HCAIs.

Hand hygiene

Hand hygiene is seen as the single most important activity for minimising the likelihood of infection, so it is an important activity in every setting. Pathogens on the hands of clinical practitioners can be removed by hand washing. Infection involves a cycle of events that promotes the spread (transmission) of infection (Figure 12.1).

Healthcare workers have the greatest potential to spread micro-organisms that may result in infection; this is related to the number of times that they have contact with patients or the patient environment. Hands therefore are a very effective vehicle for transmission of micro-organisms.

Hands should be decontaminated before direct contact with patients and after any activity or contact that contaminates the hands; this includes after the removal of gloves. Alcohol hand gels and rubs are a practical alternative to soap and water but alcohol is not a cleaning agent. Hands that are visibly dirty or potentially grossly contaminated must be washed with soap and water and dried thoroughly. Hand preparation increases the effectiveness of decontamination. Whenever feasible, staff should have access to the means to clean their hands at the point of care and where possible, soap and water should be used. However, this is not always possible with the placement of sinks. The ability to clean the hands is possible when the nurse uses other alternatives.

Detergent wipes should be used if soap and water are not available and this should be followed by drying the hands thoroughly with paper towels or air drying, then alcohol gel can be used. Only use alcohol gel if the hands are visibly clean, as using alcohol gel on contaminated hands renders the solution ineffective. Detergent wipes and hand rubs should be readily available at the point of care; if they are not then the chance of using them will be lost and hands will retain potentially dangerous microbes. Alcohol gel should be used between different care activities with the patient (Figure 12.2).

The nurse should keep nails short, clean and polish free and should avoid wearing wristwatches and jewellery, particularly rings with ridges or stones. Artificial nails must not be worn and any cuts and abrasions must be covered with a waterproof dressing.

Wristwatches and any bracelets should be removed and long sleeves rolled up before washing the hands and wrists. The NHS has implemented a 'Naked below the elbows' rule that has banned healthcare workers from wearing long sleeves, wristwatches and jewellery to promote effective hand and wrist washing; this includes the avoidance of ties when carrying out clinical activity.

Hospitals are unique places that differ considerably in the risk of potential infection spread from a 'normal' home environment. While risks occur wherever direct contact between people or equipment happens, inpatient hospitals have a large number of people living in a small physical area. Moreover, patients may have direct contact with a large number of people (staff) as a result of their ongoing care needs, allowing for many more opportunities for micro-organisms, some of which may be resistant to antibiotics, to spread from one person to another than would normally happen at home.

Figure 12.3 outlines the correct technique for hand washing and gel application.

Transmission of infection

Understanding the modes of transmission of infectious organisms and knowing how and when to apply the basic principles of infection prevention are essential in controlling infection (Table 12.1). This responsibility applies to everybody working in and visiting a healthcare facility.

Infectious agents are biological agents causing disease or illness to their hosts. Many infectious agents are present in healthcare settings. Patients and healthcare workers are the most likely sources of infectious agents and are also the most common susceptible hosts. Infection requires three main elements: a source of the infectious agent, a mode of transmission and a susceptible host. The chain must be broken to prevent transmission of infection.

13 Infection Prevention and Control: II

Table 13.1 The modes of transmission

Contact transmission	Occurs when the transfer of microorganisms results from direct physical contact between an infected or colonised individual and a susceptible host. Indirect transmission involves the passive transfer of an infectious agent to a susceptible host via an intermediate object or fomite (instruments, bed rails, bed tables and other environmental surfaces)
Droplet transmission	Occurs when respiratory droplets via coughing, sneezing or talking contact susceptible mucosal surfaces, such as the eyes, nose or mouth. Can also occur indirectly via contact with contaminated fomites with hands and then mucosal surfaces. Respiratory droplets are large and are not able to remain suspended in the air, they are usually dispersed over short distances
Airborne transmission	Refers to infectious agents spread via droplet nuclei (residue from evaporated droplets) containing infective microorganisms. These organisms can survive outside the body, remaining suspended in the air for long periods of time. Infecting others via the upper and lower respiratory tracts

Table 13.2 The principles underpinning asepsis

- Ensure the area where the procedure is to take place is as clean as possible
- Make sure there is as little disturbance as possible occurring during the procedure that might cause air turbulence and the distribution of dust, i.e. bed making, floor sweeping or buffing
- Carry out hand hygiene prior to and during the procedure as required
- Use sterile equipment
- Reduce contamination of the vulnerable site by using forceps or sterile gloves, do not touch sterile parts of the equipment (the non-touch technique)

Medical-Surgical Nursing at a Glance, First Edition. Ian Peate. © John Wiley & Sons, Ltd. Published 2016 by John Wiley & Sons, Ltd.
Companion website: www.ataglanceseries.com/nursing/medsurg

Infection can occur when micro-organisms are transferred from one patient to another, from equipment or the environment to patients or between staff. Disorders to the patient's 'normal bacterial flora' can also predispose a person to infection. If bacteria are transferred from one part of the body to another where they are not usually resident, for example, moving faecal bacteria from the perineum to the face during washing or administering oral hygiene without performing hand hygiene or changing gloves, this puts the patient at risk.

Modes of transmission

Infectious agents are biological agents that cause disease or illness to their hosts. Most infectious agents are present in healthcare settings. Patients and healthcare workers are usually the most likely sources of infectious agents and are also the most common susceptible hosts. Others visiting and working in healthcare can also be at risk of both infection and transmission.

There are three modes of transmission: contact, droplet and airborne (Table 13.1).

Methods of reducing the spread of infection

Standard Precautions

Standard Practices are work practices applied to everyone, regardless of their perceived or confirmed infectious status, and ensure a basic level of infection prevention and control. Implementing Standard Precautions as a first-line approach to infection prevention and control minimises the risk of transmission of infectious agents from person to person, even in high-risk situations.

Transmission-based precautions

The first line of prevention of infection is the use of Standard Precautions.

Transmission-based precautions are additional work practices for specific situations where Standard Precautions are not sufficient to interrupt transmission. These precautions are tailored to the particular infectious agent and its mode of transmission.

Personal protective equipment

Personal protective equipment (PPE) is used to protect healthcare workers and patients from risk of infection. The risk of infection is reduced by preventing the transmission of micro-organisms to the patient via the hands of staff or vice versa. Gloves are also required for contact with hazardous chemicals and some pharmaceuticals, such as disinfectants or cytotoxic drugs. PPE includes items such as gloves, aprons, masks, goggles or visors.

Sharps

Safe handling and disposal of sharps are essential aspects of infection prevention and control. Sharps include needles, scalpels, stitch cutters, glass ampoules, bone fragments and any sharp instrument. The main hazards of a sharps injury are bloodborne viruses, for example, hepatitis B, hepatitis C and HIV.

Unsafe or poor practice can result in injury to the individual or others, for example, cleaners who experience injuries as a result of sharps being misplaced in waste bins. Sharps injuries are preventable and learning following incidents can help to avoid repeat accidents. To reduce the risk of injury and exposure to bloodborne viruses, it is essential that sharps are used safely and disposed of carefully; agreed policies on the use of sharps should be adhered to.

Waste disposal

Waste generated by healthcare staff in the line of their work may include sharps, hazardous, offensive, municipal (household) and pharmaceutical (medicinal) waste. Reducing waste, segregation and disposal are essential to sustaining a healthy environment and reducing subsequent public health implications.

Healthcare institutions have policies on waste segregation and disposal, providing guidance on all aspects, including special waste, such as pharmaceuticals and cytotoxic waste and segregation of waste. This includes the colour coding of bags used for waste.

Spillage

Where blood and bodily fluids have been spilt, these should be dealt with quickly and in adherence to local policy and procedure for dealing with spillages. Policy and procedure will dictate the chemicals that should be used to ensure that any spillage is disinfected properly, taking into account the surface where the incident occurred, for example, a carpet in a patient's home or a hard surface in a hospital.

Asepsis and aseptic technique

Asepsis seeks to prevent or reduce micro-organisms from entering a vulnerable body site such as a surgical wound or an intravenous catheter, or during the insertion of an invasive device, such as a urinary catheter. Asepsis decreases the risk of an infection developing as a result of the procedure being undertaken.

Aseptic technique includes a set of specific actions or procedures that are performed under controlled conditions. The ability to control conditions varies according to the care setting but the principles outlined in Table 13.2 should be applied in all cases.

Indwelling devices

Common intravascular devices (urinary catheters, IV cannulae or central venous catheters) are frequently responsible for HCAIs such as urinary tract infection, insertion site or bloodstream infections. These devices when used appropriately provide valuable assistance to promote patient care and positive patient outcomes. They are not, however, without risk and the development of infection is common as they bypass the body's natural defence mechanisms such as skin and mucous membranes.

In order to assess patency (that the device is open and unrestricted) and to detect any signs or symptoms of infection, day-to-day management is essential and local policies and procedures must be adhered to; this may include, at a minimum, a daily review assessing the continuing need for the device. This should be documented. There should be regular documented checks for patency of the device, signs of infection and dressing, implementation of hand hygiene before any contact with the device or associated administration sets occurs, cleaning/disinfection of any add-on devices/attachments and the replacement of peripheral intravascular devices after 72 hours (or as per local policy) or sooner according to clinical indications.

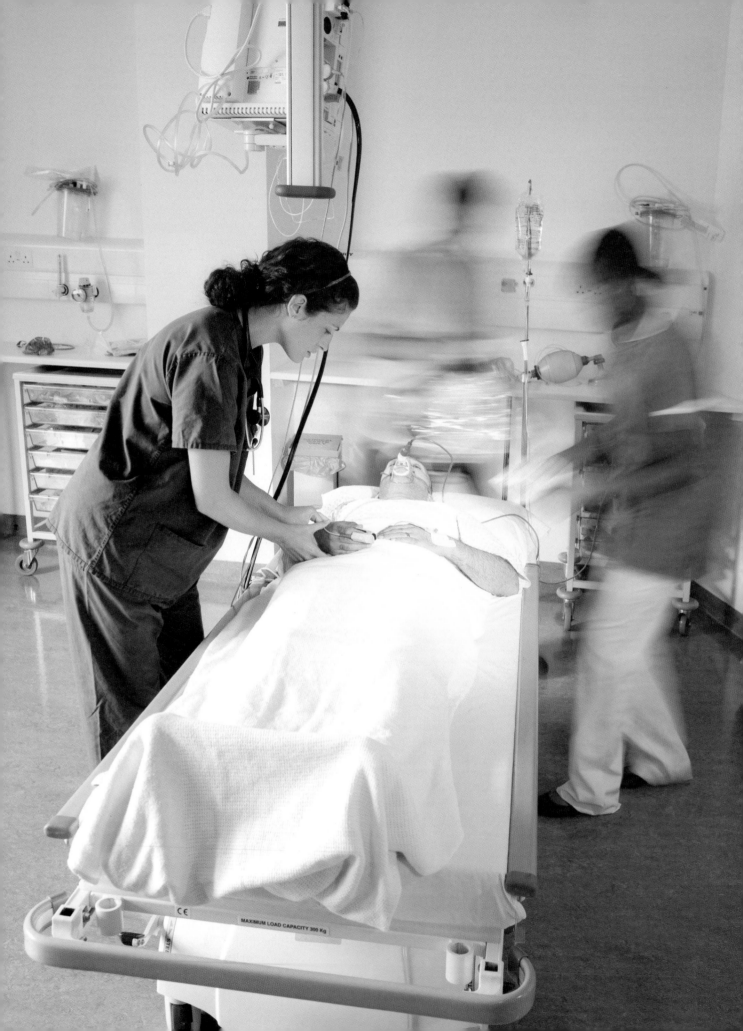

Medical nursing

Part 3

Chapters

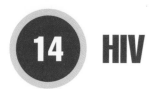

HIV

Table 14.1   The signs and symptoms of late HIV

- Rapid weight loss
- Recurring fever or profuse night sweats
- Extreme and unexplained tiredness
- Prolonged swelling of the lymph glands (lymphadenopathy)
- Diarrhoea lasting longer than a week
- Sores of the mouth, anus or genitalia
- Pneumonia
- Red, brown, pink, or purplish blotches on or under the skin or inside the mouth, nose or eyelids
- Loss of memory, depression and other neurological disorders

Figure 14.1   The main symptoms of acute HIV

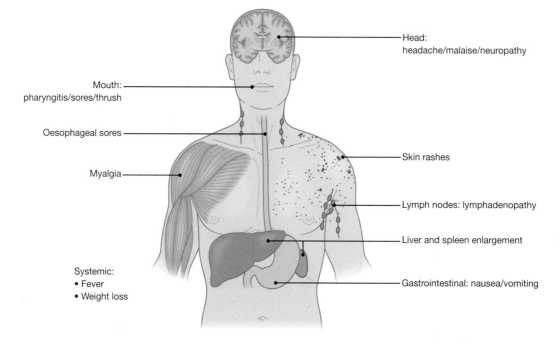

Head:
headache/malaise/neuropathy

Mouth:
pharyngitis/sores/thrush

Oesophageal sores

Myalgia

Skin rashes

Lymph nodes: lymphadenopathy

Liver and spleen enlargement

Gastrointestinal: nausea/vomiting

Systemic:
- Fever
- Weight loss

Table 14.2   Risk factors associated with HIV

- Engages in unprotected anal, vaginal, or oral sex with men who have sex with men, multiple partners, or anonymous partners
- Injects drugs or steroids where needles/syringes are shared
- Has a sexually transmitted infection, such as syphilis, genital herpes, chlamydia, gonorrhoea, bacterial vaginosis or trichomoniasis
- Has been diagnosed with hepatitis, tuberculosis, or malaria
- Exchanges sex for drugs or money
- Is exposed to the virus as a foetus or infant before or during birth or through breastfeeding from a mother infected with HIV
- Has received a blood transfusion or clotting factor anytime from 1978 to 1985
- Engages in unprotected sex with someone who has any of those risk factors listed above

Medical-Surgical Nursing at a Glance, First Edition. Ian Peate. © John Wiley & Sons, Ltd. Published 2016 by John Wiley & Sons, Ltd.
Companion website: www.ataglanceseries.com/nursing/medsurg

The human immunodeficiency virus (HIV) is the virus causing acquired immune deficiency syndrome (AIDS). HIV damages an individual's immune system by destroying CD4+ T cells; these are white blood cells essential in preventing infection. When these cells have been destroyed, this leaves people with HIV susceptible to other infections, diseases and further complications.

AIDS is the final stage of HIV infection. A person who has HIV is diagnosed with AIDS when they have one or more opportunistic infection, for example, pneumonia or tuberculosis and a CD4+ T cell count less than 200 cells per cubic millimetre of blood.

Human immunodeficiency virus

The human immunodeficiency virus is a retrovirus, which binds to CD4 receptors on the T helper cell membrane with a chemokine (CCR5) co-receptor and 'injects' RNA and associated enzymes. The virus contains two RNA strands and on one strand, uses the enzymes reverse transcriptase to incorporate (reverse transcribe) the RNA coding into a single, then a double DNA strand in the host cell and then integrase to integrate it into the host DNA, in the nucleus of the cell.

HIV cannot survive for very long outside the body. It is a fragile virus, which cannot be transmitted through activities such as using a toilet seat, sharing food utensils or drinking glasses, shaking hands or through kissing. The virus can only be transmitted from person to person, it cannot be transmitted through animals or insect bites.

Those infected with HIV and who are taking antiretroviral therapy can still infect others through unprotected sex as well as when sharing needles.

HIV risk factors

The human immunodeficiency virus has been found in blood, semen and vaginal fluid of those infected with the virus. Factors increasing the risk of becoming infected with HIV are shown in Table 14.2.

Signs and symptoms of HIV

Early stage

In the early stages of HIV infection, most people will have very few, if any symptoms; they may be asymptomatic. Within a month or two after infection (being exposed to the virus), they may experience a range of flu-like symptoms; these include fever, sore throat, headache, tiredness, enlarged cervical and femoral lymph nodes.

Often these symptoms disappear within a week to a month and are usually mistaken for another viral infection, such as influenza. During this period, however, people are highly infectious as HIV is present in large quantities in genital fluids and the blood (viral load). Some people with HIV can have more severe symptoms at first or symptoms that may last a long time, whilst others may have no symptoms for 12 years or longer. The symptoms of acute HIV are outlined in Figure 14.1.

Late stage

During the late stages of HIV infection, the virus weakens the immune system severely as viral load increases; people infected with HIV can then experience the signs and symptoms highlighted in Table 14.1.

However, it must be remembered that those signs and symptoms may also be related to other illnesses.

HIV testing

The only way to determine if a person is HIV positive is to undertake an HIV test. HIV screening provides healthcare workers with the ability to identify those who are not aware that they are HIV positive, in order to provide information on the need to avoid high-risk behaviours, safer sex practices and antiretroviral therapy. In the UK, HIV testing can be performed anonymously.

Treatment

Those with HIV infection (as well as their families) need a great deal of support, as well as monitoring and drug treatment for the patient. Management will also include the treatment of any specific complications of HIV infection.

Antiretroviral therapy (ART) is recommended for all those with established HIV infection if they have a CD4 cell count of ≤350 cells/mm^3 or signs of nervous system involvement or an AIDS-defining condition present.

The advent of ART has radically reduced the risk of developing AIDS. Antiretroviral drugs are now available to inhibit the replication of the HIV, helping to prolong life, restoring the patient's immune system to near normal activity and reducing the chances of opportunistic infections developing. Combinations of three or more drugs are usually given to reduce the possibility of resistance.

Antiretroviral treatment has side effects and may cause lipodystrophy syndrome which includes fat redistribution, insulin resistance and dyslipidaemia. Careful monitoring of the person's condition is required as well as their response to the treatment.

Postexposure prophylaxis

Postexposure prophylaxis (PEP) is a course of anti-HIV medication, also known as emergency HIV medication. The treatment must be commenced as soon as possible after exposure to HIV, ideally within a few hours. The medicines must be taken every day for 4 weeks. PEP is unlikely to work if it is commenced after 72 hours. PEP makes infection with HIV less likely but it is not a cure for HIV and may not work in all cases. PEP is usually available from:

- sexual health clinics or genitourinary medicine (GUM) clinics
- hospitals – usually accident and emergency (A&E) departments.

HIV prevention

Currently, there is no vaccine to prevent HIV infection; there is no cure for HIV. To reduce the risk of becoming infected with HIV or transmitting the virus to others, healthcare workers should implement standard isolation procedures for all patients.

Pre-exposure prophylaxis

The provision of antiretroviral therapy to people who are not infected with HIV (known as pre-exposure prophylaxis (PrEP)) but who are at high risk of getting HIV infection can help to prevent the onward transmission of HIV.

15 Systemic Lupus Erythematosus

Figure 15.1 A range of symptoms associated with SLE

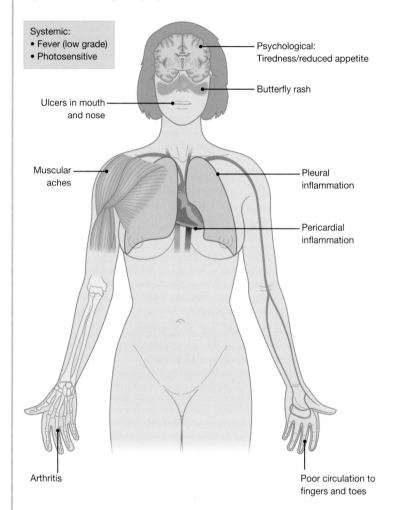

Systemic:
- Fever (low grade)
- Photosensitive

Psychological:
Tiredness/reduced appetite

Butterfly rash

Ulcers in mouth and nose

Muscular aches

Pleural inflammation

Pericardial inflammation

Arthritis

Poor circulation to fingers and toes

Table 15.1 SLE general manifestations

Dermatological: Butterfly rash, photosensitivity, subcutaneous lesions, mucosal ulcers, alopecia, pain and discomfort, pruritus, bruising

Musculoskeletal: Arthralgia, arthritis, other joint complications

Haematological: Anaemia, decreased WBC count, thrombocytopenia, elevated ESR

Cardiopulmonary: Pericarditis, myocarditis, myocardial infarction, vasculitis, pleurisy, valvular heart disease

Renal: Asymptomatic microscopic renal involvement, renal failure, fluid and electrolyte imbalance, urinary tract infection

Central Nervous System (CNS): General CNS symptomology, cranial neuropathies, cognitive impairment, mental changes, seizures

Gastrointestinal: Anorexia, ascites, pancreatitis, mesenteric or intestinal vasculitis

Ophthalmological: Eyelid problems, conjunctivitis, cytoid bodies, dry eyes, glaucoma, cataracts, retinal pigmentation

Other key issues

Pregnancy: Lupus flare, miscarriage or stillbirth, pregnancy-induced hypertension, neonatal lupus

Infection: Increased risk of respiratory tract, urinary tract, and skin infections; opportunistic infections

Nutrition: Weight changes; poor diet; appetite loss; problems with taking medications; increased risk of cardiovascular disease, diabetes, osteoporosis, and kidney disease

Table 15.2 A person may be classified as having lupus if 4 or more of the 11 criteria below are present

- Macular rash

- Discoid lupus

- Photosensitivity

- Oral or nasopharyngeal ulcers

- Non-erosive arthritis involving 2 or more peripheral joints

- Pleuritis or pericarditis

- Renal involvement

- Seizures or psychosis

- Haematological disorders

- Immunological disorder

- A positive antinuclear antibody

Medical-Surgical Nursing at a Glance, First Edition. Ian Peate. © John Wiley & Sons, Ltd. Published 2016 by John Wiley & Sons, Ltd.
Companion website: www.ataglanceseries.com/nursing/medsurg

Systemic lupus erythematosus (SLE) is a unique, complex disease with a range of symptoms. This condition affects individuals differently, no two cases of SLE are alike and because of this caring for people with SLE can be a challenge, drawing on all available resources, knowledge and strengths that the nurse and the multidisciplinary team have to offer.

Systemic lupus erythematosus

Systemic lupus erythematosus is a chronic, inflammatory, multisystem disorder of the immune system, in which the body develops antibodies that react against the individual's own normal tissue. These antibodies are markers for SLE, and are one indicator of many immune system abnormalities leading to clinical manifestations.

Systemic lupus erythematosus is not contagious, infectious or malignant. Often it develops in young women of childbearing years, but men and children also develop lupus. SLE also appears in the first-degree relatives of those with lupus, indicating a hereditary component. Most cases of SLE occur sporadically, suggesting that genetic and environmental factors play a role in the development of the condition.

Lupus erythematosus describes the characteristic rash of SLE and the term 'systemic' highlights the potential for multiorgan involvement. The cause of SLE is not known.

Risk factors

Certain human immunopathological factors are more common in lupus patients.

Environmental factors include ultraviolet light and viruses, such as the Epstein–Barr virus. Some drugs are known to cause drug-induced lupus, such as chlorpromazine, methyldopa, hydralazine, isoniazid, penicillamine and minocycline.

Signs and symptoms

The onset may be acute, resembling an infectious process, or it may be a progression of vague symptoms over several years. SLE is a remitting and relapsing illness. Often symptoms and signs are non-specific; see Figure 15.1 for the general manifestations.

The symptoms of lupus may range from minor aching pains and rash to life-threatening disease. Any major organ involvement usually develops within 5 years of disease onset. It is common for the person to complain of joint and muscle pains, usually with early morning stiffness.

There may be a photosensitivity rash. The classic feature is the malar (butterfly) rash which is often caused by sunlight. This is erythematous and may be raised and pruritic.

Pleurisy may be a feature with dyspnoea, with an increased risk of pulmonary embolism. There can be pericarditis and hypertension with an increased risk of coronary heart disease. The kidneys may be affected and nephritis can occur with proteinuria and haematuria; there may be glomerulonephritis. The person may be anxious and experience depression. SLE can be associated with almost any neurological manifestation. Vasculitis or thrombosis may cause strokes. Table 15.1 lists a range of clinical symptoms associated with SLE.

Investigations and diagnosis

A person may be classified as having lupus if four or more of the 11 criteria listed in Table 15.2 are present (these do not have to occur at the same time but can accumulate over a number of years).

A detailed patient history is obtained and a thorough physical examination undertaken in order to make an accurate diagnosis.

There is no single laboratory test that can definitely prove or disprove SLE. Initial screening includes a full blood count, liver and renal screening, laboratory tests for specific autoantibodies (such as antinuclear antibodies), an antiphospholipid antibody test, urinalysis, blood chemistries and erythrocyte sedimentation rate (ESR). Abnormalities in these test results will guide further evaluations. Biopsies of the skin or kidney can support a diagnosis of SLE. X-rays and other diagnostic tools are used to rule out other pathological conditions and to determine the involvement of specific organs. The nurse will be required to offer care to the patient before, during and after these tests are undertaken.

Management and care

Lupus symptoms often present according to the body system affected. To effectively care for a person with lupus, the nurse needs up-to-date knowledge and understanding of the disease, its many manifestations and its changing and often unpredictable course.

As a care plan is developed, the nurse should keep in mind the importance of frequently reassessing the patient's status, adjusting treatment to accommodate the variability of SLE manifestations. The nurse should incorporate the patient's needs and routines in the care plan, adjusting nursing interventions and medical protocols. Working together, the nurse and the patient have much to offer each other.

The person with SLE will require physical and psychological care; they may need counselling about their prognosis and symptoms. The person should be encouraged to rest, have a balanced diet and engage in exercise. The nurse needs to assist the person with the activities of living that they are unable to perform for themselves, and attention should be paid to any psychosocial issues. The person should be advised to avoid sun exposure as much as possible and use sunscreens.

Underlying causes such as anaemia and depression should be identified and treated. Simple analgesics and non-steroidal anti-inflammatory drugs (NSAIDs) can be prescribed for joint and muscle pains, headaches and musculoskeletal chest pains (NSAIDs should be used with caution because of gastrointestinal, renal and cardiovascular risks). If pain is not controlled then additional treatment may be needed to control symptoms, depending on the individual systems involved.

Other medications include corticosteroids. Hydroxy-chloroquine is effective for skin lesions, arthralgia, myalgia and malaise; this is first-line treatment for those with mild SLE. Immunosuppressive agents can be given such as methotrexate and ciclosporin.

With earlier recognition and improved management, the prognosis for this condition has improved. Morbidity and mortality are usually higher in those with extensive multisystem disease and multiple autoantibodies.

16 Irritable Bowel Syndrome

Figure 16.1 Irritable bowel syndrome

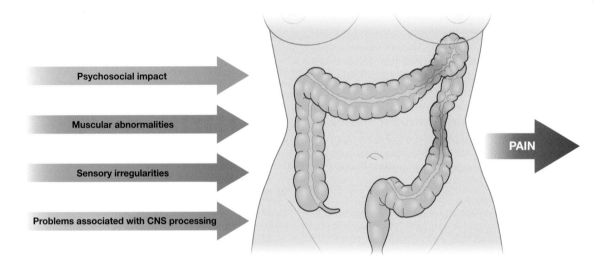

Psychosocial impact

Muscular abnormalities

Sensory irregularities

Problems associated with CNS processing

PAIN

Figure 16.2 Areas of spasm associated with irritable bowel syndrome

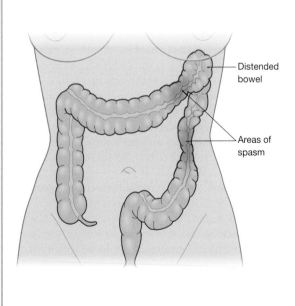

Distended bowel

Areas of spasm

Figure 16.3 Some signs and symptoms of irritable bowel syndrome

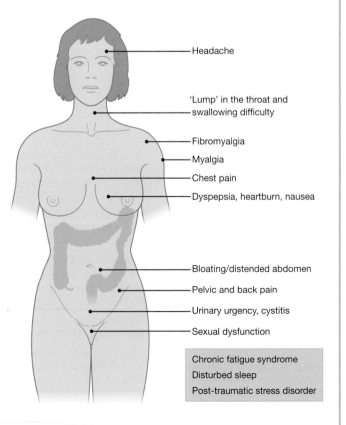

Headache

'Lump' in the throat and swallowing difficulty

Fibromyalgia

Myalgia

Chest pain

Dyspepsia, heartburn, nausea

Bloating/distended abdomen

Pelvic and back pain

Urinary urgency, cystitis

Sexual dysfunction

Chronic fatigue syndrome
Disturbed sleep
Post-traumatic stress disorder

Medical-Surgical Nursing at a Glance, First Edition. Ian Peate. © John Wiley & Sons, Ltd. Published 2016 by John Wiley & Sons, Ltd.
Companion website: www.ataglanceseries.com/nursing/medsurg

Irritable bowel syndrome comprises an assortment of gastrointestinal symptoms also known as irritable bowel disease, irritable colon, spastic colon or mucous colitis. In the UK, one-third of the population experience symptoms at some time, occurring at any age, predominantly between 20 and 40 years. Women are more affected than men, also experiencing more severe symptoms than men. IBS costs in the region of £45.6 million in the UK, and between 7 and 13 days per year are taken off work. The condition can have a negative influence on a person's health and well-being. The cause of IBS is unknown. There is no cure for IBS but symptoms can often be alleviated with treatment.

Irritable bowel syndrome is described as abnormally increased motility of the bowel, usually associated with emotional stress (Figure 16.1). IBS causes the bowel to become oversensitive, which can result in a number of abdominal and bowel symptoms including spasm; there may be a loss of peristaltic activity (Figure 16.2). IBS is a chronic, unremitting, long-term condition which may have a genetic link.

Signs and symptoms

Irritable bowel syndrome is a combination of abdominal symptoms which can be variable, may flare up, lasting 2–4 days, and are often followed by remission, although some people feel the pain continuously. There is significant variability in signs and symptoms. Some of the signs and symptoms associated with IBS are detailed in Figure 16.3. Altered bowel habit features widely. There may be abnormal stool frequency, diarrhoea or constipation, while stool form may be lumpy, hard, small pellet-like, loose or watery. The person may strain at stool, experience urgency or feel there may have been an incomplete bowel movement. Mucus may be passed per rectum.

Investigations and diagnosis

A detailed health history must be undertaken. The person will be physically examined. The nurse should ensure that this is done with sensitivity, assisting the person with regard to the physical examination. A number of other investigations will be undertaken based on the person's unique needs, clinical judgement and the symptoms associated with IBS. Investigations, imaging and laboratory studies must be tailored to the individual in order to make a diagnosis. Gastroscopy, colonoscopy, ultrasound, barium studies and computed tomography (CT) colonography may be indicated.

Symptoms associated with IBS should be present for at least 6 months to distinguish them from those caused by other conditions. If, for example, the person has been experiencing rectal bleeding, anaemia, pyrexia or weight loss, other investigations may be considered appropriate as other conditions may mirror IBS.

Screening studies needed to rule out other disorders include a full blood count to detect anaemia, inflammation and infection, and stool examinations for ova, parasites and enteric pathogens.

The use of hydrogen breath testing can exclude bacterial overgrowth in people with diarrhoea to screen for lactose and/or fructose intolerance. Thyroid function tests are needed. C-reactive protein is measured; this is a non-specific screening test for the presence of inflammation. Specific antibody testing and small bowel biopsy can lead to coeliac disease diagnosis.

Care and management

Most people with IBS self-manage the condition. Most are cared for in the primary care setting, and it is unusual to be admitted to a secondary care setting.

The person should be considered from a biopsychosocial perspective utilising a multidisciplinary approach. Treatment must be undertaken on an individual basis so that the person can develop an understanding of what may trigger an attack of IBS.

For the majority of people with IBS, lifestyle modification is usually the best way to improve and prevent symptoms; pharmacological treatment is adjunctive and should be directed at symptoms. Avoiding tea, coffee, alcohol, spicy foods and the artificial sweetener sorbitol may help if the person's main symptom is diarrhoea. An increase in foods that are fibre rich, such as bran, fruit and vegetables, may help if constipation is problematic. It is important to reduce or cut those foods that may cause an accumulation of flatus in the intestine, for example, beans and green vegetables. Another factor that triggers IBS is stress and if this is the case, stress management or relaxation techniques can be suggested. The advice of a dietician and psychologist may be needed.

Pharmacological and psychological interventions

A number of medications can be purchased over the counter to help relieve some IBS symptoms. Ibuprofen or aspirin can make symptoms worse but paracetamol is less likely to. Antidiarrhoeal medications may help, for example, loperamide (Imodium) and laxatives such as isphaghula husk (Fybogel). Antispasmodic medications such as mebeverine (Colofac), hyoscine butylbromide (Buscopan) and charcoal tablets can help to treat excess flatulence. Antidepressant medications in small doses may also help, such as amitriptyline (Triptafen).

There are some psychological interventions available on the NHS such as stress counselling, cognitive behavioural therapy, psychotherapy and hypnotherapy.

When caring for people with IBS, the nurse must take into account the individual's personal needs and preferences; the person should be considered as a partner in their care, working alongside the healthcare team. The aim is to fully inform about all proposed interventions, procedures and planned treatment. It is essential that respect and sensitivity are maintained at all times and any information that is required by the person be provided in such a way that they will be confident in making informed decisions.

A healthy lifestyle may improve the symptoms connected to IBS. Explaining the nature of the condition can assist people in understanding issues concerning lifestyle, such as diet, smoking, avoiding constipation, managing diarrhoea and controlling pain, and referring the person to self-help groups can help. As many people with IBS will either self-manage their condition or be cared for in a primary care setting, focusing on patient teaching is vital.

Reassurance and explanation are vital, including an open explanation of the probable course of the condition. Patients may have a dread of cancer; the nurse can help to reduce this by careful and repeated explanations of the nature of the illness.

17 Asthma

Figure 17.1 Changes in the airways from asthma

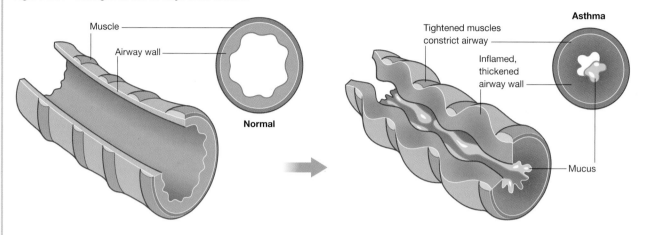

Muscle
Airway wall
Normal

Asthma
Tightened muscles constrict airway
Inflamed, thickened airway wall
Mucus

Table 17.1 Key nursing actions

- Ongoing monitoring of vital signs until stabilised

- Administration of prescribed oxygen to maintain oxygen saturation above 92%

- Safe administration of prescribed bronchodilators and steroids – to relieve dyspnoea

- Communication – use closed questions, observe body language. Verbal communication can cause acute breathlessness patients only able to talk for very short periods, inability to complete a sentence, provides a measure of the extent of respiratory distress

- Regular peak expiratory flow rate (PEFR) – singular or infrequent does not accurately reflect the patient's status. PEFR should be measured every 15–30 minutes after commencement of treatment until stabilised. PEFR can also measure the effectiveness of bronchodilator therapy (measure pre- and post-inhaled or nebulised beta-2 agonists at least 4 times a day)

- Comfort and re-assurance – dyspnoea can increase fear and anxiety as well as hyperventilation. Listening to anxieties and providing explanations for interventions can alleviate this

- Sputum collection – yellow or green sputum can signify infection

- Health promotion – avoid triggers, take prescribed pharmacological therapies as directed, stop smoking and reduce weight

Table 17.2 Overview of bronchodilator therapies used for asthma

Type	Actions	Examples	Routes	Nursing considerations
Beta-2 agonists	Similar to the actions of adrenaline. Beta-2 agonists stimulate beta-2 receptor to sites in the airways encouraging rapid bronchodilation within 15 minutes, with a duration of 4–8 hours – contingent on dose	Salbutamol Terbutaline Fenoterol Salmeterol	Inhaler Nebuliser Oral Subcutaneous	Patient will need to be advised of the possibility of tachycardia and hand tremor
Anticholergenics	Blocks the action of acetylcholine, a neurotransmitter released by the parasympathetic nervous system. Acetylcholine causes broncho-constriction and bronchial secretion. Peak bronchodilator effects within 1 hour, with a duration similar to beta-2 agonists	Ipratropium bromide	Inhaler Nebuliser	Patient may need frequent mouthwashes as can cause dry mouth and a bitter taste
Methylxanthines	Increases intensity of intracellular cyclic adenosine monophosphate (cAMP). Increased cAMP results in bronchodilation	Theophylline	Oral Intravenous (as aminophylline)	Ideal effects happen when plasma theophylline levels are between 10 and 20 mg/L. Regular blood tests are needed

Medical-Surgical Nursing at a Glance, First Edition. Ian Peate. © John Wiley & Sons, Ltd. Published 2016 by John Wiley & Sons, Ltd.
Companion website: www.ataglanceseries.com/nursing/medsurg

A sthma is caused by inflammation of the airways; this is a common condition that is associated with the immune system. In asthma, the bronchi are inflamed and become constricted and this can result in the characteristic wheeze. The condition is known as an obstructive lung disorder. The person with asthma has an actual or potential problem associated with oxygenation. Where there is oxygen depletion (hypoxia), the person will be unable to maintain a safe environment internally and externally. There is rarely a cure for asthma (as is the case with other immune disorders) and people live with the condition for all their lives.

Causes of asthma

In asthma there is an exaggerated response (hyperresponsiveness or bronchial hyperreactivity) to exogenous and endogenous stimuli (internal or external triggers); this then results in direct stimulation of airway smooth muscle as well as indirect stimulation. The degree of airway hyperresponsiveness is usually related to the clinical severity of asthma, leading to a decreased ability to expel air, and can result in hyperinflation (Figure 17.1).

There are a number of risk factors but many people develop the disease in the absence of known risk factors. Allergies play a role in childhood asthma, not so much in adults. There is a strong genetic component to the disease. Active and passive smoking as well as environmental factors, including air pollution and occupational exposure, can contribute. Respiratory viruses, for example, rhinovirus and influenza, and chest infection can bring on attacks.

Signs and symptoms of acute asthma

These include:

- chest tightness
- cough
- dyspnoea
- wheezing
- tachypnoea
- tachycardia
- anxiety and fear.

Frequency of attacks and severity of symptoms vary. Whilst some people have infrequent, mild episodes, others can experience continuous signs and symptoms of cough, dyspnoea on exertion and wheezing with episodic severe exacerbations. Status asthmaticus is severe, prolonged asthma that does not respond to routine treatment; this can lead to respiratory failure with hypoxaemia, hypercapnia and acidosis.

In the UK a significant number of people die from asthma each year and therefore the nurse must be aware of and alert to the signs and symptoms of asthma or an impending asthmatic attack.

Investigations and diagnosis

Presentation of wheezing and shortness of breath is not specific to asthma alone. Diagnosis is made from a combination of a detailed history and the results of objective lung function tests. Objective lung measurements will commonly include peak flow measurement and spirometry.

Assessment must be focused and timely. The diagnosis of asthma is based on the recognition of the characteristic signs and symptoms that will eliminate any other problems. A careful clinical history is essential.

Care and management

The condition is reversible and nursing management should focus on close monitoring and health promotion. The essential nursing goals include those outlined in Table 17.1. Acute exacerbations of asthma can produce significant anxiety. Fear of being unable to breathe and feelings of suffocation associated with acute asthma are significant. Increasingly frequent and severe episodes may cause fear for the future. Hypoxia contributes to anxiety as well, stimulating the sympathetic nervous system and the fight-or-flight response.

The majority of medications for asthma are administered via inhalation. This allows treatments to be in direct contact with the affected airways, reducing the use of systemic medicines and side effects. Table 17.2 provides an overview of the bronchodilator therapies used for asthma.

Inhaled corticosteroids are central to asthma treatment; they reduce oedema in the airways, reducing bronchial hyperreactivity. Inhaled corticosteroids should be administered after bronchodilators to facilitate transit of the medication to distal airways. Sore throat, hoarseness and oropharyngeal or laryngeal *Candida albicans* infection are common side effects. The person should be advised to rinse the mouth after using the inhaler, reducing the risk of fungal infections. These medications should not be used to ease the symptoms of an acute attack. Several weeks of continued therapy may be required before a favourable effect is noticed.

The nursing care needs of people with asthma must be tailored to the person's unique needs using an evidence-based approach. Priorities during an acute attack focus on improving the airway and reducing fear and anxiety. Offer advice about prevention of future attacks; the person is not discharged until adequate ventilation has been restored. The management and care pathway for asthma is based on published national guidance.

A 'stepwise' approach is advocated, from step 1 (mild symptoms) to step 5 (most severe). After assessment, treatment commences at the step most appropriate to the initial severity of the person's asthma. A person with severe symptoms, for example, would be placed on step 4 of the protocol; when symptoms improve, the person steps down the protocol of treatment options.

Aftercare

Once acute asthma is under control and effective ventilation has been re-established, the nurse helps the person to identify factors contributing to the attack. This helps the person to prevent future episodes.

Assess the person's level of understanding about their asthma and their prescribed treatment. Offer additional information and teaching as indicated. Assist the person to identify factors that may have contributed to the acute episode and contributing factors that may increase awareness of the condition and strategies to prevent future exacerbations.

Lifestyle changes may be required that can have a significant impact on the person and their family; for example, there may be a need to eliminate cigarette smoking or pets from the household, removing carpets or daily damp-dusting to remove dust mites. The person's working environment and any potential triggers need to be assessed.

The person should be provided with verbal and written instructions concerning the condition and the medications they will require. This includes when to take the medication and how to take it effectively.

18 Pulmonary Embolism

Figure 18.1 Pulmonary embolism

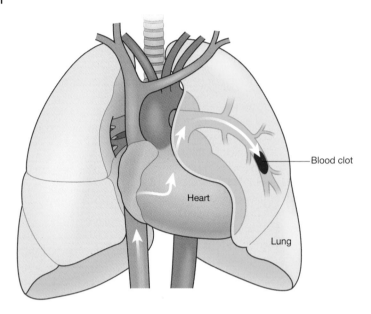

Blood clot

Heart

Lung

Table 18.1   Risk factors associated with pulmonary embolism

High risk factors	
Surgery • Major abdominal/pelvic surgery • Hip/knee replacement • Being cared for in an intensive care unit postoperatively	**Cancer** • Abdominal/pelvic cancer • Advanced/metastatic cancer
	Reduction in mobility • Hospitalisation • Being cared for in institutional settings
Obstetrics • Late pregnancy • Puerperium • Caesarean section	**Previous venous thromboembolism** • Previous venous thromboembolism
Problems of the lower limbs • Fracture • Varicose vein surgery • Superficial thrombophlebitis	**Other** • Major trauma • Spinal cord injury • Central venous lines

Low risk factors	
Cardiovascular • Congenital cardiac disease • Congestive cardiac failure • Hypertension • Stroke	**Renal** • Nephrotic syndrome • Chronic dialysis
Hormones (oestrogens) • Pregnancy • Combined oral contraceptive pill • Hormone replacement therapy	**Other** • Chronic obstructive pulmonary disease • Neurological disability • Hidden malignancy • Long-distance sedentary travel • Obesity
Blood disorders • Thrombotic disorders • Myeloproliferative disorders	

Table 18.2   Tests used in making a diagnosis of pulmonary embolism

Test	Comment
Leg ultrasound	In those with co-existing clinical DVT, ultra sound of the lower limb is the initial imaging test, this is usually sufficient to confirm VTE and as such to commence treatment
Isotope lung scanning (also called V/Q scan)	Reliable enough to exclude or confirm pulmonary embolism. However, if the result is 'uncertain', then further imaging is needed
CT pulmonary angiogram (CTPA)	Quick to perform and is often accurate in making a diagnosis. A special dye is injected before a CT scan is performed. The scan involves taking a series of X-rays showing the presence of a pulmonary embolism
If pulmonary embolism is suspected and the result of tests are negative there may still be a need for follow up. Referral to a respiratory physician and radiologist may be needed.	

A pulmonary embolism can lead to respiratory failure. When respiratory failure occurs, the lungs are unable to oxygenate the blood and remove carbon dioxide adequately to meet the body's needs, even when at rest.

Causes of pulmonary embolism

Pulmonary embolism (PE), also known as a thromboembolism, is the obstruction of blood flow in a part of the pulmonary vascular system by an embolus. Thromboemboli, or blood clots, that have developed in the venous system (deep venous thrombosis or DVT) or right side of the heart are the most common cause of pulmonary embolism (Figure 18.1). Some risk factors for PE are detailed in Table 18.1.

Other sources of emboli can include tumours that have invaded venous circulation, fat or bone marrow that enters the circulation as a result of fracture or other trauma, amniotic fluid released into the circulation during childbirth and intravenous injection of air or other foreign substances.

Pulmonary embolism is a medical emergency. Over half the deaths from pulmonary embolism happen within the first 2 hours after embolisation. In a number of cases, DVT has not been recognised or treated and embolisation can go undetected. The most effective treatment strategy for pulmonary embolism is prevention.

Signs and symptoms of pulmonary embolism

As this condition may present with very few clinical signs and/or symptoms, it can be easily missed. The signs and symptoms are not specific; in severe cases this can lead to collapse and sudden death.

Signs and symptoms will depend on the location; small emboli may be asymptomatic. There may be dyspnoea, pleuritic chest pain, retrosternal chest pain (these are the most common symptoms), cough and haemoptysis, dizziness or syncope, tachypnoea, tachycardia, hypoxia leading to anxiety, restlessness, agitation and impaired consciousness, pyrexia, raised jugular venous pressure, arrhythmia, abnormal heart sounds, hypotension and cardiogenic shock.

Investigations and diagnosis

National guidelines have been produced concerning the investigations required in order to make the diagnosis.

In some cases, in order to save life, treatment may be carried out before any investigations are undertaken. The investigations and the order in which they are carried out will depend on the clinical likelihood of pulmonary embolism, the person's condition and the availability of the proposed tests.

Baseline investigations include oxygen saturation, full blood count, biochemistry and baseline clotting screen. Troponin (a cardiac enzyme) and brain natriuretic peptide levels will also be assessed as these may be elevated which may help to make a diagnosis. An ECG may be normal but it can also reveal some changes. ECG characteristics associated with a large PE show changes that are consistent with acute cardiac ischaemia, and sometimes it is difficult to distinguish a diagnosis of pulmonary embolism from myocardial infarction.

A chest X-ray is undertaken to exclude other chest disease (such as pneumonia) and is needed for interpreting other specific investigations. Often the chest X-ray is normal but it can show some abnormalities. Analysis of arterial blood gases may show a reduction in oxygen and carbon dioxide. Results provide information about oxygenation, adequacy of ventilation and acid–base levels. An echocardiograph may show the presence of a thrombus in the pulmonary arteries as well as information about the structure and function of the heart.

D-dimer fibrin (the breakdown product of a blood clot) is another type of investigation. In those with venous thromboembolism, the concentration increases and this offers a very sensitive test to exclude an acute deep vein thrombosis or pulmonary embolism. The d-dimer test is used to rule out active blood clot formation, and a negative (normal) d-dimer result can rule out the chance that there is a blood clot actively forming. Tests outlined in Table 18.2 can help to make diagnosis.

Care and management

In the initial stages (initial resuscitation), the person will require 100% oxygen (this is a drug and must be prescribed). Intravenous access is required; the person should be monitored closely (ECG, oxygen saturation, vital signs). All observations must be recorded and if there is any cause for concern then this should be raised immediately with more senior members of staff. Local protocols and procedures must be adhered to.

An effective way of preventing venous stasis and decreasing the frequency of pulmonary embolism is early mobilisation. External compression of the legs with antiembolic stockings is effective for people undergoing surgery, or when anticoagulant therapy is contraindicated. Elevating the legs and active and passive leg exercise are also preventive measures.

The usual treatment to prevent pulmonary emboli is anticoagulant therapy. Anticoagulation therapy should be given to those who have a confirmed pulmonary embolism but there are exceptions, for patients with severe renal impairment or established renal failure and for those with an increased risk of bleeding. It is often used in those who are seen as high risk, who have no evidence of pulmonary embolism, to prevent possible harmful effects. In the person with pulmonary embolus, anticoagulants are given to prevent further clotting and embolism. For pulmonary embolus, heparin therapy is usually used for 5 days or until oral anticoagulant therapy has become fully effective.

Those receiving anticoagulation therapy must be provided with an anticoagulant information booklet and an anticoagulant alert card; the alert card should be carried with the person at all times.

An analgesic such as morphine may be required. This helps to control pain and reduce anxiety. Providing information and an explanation of all interventions can also result in a reduction of anxiety. Time should be made available to allow the patient to ask questions or raise any concerns they may have.

An important aspect of the role and function of the nurse is to offer support which may be required before, during or after the procedure, test or investigation. There may be a need to offer physical and psychological support to the patient and their family.

The nurse may be required to provide assistance to the person, helping them to carry out the activities of living. Any care provided should be kind, compassionate and caring, underpinned by a sound evidence base. Care provided (or omitted), any observations undertaken and the response to treatment interventions must be documented in line with local policy and procedure.

19 Pneumonia

Figure 19.1 Signs and symptoms of pneumonia (main symptoms in bold)

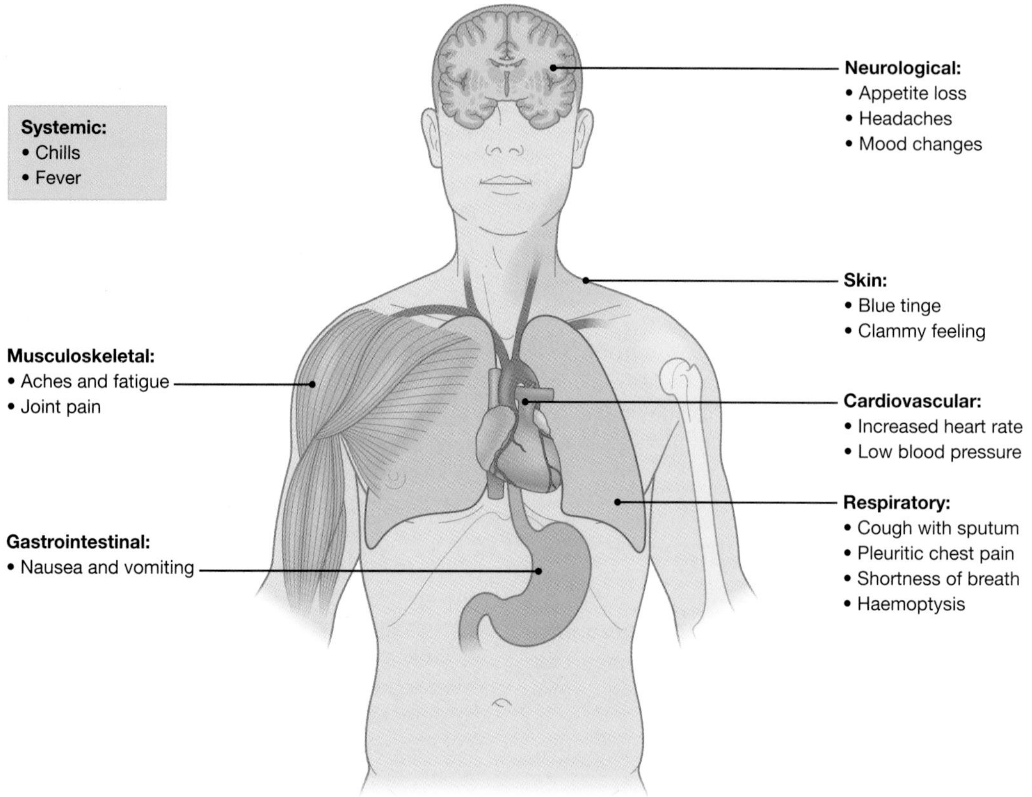

Systemic:
• Chills
• Fever

Neurological:
• Appetite loss
• Headaches
• Mood changes

Skin:
• Blue tinge
• Clammy feeling

Musculoskeletal:
• Aches and fatigue
• Joint pain

Cardiovascular:
• Increased heart rate
• Low blood pressure

Respiratory:
• Cough with sputum
• Pleuritic chest pain
• Shortness of breath
• Haemoptysis

Gastrointestinal:
• Nausea and vomiting

Pneumonia is an acute inflammation in and around the alveoli and the terminal bronchioles. There may be segmental aspects of the lung affected or the entire lobe may be consolidated as a result of the inflammation and oedema. Pneumonia can be infectious or non-infectious. Bacteria, viruses, fungi, protozoa and other microbes can lead to infectious pneumonia. Aspiration of gastric contents and inhalation of toxic or irritating gases are causes of non-infectious pneumonia.

Older people are especially at risk of pneumonia, as well as people in hospital due to a combination of general illness, immobility and the presence of many bacteria in the hospital environment. Inhalation pneumonia is due to inhalation of foreign material, for example food or vomit (if a person is unconscious or has a stroke and loses the normal control protecting the airway). Chronic illness can also be a cause of inhalation pneumonia, for example in those where the cough reflex may be limited.

Risk factors for pneumonia include:

- extremes of age: infants and the elderly
- lifestyle factors: smoking, alcohol
- preceding viral infections: influenza
- respiratory conditions: asthma, chronic obstructive pulmonary disease, malignancy, tuberculosis
- immunosuppression: HIV, cytotoxic therapy
- intravenous drug abuse
- hospitalisation
- aspiration pneumonia
- underlying predisposing disease: diabetes mellitus, cardiovascular disease.

Signs and symptoms

The signs and symptoms will depend on the cause. Symptoms in the older person may be vague; for example, they may have a borderline pyrexia or may even appear normal. The only clue that something is amiss may be confusion or disorientation. The person may have a pyrexia, which may lead to dehydration, tachycardia, hypoxaemia, tachypnoea and dyspnoea. There may be difficulty in expanding the lung due to consolidation, making it difficult to breathe normally. Pleuritic pain may occur as a result of inflammation spreading to the pleura; the person may complain of sharp localised pain increasing with breathing and coughing. There can be malaise. Sputum may be purulent, blood-stained or rust-coloured, and the person may be breathless or exhibit tachypnoea or bronchial breathing. Listening to the chest can reveal crepitations or pleural rub; dullness with percussion may be evident. See Figure 19.1 for the signs and symptoms of pneumonia.

Investigations and diagnosis

For the majority of patients who are managed in the community, i.e. those who attend the general practice, general investigations are not usually necessary. In the general practice, pulse oximeters permit simple assessment of oxygenation. When a patient is admitted to hospital, a full blood count with differential white cell count is undertaken. C-reactive protein to aid diagnosis is assessed as well as using this as a baseline measure. Renal function tests and estimation of electrolytes along with liver function tests are required. If appropriate, blood cultures are taken. A chest X-ray is required with a follow-up 6 weeks after recovery from pneumonia. A sputum specimen is obtained for examination and culture. Pulse oximetry and blood gas analysis are undertaken. There may be a need to aspirate pleural fluid for biochemistry and culture.

Care and management

The decision to admit the person to hospital (patients with community-acquired pneumonia) is based on a number of things, including the severity of illness, the age of the person, underlying health problems and the person's social circumstances.

In order to help the patient stay calm, to reduce anxiety and to encourage concordance to treatment and care, the nurse should develop a therapeutic nurse–patient relationship. This means the nurse has to explain all actions in such a way that the patient (and, if appropriate, the patient's family) will understand. Provide time to answer any questions asked and to anticipate the person's needs based on an in-depth nursing assessment.

The nurse should observe for obvious signs of respiratory distress, the respiratory rate, rhythm, depth should be observed, and note if the person is using the accessory muscles of respiration. Heart rate, temperature and blood pressure should be taken and recorded with any abnormality reported. Oxygen saturation levels will be measured with a pulse oximeter and recorded.

It is important to place the person in a comfortable upright position with the intention of promoting diaphragm and intercostal muscle movement which will help the person to breathe more easily. If the person complains of pain, a reliable and valid pain assessment tool should be used to assess pain levels. Efficient pain management can help the person relax and enhance ventilation. The nurse should administer prescribed oxygen therapy according to local policy and procedure with the intention of increasing oxygen saturation levels above 90% as well as correcting any hypoxia. Prescribed antipyretic and antibiotic therapy should be administered to reduce temperature and to manage bacterial infection.

Vital signs should be observed and recorded hourly in order to detect any deterioration in condition, which could be indicated by a fall in the person's blood pressure and the start of mental confusion. The nurse should note that a rising respiratory rate is a sensitive indicator of a deteriorating condition. A modified early warning score can be used to quickly highlight a deteriorating patient.

In order to encourage the person to expectorate sputum and to address the effects of a high temperature and sweating, attention to hydration is essential. Intravenous fluids may be prescribed, and a fluid balance chart will be needed to assist with assessment of hydration status. The person should be offered a light balanced diet with assistance from the nurse, encouraging independence as symptoms subside. The person should be encouraged to rest. The nurse should place the nurse call bell within easy reach of the patient as well as a sputum pot, tissues and a receptacle to place used tissues in for safe disposal.

Prevention

Early appropriate antibiotic therapy has the ability to reduce mortality and morbidity. Influenza and pneumococcal vaccines should be given to those who are at risk, but this should be in line with national guidelines. Ongoing targeted risk reduction in areas such as smoking cessation is required using a multidisciplinary approach.

20 Iron Deficiency Anaemia

Table 20.1   Classifications of anaemia

Anaemia as result of reduced erythropoiesis	Anaemia as result of excessive haemolysis	Anaemia as result of blood loss
• Aplastic anaemia	• Sickle cell disease	• Gastric haemorrhage
• Vitamin B_{12} deficiency	• Thalassaemia syndromes	• Menorrhagia
• Folate deficiency	• Hereditary spherocytosis	• Oesophageal varicies
• Iron deficiency	• Glucose-6-phosphate-dehydrogenase	• Inflammatory bowel disease
• Cronh's disease	• Disseminated intravascular coagulation	• Haemorrhoids
• Myelodysplastic syndrome	• Thrombocytic thrombocytopenia purpura	• Uterine fibroids
	• Burns	
	• Drugs (i.e. primaquine)	

Figure 20.1   Signs and symptoms of IDA

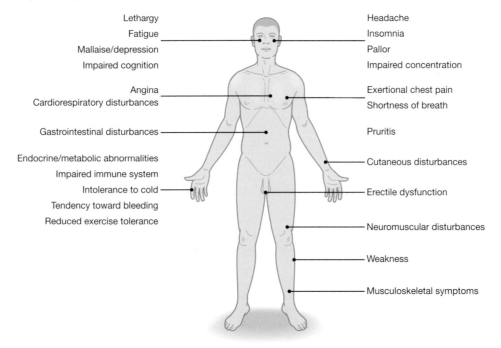

Lethargy
Fatigue
Mallaise/depression
Impaired cognition

Angina
Cardiorespiratory disturbances

Gastrointestinal disturbances

Endocrine/metabolic abnormalities
Impaired immune system
Intolerance to cold
Tendency toward bleeding
Reduced exercise tolerance

Headache
Insomnia
Pallor
Impaired concentration

Exertional chest pain
Shortness of breath

Pruritis

Cutaneous disturbances

Erectile dysfunction

Neuromuscular disturbances

Weakness

Musculoskeletal symptoms

Table 20.2   Other possible investigations needed to confirm the cause of IDA

• Faecal occult blood testing
• Upper and lower endoscopy to determine if there is a diagnosis of coeliac abnormality in the gastrointestinal tract
• Barium enema, barium swallow
• Small bowel biopsy
• CT scan of the abdomen
• Urinalysis for the presence of blood
• A gynaecological examination and investigations to establish the cause of menorrhagia can include a pelvic ultrasound or uterine biopsy
• To diagnose coeliac disease a blood test may be taken (a biopsy of the lining of the intestine to confirm a diagnosis coeliac disease)
• A stool specimen to exclude hookworm if the person has recently travelled to the tropics

Medical-Surgical Nursing at a Glance, First Edition. Ian Peate. © John Wiley & Sons, Ltd. Published 2016 by John Wiley & Sons, Ltd.
Companion website: www.ataglanceseries.com/nursing/medsurg

A dysfunction of the erythrocytes will result in inability to transport and distribute oxygen to tissues. The size and shape of red blood cells (morphology) are usually altered in erythrocyte disorders, including iron deficiency anaemia. The most common problem of erythrocytes is anaemia; this is defined as a reduction in either the number of circulating red blood cells (RBCs) or in haemoglobin concentration, or both.

Anaemia can be classified into three categories as shown in Table 20.1. The type and severity of the anaemia determine the treatment and interventions required to manage it. The most common form of anaemia in the UK is iron deficiency anaemia (IDA); iron is required to create haemoglobin.

Iron deficiency anaemia

There are a number of key nutrients required for erythropoiesis. Iron is crucial for haemoglobin. Vitamin B_{12} (cobalamin) is essential for nucleic synthesis in the pro-erythroblast stage. Folic acid helps with maturation of red blood cells and RNA synthesis. Copper acts as a catalyst for iron to be utilised by haemoglobin. Protein is key for red cell membrane and globin manufacture. Vitamin C aids in iron absorption and vitamin E, an antioxidant, helps to protect cells from damage and oxidation. Without these components erythropoiesis is compromised.

When there is not enough iron in the body, IDA occurs, reducing the quantity of RBCs. The body uses iron to manufacture haemoglobin, which helps store and carry oxygen in RBCs. Excess iron is readily available for the production of RBCs and is stored in the liver and muscle cells.

There are some inflammatory disorders, for example Crohn's disease, that affect the absorption of iron from the gastrointestinal tract, negatively impacting on the synthesis of RBCs. The most common cause of lack of iron in the UK is heavy menstrual periods. The amount of iron eaten may not be enough to replace the iron lost during each menstrual period. In pregnancy, anaemia is common, and is more likely to develop in pregnancy if the diet has little iron in it.

Other gastrointestinal conditions can lead to bleeding. For example, after a duodenal ulcer bleeds, a constant trickle of blood into the gastrointestinal tract and can appear unnoticed in the faeces. Iron loss may indicate more than haemorrhoids; cancer of the bowel and other bowel disorders can also result in iron deficiency. In the early stages there may be no symptoms and anaemia may be the first thing noticed.

Some medicines may cause gastrointestinal bleeding. Aspirin is the most common example. Others include ibuprofen, naproxen and diclofenac. These medications may trigger bleeding by irritating the gastric mucosa, leading to a bleed.

IDA can also be caused by not eating foods containing iron.

Signs and symptoms

Iron deficiency anaemia can be so mild that it goes unnoticed. However, as the deficiency worsens, the signs and symptoms intensify (Figure 20.1). The symptoms experienced as a result of the reduction in the amount of oxygen in the body can include fatigue, tiredness, feeling faint and becoming short of breath. There can be headaches, arrhythmias, glossitis and tinnitus. The person may appear pale.

As the condition develops untreated, the person's nails may become fragile and broken, there may be alopecia and cardiac

failure. IDA may also compromise the immune system and as such the person is more susceptible to infections.

Investigations and diagnosis

A person suspected of having IDA should undergo a full assessment; the aim is to determine if there is an underlying cause of the IDA and if the person has any complications. A history, physical examination and investigations will help to determine this.

The most common investigation undertaken is a full blood count; another is a blood smear (a thin film of blood is examined under a microscope to look for abnormal shapes of cells and cells with pale centres).

Measurement of ferritin (a protein) is required to confirm that the cause of the anaemia is iron deficiency. To determine the cause of the iron deficiency, the investigations in Table 20.2 may be undertaken.

Care and management

Undertaking a holistic assessment of needs with the person can help to identify actual and potential problems from a psychological and physical perspective. Address underlying causes as necessary, for example treat menorrhagia, and if possible, non-steroidal anti-inflammatory medications should be stopped.

As IDA can cause weakness and shortness of breath on exertion due to decreased circulating oxygen as a result of low haemoglobin levels, care provision should be adapted to meet the individual's needs. The nurse should aim to relieve symptoms, expand oxygen-carrying capacity of RBCs and prevent complications. Assessment and effective care planning are key in addressing and identifying the help and advice that patients may require. Assisting the person to maintain a safe environment is a key aspect of the role and function of the nurse.

The aim of treatment should be to restore haemoglobin concentrations and red cell levels to normal and to replenish iron stores. The condition is primarily treated with oral iron medication. Ferrous gluconate (300 mg) three times a day or ferrous sulphate (200 mg) three times a day are the usual drug regimens. Before administering oral iron, the nurse should be aware of drugs that could adversely interact with iron. When given in syrup form, ferrous sulphate may stain the teeth, so to avoid this a straw should be used. Parenteral administration of iron by injection should be considered if oral iron is not being absorbed from the gut, the iron balance remains unresolved with maximum oral dosage being prescribed, or malabsorption reduces the absorption of iron.

The nurse should note and discuss with the patient that constipation, black stools and dysphagia are some side effects of iron medication. Increasing fibre intake and fluids can help minimise the discomfort of constipation.

Helping people to understand that continuing their iron medication for the specified period of time (3–6 months) is important as it may take 3 months for the body to replenish its stores. Some people feel much better after a short period of taking iron supplementation and may discontinue before replenishment of the body stores has occurred, at which point IDA could return.

21 Thrombocytopenia

Figure 21.1   Components of platelet plug formation

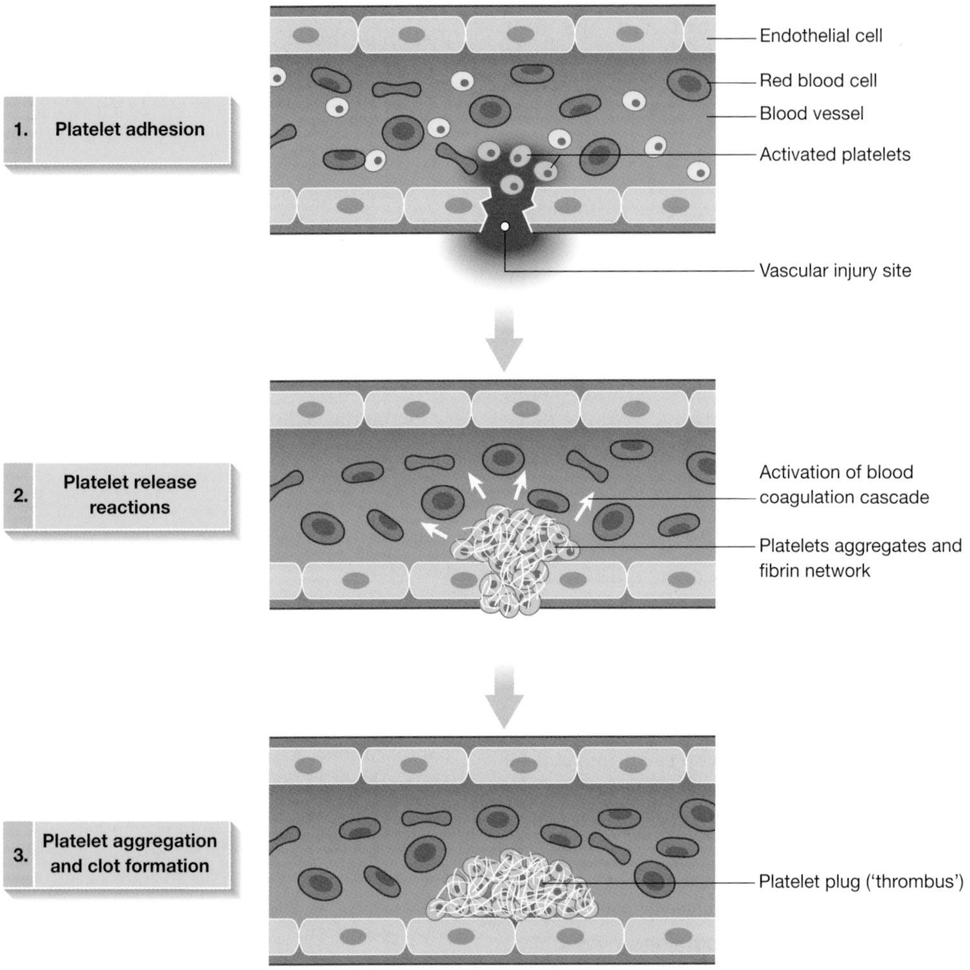

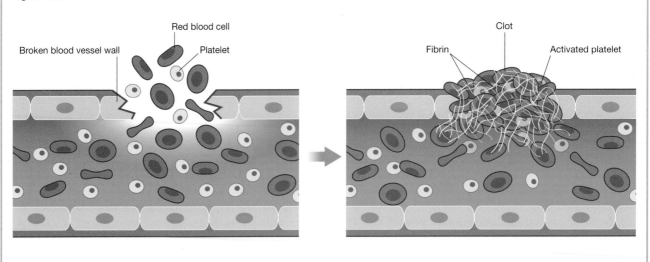

Figure 21.2   Blood clot

Medical-Surgical Nursing at a Glance, First Edition. Ian Peate. © John Wiley & Sons, Ltd. Published 2016 by John Wiley & Sons, Ltd.
Companion website: www.ataglanceseries.com/nursing/medsurg

Any platelet or coagulation disorder will affect haemostasis, and these conditions can be acquired or inherited. Haemostasis sustains a fairly steady state of blood volume, blood pressure and blood flow. Bleeding disorders can result from deficient, defective platelets or disruption of the clotting cascade. Figure 21.1 provides an overview of the various steps and stages of platelet plug formation.

Thrombocytopenia

This is a condition in which the blood has a lower than normal number of blood cell fragments (platelets). Platelets are manufactured in the bone marrow. They travel through the blood vessels and come together to form a clot to stop any bleeding that occurs if a blood vessel is damaged. Platelets are also called thrombocytes, and a clot is a thrombus. See Figure 21.2.

When the blood has too few platelets, mild to serious bleeding can occur. Internal bleeding may occur or bleeding underneath the skin or from the surface of the skin. Bleeding due to thrombocytopenia often occurs in small vessels, causing petechiae and purpura. The mucous membranes of the nose, mouth, gastrointestinal tract and vagina often bleed. A platelet count of less than $150 \times 10^9/L$ is deemed thrombocytopenia. The risk for serious bleeding does not occur until the count becomes very low, less than 10,000 or $20,000 \times 10^9/L$. Mild bleeding sometimes occurs when the count is less than $50,000\ 10^9/L$.

Causes of thrombocytopenia

There are many factors that can cause a low platelet count. How long the condition lasts depends on its cause. It may last from days to years.

Causes include certain congenital disorders: decreased production (disorders of bone marrow), for example, malignancy (leukaemia, lymphoma), certain drugs such as chemotherapy, some anaemias. Decreased platelet survival, for example, immune disorders, idiopathic thrombocytopenia, drug induced (heparin). Dilutional thrombocytopenia is caused by the transfusion of large volumes of blood which may be depleted of functioning platelets, as a result of prolonged storage. An enlarged spleen (splenomegaly) may retain too many platelets, and this causes a decrease in the number of platelets in circulation.

Signs and symptoms

There may be no symptoms, particularly if the condition is mild, and it may only be detected incidentally on routine blood analysis carried out for other reasons. Signs and symptoms of thrombocytopenia may include the following.

- Easy or excessive bruising.
- Superficial bleeding into the skin that appears as a rash of pinpoint-sized, reddish-purple spots (petechiae), often on the lower legs.
- Prolonged bleeding from cuts (such as after a graze, after shaving).
- Spontaneous bleeding from the gums or nose (epistaxis).
- Blood in the urine indicates bleeding within the urinary tract.
- Blood in the stools suggests bleeding in the gastrointestinal tract.
- Unusually heavy menstrual periods.
- Profuse bleeding during surgery or after dental work has been performed.

Investigations and diagnosis

A detailed medical history is obtained and any underlying medical conditions must be considered that may give an indication of the possible cause of the condition. A physical examination is undertaken to determine if there are any signs of bleeding, such as excessive bruising or petechiae. The abdomen may also be palpated to establish if there is any evidence of splenomegaly.

A full blood count is obtained to assess the extent of the thrombocytopenia; this also helps in establishing the underlying cause. After the history and examination have been undertaken, investigations for any underlying cause will be evident.

Investigations regarding platelet function, for example clotting time, are carried out. There may be a need to undertake a bone marrow biopsy. If there is any possible complication of thrombocytopenia identified, such as an intracranial haemorrhage, a CT scan of the head may be needed.

Care and management

The treatment for this condition will also depend on its cause and severity. Often mild thrombocytopenia does not require treatment. The key aim is to prevent death and disability caused by bleeding. If the condition causes or puts the person at risk of serious bleeding, medication or transfusion of platelets may be required; in some instances the spleen may need to be removed. The condition often improves when the underlying condition has been treated.

As bleeding is a serious complication, 4-hourly monitoring of vital signs and frequent assessment for signs of bleeding should be undertaken; the frequency may increase depending on the person's condition. The skin and mucous membranes should be assessed for petechiae, ecchymoses and haematoma formation. The nasal membranes and conjunctiva should also be assessed for bleeding. Stools should be observed for occult blood and urine tested for haematuria. Individuals should be advised to inform the nurse of any vaginal bleeding. Nurses should observe puncture sites, such as where intravenous cannulae have been inserted, or wounds for prolonged bleeding. Thrombocytopenia may result in neurological problems due to intracranial bleeding, for example, headaches, blurred vision, confusion, seizures, decreasing level of consciousness.

If venepuncture is required, pressure should be applied for 3–5 minutes and 15–20 minutes to arterial puncture sites to promote haemostasis and clot formation. Patients should be advised to avoid forcefully blowing the nose or picking crusts from the nose, straining to have a bowel movement and forceful coughing or sneezing. There is the risk that these activities may cause external and internal bleeding.

Thrombocytopenia often causes the gums and oral mucosa to bleed. This poses a risk for infection and impaired nutrition. Oral care should be offered in alignment with local policy and patient preference.

All care interventions and observations must be documented in the person's notes and any concerns raised immediately. The nurse should spend time with the patient and, if appropriate, the family, explaining the condition and the reason why the person is experiencing the signs and symptoms, i.e. the easy or excessive bruising.

22 Leukaemia

Figure 22.1 Signs and symptoms of leukaemia

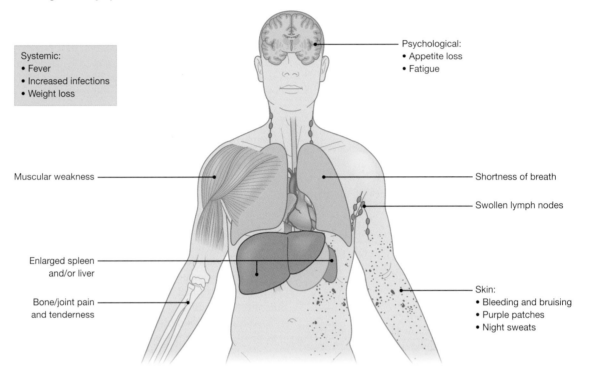

Systemic:
- Fever
- Increased infections
- Weight loss

Psychological:
- Appetite loss
- Fatigue

Muscular weakness

Shortness of breath

Swollen lymph nodes

Enlarged spleen and/or liver

Bone/joint pain and tenderness

Skin:
- Bleeding and bruising
- Purple patches
- Night sweats

Table 22.1 Four general classifications of leukaemia

- Acute myeloid leukaemia (AML)
- Chronic myeloid leukaemia (CML)
- Acute lymphoblastic leukaemia (ALL)
- Chronic lymphoblastic leukaemia (CLL)

Table 22.2 Investigations and tests

• Full blood count	• Cytogenetic screening
• Bone marrow aspiration	• Clotting screening
• Bone marrow trephine	• Lumbar puncture
• Biochemistry tests	• Chest X-ray

Table 22.3 Key nursing considerations

Inadequate nutrition	Chemotherapy and radiotherapy takes a significant toll on the body and nutritional support is essential in aiding recovery. Nausea and vomiting are other debilitating side-effects, administer and record impact of antiemetics. Stomatitis is a major complication. Assessment of nutritional needs is required. The provision of evidence based oral hygiene is essential if complications are to be avoided and comfort enhanced
Impaired skin integrity	Can be compromised due to radiation and chemotherapy on the skin can cause dryness, blisters and rashes. Insertion of central venous catheter creates possible entry sites for infective organisms. Assessment of risk of skin damage is needed. Use pressure relieving aids if indicated
Sexual dysfunction	Chemotherapy and radiotherapy can cause reduction in the sex hormones loss of libido, vaginal dryness, amenorrhoea and dyspareunia. In men loss of libido, erectile dysfunction, premature ejaculation, azoospermia and gynaecomastia are significant problems. Referral to psychosexual therapist may be needed
Altered body image	The loss of weight, alopecia, nausea and vomiting, loss of sexuality are some issues which can lead to negative self esteem. Discuss the risks for and measures to cope with alopecia, suggest wigs, scarves, hats or caps. Scalp care using baby shampoo or mild soap, a soft brush, sunscreen and mineral oil to reduce itching should be encouraged. Teach eye protection, for example, wearing spectacles and caps with wide brims if eyelashes and eyebrows are lost
Psychological support	There may be a sense of fear, anxiety and dread. Fear of an unknown future, issues regarding survivorship, how will family cope, these are major areas of concern. Provide support for the individual and family through the treatment (holistic care). Effective interpersonal skills are key in creating an environment that encourages communication. Provide information concerning charitable organisations such as Macmillan

Medical-Surgical Nursing at a Glance, First Edition. Ian Peate. © John Wiley & Sons, Ltd. Published 2016 by John Wiley & Sons, Ltd.
Companion website: www.ataglanceseries.com/nursing/medsurg

There are approximately 7000 new cases of leukaemia per year in the UK; it is more common in males than females.

Leukaemia

Leukaemia is an abnormal rise in the number of white blood cells (WBCs), it is a malignant pathology. The WBCs crowd out other blood cell elements such as red blood cells and platelets. The increased WBCs are immature and fail to function effectively; for example, they are unable to fight off infection, a key function of the WBCs.

There are four general classifications of leukaemia (Table 22.1). They are classified as acute or chronic. Chronic leukaemia progresses more slowly and the leukaemia cells develop to full maturity. Leukaemia is further classified according to the type of WBCs involved, most commonly myeloid or lymphoid.

Acute lymphoblastic leukaemia (ALL) is more widespread in children but acute myeloid leukaemia (AML) is more common in adults. Chronic lymphoblastic leukaemia (CLL) has a higher incidence in adults over 70 years but chronic myeloid leukaemia (CML) is more prevalent in young adults. Leukaemias are more commonly found in Caucasians in western European and American populations and less commonly in Afro-Caribbean, South East and Far East Asians.

The abnormally produced WBCs tend to live well beyond their normal life span; they inhibit vital organ functions, reduce the body's supply of oxygen and interfere with platelet production to ensure proper clotting. The WBCs that are produced fail to fight infection. Those with leukaemia may be anaemic as well as increasing their risks of bruising, bleeding and infection.

Risk factors for leukaemia

The exact cause of leukaemia is unknown. Some chromosomal abnormalities have been associated with leukaemia, but they do not cause it. Nearly all people with CML and some with ALL have an abnormal chromosome known as the Philadelphia chromosome.

Genetic disorders are associated with AML such as Downs syndrome. Environmental factors appear to influence the risk of developing leukaemia. Smokers are more prone to certain leukaemias. Prolonged exposure to radiation, numerous chemicals in the home and at work and non-ionizing radiation are associated with leukaemia. Leukaemia is also a rare complication of chemotherapy and radiation. A family history is a risk factor for leukaemia as well (genetic predisposition). Viruses such as HIV and bone marrow disease are also risk factors.

Signs and symptoms

The signs and symptoms associated with acute leukaemia are marked. Chronic leukaemia progresses more slowly and there may be fewer symptoms until the condition is advanced, so diagnosis may be incidental. Figure 22.1 outlines some of the signs and symptoms associated with leukaemia.

Investigations and diagnosis

A number of blood tests are commonly undertaken to aid diagnosis as well as additional tests that may confirm and establish the severity or the stage of the illness (Table 22.2).

Care and management

The basis of the clinical management of leukaemia includes chemotherapy, radiotherapy, growth factors, steroids, monoclonal antibodies and stem cell transplant. The treatment of leukaemia can cause a number of problems for the person; the nurse needs to be aware of these actual and potential problems in order to make patient-centred responses to care provided, for the patient and the family.

The treatment of choice for most types of leukaemia is chemotherapy. The type of treatment, dose used, the route of administration and duration of treatment depend on the type of leukaemia (the classification), stage and subtype, presence or absence of genetic abnormalities, age, and any co-morbidities (liver, renal or cardiac dysfunction). The overall aim is to eradicate malignant cells, re-establish normal bone marrow function and improve the person's overall health and well-being.

In the case of acute leukaemia, because of its aggressive behaviour, combination chemotherapy is offered. Combination chemotherapy can attack malignant cells at all stages of the cell cycle, it reduces the ability of the malignant cell to develop resistance and it assists in improving remission rates. It also reduces the need for and attendant danger of giving a very high dosage of a single drug. Combination chemotherapy is generally given in 'cycles' allowing for the normal marrow to recover as well as attacking the malignant cells.

Leukaemia, a life-threatening illness, is compounded by the treatment required to manage or possibly cure the condition. The nurse should be skilled in managing the potential effects of the illness and side effects of the treatment. Chemotherapy and radiotherapy cause systematic damage to cells, mainly the rapidly dividing cells, for example, mucosal cells, hair follicles, gonads and gastrointestinal system. This affects the physical, emotional and psychological health and well-being of the individual and their family.

Managing the risk of infection and haemorrhage, managing the side effects of chemotherapy and radiation therapy and psychological support are key areas of nursing care.

Infections are a major risk and the main cause of mortality. There is a need to provide meticulous care in reducing the risk of cross-infection. Antimicrobial medication is prescribed to reduce the risk of infections and treat any infection that may develop. The individual is usually nursed in protective isolation, in a single room. Temperature observation is key in providing an early indication of infection. Tachypnoea, tachycardia, restlessness and change in PaO_2 are early signs of sepsis. Fever, cough or chills should be investigated immediately.

Bleeding is the second most common cause of death in leukaemia. Daily assessment includes observing for signs of bruising or easy bleeding. The patient should be advised to inform nurses of any bleeding episodes.

Table 22.3 outlines other key nursing considerations. The nurse must work in partnership with the patient and family (if appropriate), offering physical and psychological support. Referral to other members of the multidisciplinary team may be required.

23 Myocardial Infarction

Figure 23.1 Signs and symptoms of acute myocardial infarction (women)

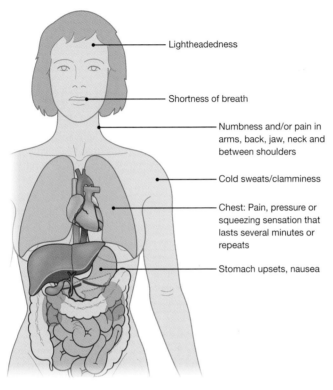

Lightheadedness

Shortness of breath

Numbness and/or pain in arms, back, jaw, neck and between shoulders

Cold sweats/clamminess

Chest: Pain, pressure or squeezing sensation that lasts several minutes or repeats

Stomach upsets, nausea

Other signs:
Some people may feel very tired, sometimes for days or weeks prior to an MI. There may be heartburn, a cough, palpitations and loss of appetite

Figure 23.2 Typical distribution of referred pain

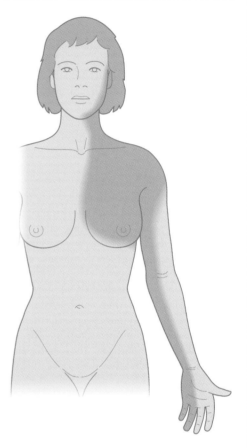

Table 23.1 The PQRST mnemonic for assessing chest pain

P – Precipitating and palliative factors
- What was occurring when the pain began?
- Is there anything that worsens or eases the pain?
- Does taking a deep breath influence the pain?

Q – Quality
- What does the pain feel like? – Descriptors, e.g. sharp, tight, vice like, burning, heavy, deep

R – Region and radiation
- Exact location of pain
- Does it extend or travel to any other areas

S – Severity
- On a scale of 1–10; rating pain where 10 is the worst pain ever experienced

T – Time
- Since the pain started, is it passing?
- Has it happened before?

Medical-Surgical Nursing at a Glance, First Edition. Ian Peate. © John Wiley & Sons, Ltd. Published 2016 by John Wiley & Sons, Ltd.
Companion website: www.ataglanceseries.com/nursing/medsurg

Acute myocardial infarction (MI) is caused by necrosis of myocardial tissue as a result of ischaemia, often due to occlusion of a coronary artery by a thrombus. Most MIs are anterior or inferior but may affect the posterior wall of the left ventricle, causing a posterior MI.

Myocardial infarction

Myocardial infarction is part of a spectrum known as acute coronary syndrome, an umbrella term for a collection of conditions that result from coronary artery disease.

In MI, blood flow to a portion of cardiac muscle is completely blocked, resulting in prolonged tissue ischaemia and irreversible cell damage. This causes a risk of dysrhythmias, myocardial contractility decreases, reducing stroke volume, cardiac output, blood pressure and tissue perfusion.

Signs and symptoms

The key symptom is chest pain, more severe than anginal pain. The pain can be explained as crushing, severe, heavy pressure, a vice-like sensation, chest tightness or burning. Often the pain starts in the centre of the chest and can radiate to the shoulders, neck, jaw or arms. It is not relieved by rest or prescribed vasodilators such as glyceryl trinitrate (GTN). There may be anxiety, tachycardia and vasoconstriction, tachypnoea, pyrexia, nausea and vomiting, hypotension, hiccupping, a sense of impending doom and death, cold and mottled skin. There will also be changes in the electrocardiogram (ECG). Figure 23.1 provides a review of the signs and symptoms associated with MI and Figure 23.2 demonstrates the typical distribution of referred pain. Atypical presentations occur and these are seen in women, older men, people with diabetes and those from ethnic minorities. Atypical symptoms include abdominal discomfort or jaw pain; elderly people may present with altered mental state.

Investigations and diagnosis

A detailed medical history should be obtained, preferably from the patient but a secondary source may have to suffice. Issues to consider include the history of the pain, any cardiovascular risk factors, history of ischaemic heart disease and any earlier treatment, and prior investigations for chest pain.

When heart muscle is damaged, cardiac enzymes are released. In isolation, they do not provide conclusive evidence that MI has occurred; they must be considered along with the ECG. An ECG may be helpful in a prehospital setting if diagnosis is uncertain. Features may initially be normal but abnormalities may develop.

A full blood count helps rule out anaemia, assess and monitor potassium levels; renal function should be measured. A lipid profile needs to be obtained; C-reactive protein (CRP) and other markers of inflammation should be measured.

Serial ECGs and continuous ECG monitoring are required. A chest X-ray is taken to assess the heart size and the presence or absence of heart failure and pulmonary oedema. Pulse oximetry and blood gases and oxygen saturation are monitored.

Cardiac catheterisation and angiography are undertaken. Echocardiography can define the extent of the infarction and assess overall ventricular function, identifying complications, such as acute mitral regurgitation, left ventricular rupture or pericardial effusion. Myocardial perfusion scintigraphy is recommended.

Care and management

The immediate goals of care following an MI are to relieve pain, reduce degree of myocardial damage, maintain cardiovascular stability, reduce cardiac workload, prevent further complications, record an ECG and begin intravenous access.

It is essential that rapid assessment and early diagnosis be secured in treating MI; within 15 minutes, 50% of the myocardium has died and in 3 hours 80% of the muscle is affected. Rapidly restoring blood flow to the damaged myocardium surrounding the infarcted tissue increases survival and better long-term outcomes.

Blood should be restored to the damaged area of the heart as fast as possible using reperfusion strategies such as percutaneous coronary interventions or thrombolysis. Further blood clots should be prevented from developing by giving antiplatelet and anticoagulant therapy. The person should be monitored for risk factors and side effects emerging from the treatment.

Aspirin therapy halves the rate of deaths for people who experience a non-fatal MI and unstable angina. Clopidogrel (an antiplatelet) is usually given with aspirin, which improves the blood thinning effect.

GTN is given to relieve pain, morphine is administered to manage anxiety and pain and an antiemetic is usually given at the same time to reduce nausea and vomiting. See Table 23.1 for the PQRST mnemonic used for assessing chest pain.

Preperfusion using percutaneous coronary intervention (PCI) has become the primary treatment strategy, restoring patency to the artery affected in most cases. Thrombolysis (the breakdown of the blood clots) was the standard treatment prior to PCI becoming more widely available, for example, streptokinase and tissue plasma activators (alteplase, reteplase and tenectoplase), given intravenously up to 24 hours after the commencement of the chest pain.

Treatment is aimed at restoring the balance between the oxygen supply and demand to prevent further damage and death to cardiac muscle. The nurse should work with other members of the multidisciplinary team aiming to prevent and treat any complications, communicating at all times with the patient and if appropriate the family.

The person is encouraged to rest; this helps to reduce the workload on an already compromised heart. In order to improve coronary blood flow, nitrates may be given (coronary artery dilators). Diuretics encourage blood flow and help to prevent renal damage. Inotropic agents can enhance cardiac contractility. Oxygen therapy reduces the demands being made by the heart.

The nurse will be required to assist the person with the activities of living. Physical activity should be limited – chair to bed, with gradual increase in mobility depending on the individual's progress. All care should reflect that prescribed in the care plan; any care given or omitted must be documented as per local policy and procedure.

Diagnosis of MI can instill fear and anxiety in patients, family and staff. The nurse should communicate with compassion with the person and their family; care should be undertaken in a confident and competent manner. The nurse provides the person with an explanation of all activities and interventions, ensuring time is provided for any questions. Reassurance comes in the form of verbal and non-verbal communication.

24 Heart Failure

Figure 24.1   Signs and symptoms of heart failure

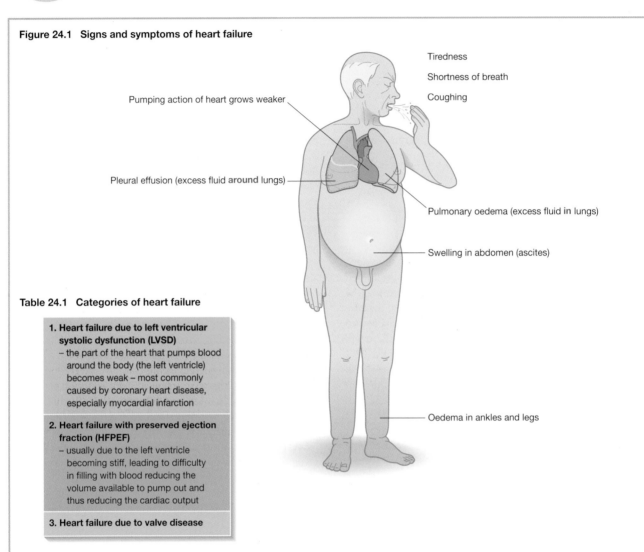

Tiredness

Shortness of breath

Coughing

Pumping action of heart grows weaker

Pleural effusion (excess fluid **around** lungs)

Pulmonary oedema (excess fluid **in** lungs)

Swelling in abdomen (ascites)

Oedema in ankles and legs

Table 24.1   Categories of heart failure

> **1. Heart failure due to left ventricular systolic dysfunction (LVSD)**
> – the part of the heart that pumps blood around the body (the left ventricle) becomes weak – most commonly caused by coronary heart disease, especially myocardial infarction

> **2. Heart failure with preserved ejection fraction (HFPEF)**
> – usually due to the left ventricle becoming stiff, leading to difficulty in filling with blood reducing the volume available to pump out and thus reducing the cardiac output

> **3. Heart failure due to valve disease**

Table 24.2   Severity of heart failure – New York Heart Association (NYHA) Functional Classification

Class	Description
Class I (mild)	No limitation of physical activity. Ordinary physical activity does not cause undue fatigue, palpitation, or dyspnoea (shortness of breath). Essentially well treated heart failure
Class II (mild)	Slight limitation of physical activity. Comfortable at rest, but ordinary physical activity results in fatigue, palpitation, or dyspnoea
Class III (moderate)	Marked limitation of physical activity. Comfortable at rest, but less than ordinary activity causes fatigue, palpitation, or dyspnoea
Class IV (severe)	Unable to carry out any physical activity without discomfort. Symptoms of cardiac failure at rest. Patient is essentially housebound

Medical-Surgical Nursing at a Glance, First Edition. Ian Peate. © John Wiley & Sons, Ltd. Published 2016 by John Wiley & Sons, Ltd.
Companion website: www.ataglanceseries.com/nursing/medsurg

Heart failure may be acute or chronic and can result from the long-term effects of coronary heart disease, acute coronary syndrome, structural defects of heart valves and hypertension. The condition is regarded as a 'syndrome' as it is a collection of associated problems primarily resulting from damage or dysfunction of the left ventricle. Synonyms associated with heart failure include congestive heart failure, left-side heart failure, right-side heart failure and cor pulmonale.

Heart failure

Heart failure is a condition in which the heart is unable to pump sufficient blood to meet the needs of the body. In some cases, the heart is unable to fill with enough blood; in other cases, it is unable to pump blood to the rest of the body with enough force. There are some people who have both problems. Categories of heart failure are outlined in Table 24.1.

Chronic heart failure can be compensated and stable, with few signs and symptoms, or decompensated with a recent clinical deterioration and physical evidence of impaired perfusion and oxygenation.

Causes of heart failure

An acute coronary problem, for example, myocardial infarction, uncontrolled hypertension, chest infection, heart valve disorders, cardiomyopathies, arrhythmias, diabetes, excessive alcohol consumption, obesity, chronic heart failure no longer responding to treatment and failure to adhere to treatment can contribute to heart failure. Men have a higher rate of heart failure than women. There will continue to be an increase in people with heart failure.

Those with this condition often face repeated hospital admissions for the remaining years of their life. It is important to understand the cause of heart failure as it impacts on treatment choices. The severity of heart failure can be classified using several systems but the most commonly used is the New York Heart Association (NYHA) Functional Classification (Table 24.2).

Signs and symptoms (Figure 24.1)

The most common signs and symptoms of heart failure are shortness of breath, dyspnoea, orthopnoea, fatigue, oedema, ascites and engorged veins in the neck. Signs of pulmonary oedema may ensue (extreme shortness of breath, a feeling of suffocating or drowning, wheezing or gasping for breath, anxiety, restlessness or a sense of apprehension, a cough that produces frothy sputum that may be tinged with blood, excessive sweating, pale skin, chest pain, tachycardia, palpitations). Jaundice may appear if there is liver involvement and the person may feel bloated and nauseous. Appetite and food intake decrease.

Investigations and diagnosis

A detailed medical history is undertaken and physical examination is performed. The nurse may need to assist the person particularly when there is shortness of breath or any concerns about maintaining a safe environment. The severity of heart failure can be classified using the NYHA Functional Classification.

The tests and investigations undertaken can include a full blood count. Other blood tests will measure C-reactive protein to ascertain if there is infection present, renal function tests, blood clotting screen, assessment of arterial blood gases, assessment of cardiac markers, troponins to establish if there has been a myocardial infarction. Echocardiography may be undertaken to determine heart function and function of heart valves, 12-lead ECG to assess for heart disease, cardiac catheterisation to assess for heart disease and to assess heart function, chest X-ray to consider heart size and for signs of pulmonary oedema, exercise tolerance test to assess for heart disease and exercise ability.

Care and management

The aim of treatment is to reduce the work of the heart (preload and afterload); there are several ways in which this can be achieved. Diuretic and vasodilator drugs can assist – furosemide along with spironolactone, an angiotensin-converting enzyme (ACE) inhibitor such as ramipril or an angiotensin-receptor blocker (candesartan) may be given. Glyceryl trinitrate (GTN) is another vasodilator which also improves diuresis. Drug regimen is tailored to meet individual needs.

A ventricular assist device is a pump fixed externally or inserted internally. External pumps are used as an interim for those awaiting cardiac transplants. Heart transplants are part of the standard care for end-stage heart disease and have a good success rate, most people returning to normal functional abilities.

Providing nursing care to the person with heart failure requires skill and attention to detail. Initially a swift response to symptoms is required as the condition can rapidly deteriorate. Whilst monitoring and measuring the physiological status of the person, care also involves the art of reassuring the person, communicating effectively to reduce anxiety and fear as well as responding to the person's individual needs such as personal hygiene. The person may find it more comfortable to be nursed upright and may prefer to sit in an armchair as opposed to lying in bed as this may make them feel more breathless. Oxygen therapy will be required which can be delivered by non-invasive positive pressure ventilation (NIPPV), continuous positive airway pressure (CPAP) or bi-level positive airway pressure (BiPAP).

When delivered this way, oxygen reduces the effort the person has to make to breathe, causing less fatigue. If these methods are ineffective, it may be necessary to mechanically ventilate the person.

Mobility will be compromised, so assistance will be needed with personal care and the nurse ensures that the person does not develop pressure ulcers (a risk assessment must be undertaken) and other complications such as thromboembolisms, respiratory and urinary tract infections and constipation.

The breathlessness and oxygen therapy result in the person having a dry mouth; frequent mouthcare is needed to prevent infection. Sucking flavoured ice or chilled pineapple chunks is refreshing and may reduce the risk of oral infection.

There may be a need to introduce fluid restriction. Strict fluid balance monitoring is needed and consider daily weights. Attention must be given to the person's nutritional status and a risk assessment tool should be used to help the nurse meet the individual's nutritional needs.

Referral to members of the multidisciplinary team will be required such as the dietician, physiotherapist and occupational therapist.

25 Angina

Table 25.1 Types of angina

Type of angina	Description
Stable angina	The most common form directly linked to increased activity or stress, exposure to cold and is relieved by rest and drugs
Prinzmetal's (variant) angina	Not necessarily related to coronary heart disease and atherosclerosis, occurs unpredictably, unrelated to activity, often at night, caused by coronary artery spasm; exact mechanism is unknown
Unstable angina	The pain is unpredictable, can occur at rest. Episodes increase in frequency, severity and duration and patients are at increased risk of myocardial infarction

Table 25.2 Severity of angina graded by the degree to which the condition limits activities

Class	Description
Class I	Angina is prompted by strenuous, rapid or prolonged physical exertion, and not normal activity
Class II	Angina develops with rapid or prolonged walking or stair climbing
Class III	Angina severely limits ordinary physical activities
Class IV	Angina occurs at rest, as well as with any physical activity

Figure 25.1 Angina

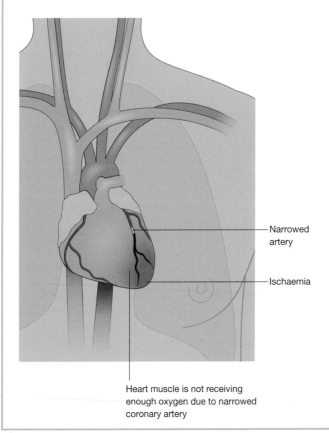

Narrowed artery

Ischaemia

Heart muscle is not receiving enough oxygen due to narrowed coronary artery

Figure 25.2 Insertion of stent to improve cardiac blood flow

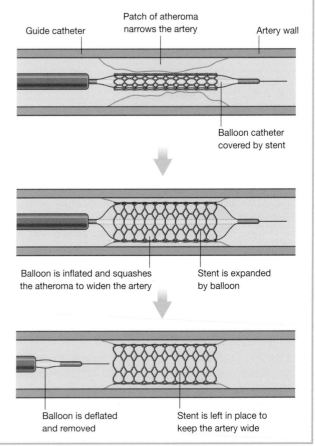

Guide catheter

Patch of atheroma narrows the artery

Artery wall

Balloon catheter covered by stent

Balloon is inflated and squashes the atheroma to widen the artery

Stent is expanded by balloon

Balloon is deflated and removed

Stent is left in place to keep the artery wide

Medical-Surgical Nursing at a Glance, First Edition. Ian Peate. © John Wiley & Sons, Ltd. Published 2016 by John Wiley & Sons, Ltd.
Companion website: www.ataglanceseries.com/nursing/medsurg

Stable angina (or angina pectoris) is chest pain or discomfort caused when the muscle of the heart does not receive sufficient blood which causes a temporary imbalance between myocardial blood supply and demand (Figure 25.1). Angina occurs when the demands made of the myocardium cannot be met by the blood supply. Often this is due to narrowing of one or more coronary artery as a result of coronary heart disease or atherosclerosis. Hypermetabolic conditions, for example, exercise, stimulant abuse (such as cocaine), hyperthyroidism and emotional stress, can increase myocardial oxygen demand, triggering angina. Anaemia, heart failure, ventricular hypertrophy or pulmonary diseases can also affect blood and oxygen supplies, prompting angina.

Three types of angina have been identified (Table 25.1).

Signs and symptoms

The key sign of angina is chest pain brought on by an identifiable event, for example, physical activity, strong emotion, stress, eating a heavy meal or exposure to cold. The usual sequence of angina is activity > pain > rest > relief. The person often describes the pain as a tight, squeezing, heavy pressure or as a constricting vice-like sensation. It typically begins beneath the sternum and can radiate to the jaw, neck, shoulder or arm; however, it can also be felt in the epigastric region or the back. Anginal pain often occurs in a crescendo–decrescendo pattern – it increases to a peak, then it gradually decreases, normally lasting 2–5 minutes. Generally, rest relieves it. There may be changes in the ECG.

Frequently women present with atypical symptoms of angina, including indigestion or nausea, vomiting and upper back pain.

The severity of angina can be graded by the degree to which it limits activities (Table 25.2).

Investigations and diagnosis

The diagnosis of stable angina is based on clinical assessment alone or clinical assessment with diagnostic testing. A detailed medical history is undertaken along with physical examination. A 12-lead ECG may demonstrate some ischaemic changes but a normal ECG does not rule out a diagnosis of angina. A full blood count is undertaken to exclude anaemia, and renal function and electrolytes are used to assess renal function. If diabetes is not known to exist, fasting blood glucose is needed; if diabetes is known and recent data are not available then glycosylated haemoglobin and microalbuminuria should be checked. Fasting blood cholesterol and triglycerides are needed and baseline liver function tests. Thyroid function should be tested. An analysis of troponins or cardiac enzymes is needed.

Echocardiography may be required to assess cardiac function or if aortic valve disease is suspected.

Care and management

Three main drugs are used to treat angina.

• Glyceryl trinitrate (GTN) is used to treat acute attacks; longer-acting nitrate preparations are used to prevent angina.

When given sublingually, GTN acts within a minute or two, by improving myocardial oxygen supply, dilating collateral blood vessels and reducing stenosis. GTN is available as an oral spray; some people find this easier to handle than the small GTN tablets. Longer-acting preparations (oral tablets, ointment or transdermal patches) are used to prevent attacks of angina, not to treat an acute attack. Common side effects include headache, nausea, dizziness and hypotension.

• First-line drugs used to treat stable angina (not Prinzmetal's angina as it may cause adverse effects) are beta-blockers as they inhibit the cardiac-stimulating effects of norepinephrine and epinephrine, preventing anginal attacks by reducing heart rate, myocardial contractility and blood pressure. Beta-blockers may be used alone or with other medications, but are contraindicated for those with asthma or severe chronic obstructive pulmonary disorder (COPD) as they can cause severe bronchospasm.

• Calcium channel blockers reduce myocardial oxygen demand and increase myocardial blood and oxygen supply, lowering blood pressure and reducing myocardial contractility and heart rate. They are also effective coronary vasodilators, increasing oxygen supply. These drugs are not usually prescribed in the initial treatment of angina. In those with dysrhythmias, heart failure or hypotension, these drugs are used cautiously.

A range of other procedures such as angiography, ventriculography and atherectomy (the shaving off of atheroma plaques from the artery wall) can be used to diagnose and treat angina (Figure 25.2). Coronary artery bypass grafting uses a section of vein or artery to create a bypass between the aorta and the coronary artery beyond the obstruction, permitting blood to perfuse the ischaemic aspect of the heart.

The management of angina includes modification of cardiovascular risk factors and specific treatment for angina. Informing the patient of the diagnosis and its implications is key to successful outcomes. The nurse should work with the multidisciplinary team, advising the patient that when an attack of angina occurs, they should stop what they are doing and rest, take GTN as instructed, take a second dose of GTN after 5 minutes if the pain has not eased, and take a third dose of GTN after a further 5 minutes if the pain has still not eased. If the pain has not eased after another 5 minutes (i.e. 15 minutes after onset of pain), or earlier if the pain is intensifying or the person is unwell, then they should call for an ambulance.

Health promotion

The majority of people with stable angina are able to manage their pain effectively, living active and productive lives. The nurse can offer the person the following advice on the condition and coronary heart disease and the relationship between the pain and reduced blood flow to the heart muscle: how to use GTN and the desired and adverse impact of prescribed medications and the importance of not discontinuing medications abruptly, especially those for hypertension; how to store and use GTN – the person should always carry some with them for use in emergency situations. GTN can be used prophylactically before activities that result in chest pain.

26 Meningitis

Figure 26.1 Signs and symptoms of meningitis

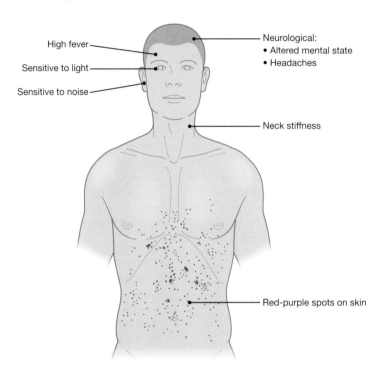

High fever

Sensitive to light

Sensitive to noise

Neurological:
• Altered mental state
• Headaches

Neck stiffness

Red-purple spots on skin

Figure 26.2 Lumbar puncture

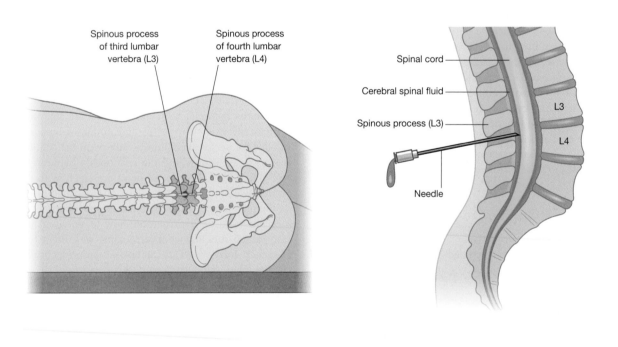

Spinous process
of third lumbar
vertebra (L3)

Spinous process
of fourth lumbar
vertebra (L4)

Spinal cord

Cerebral spinal fluid

Spinous process (L3)

Needle

L3

L4

Medical-Surgical Nursing at a Glance, First Edition. Ian Peate. © John Wiley & Sons, Ltd. Published 2016 by John Wiley & Sons, Ltd.
Companion website: www.ataglanceseries.com/nursing/medsurg

Meningitis is an inflammation of the membranes surrounding the brain and spinal cord and may be bacterial, viral, fungal or parasitic. The responsible organism has to overcome the host's defence mechanisms to attack and replicate in the cerebral spinal fluid (CSF). These include the skin barrier, the blood–brain barrier (BBB), the non-specific inflammatory response and the immune response. Once penetrated, the inflammation spreads quickly throughout the central nervous system (CNS) through the circulation of CSF around the brain and spinal cord. Concerning bacterial meningitis, purulent exudate infiltrates the CSF and cranial nerve sheaths, blocking the choroid plexus and subarachnoid villi. Increased intracranial pressure (IICP) occurs as brain tissue reacts to the pathogen and cerebral perfusion decreases and cerebral perfusion autoregulation is lost. There are two main types of meningitis: bacterial and viral.

Meningococcal disease

Often but not always, meningitis is accompanied by septicaemia. The two conditions have different kinds of symptoms. When caused by meningococcal bacteria, these two conditions together are known as meningococcal disease.

Meningitis or meningococcal septicaemia is a notifiable disease and practitioners have a duty to notify the proper officer of the local authority as a matter of urgency when they have grounds for suspecting that a person has meningitis or meningococcal septicaemia.

Bacterial meningitis

Causative organisms are varied. The person with bacterial meningitis usually presents with restlessness, agitation and irritability, and signs of meningeal irritation, which include neck stiffness, positive Brudzinski's sign and positive Kernig's sign, chills and pyrexia, raised intracranial pressure, photophobia, arthralgia, myalgia, petechial rash (in meningococcal meningitis) and seizures.

Viral meningitis

Viral meningitis is more common than bacterial meningitis and many cases go unreported as the disease is usually mild, with an uneventful recovery. There are several causative organisms which are viral in nature, such as herpes simplex, herpes zoster, Epstein–Barr virus or cytomegalovirus (CMV). Viral infection triggers the inflammatory response; the course of the disease is benign and of short duration.

The signs and symptoms of viral meningitis are akin to those of bacterial meningitis but are usually milder.

The signs and symptoms of meningitis are outlined in Figure 26.1.

Investigations and diagnosis

To confirm diagnosis or to make a differential diagnosis, a variety of tests and investigations are required. The nurse will need to assist with the taking of blood, as a full blood count is required. The white cell count may be elevated and there may be evidence of an electrolyte imbalance. Blood may be taken for culture in order to determine the causative organism if bacteraemia is present; this should be done as soon as possible. A lumbar puncture may be performed to obtain a specimen of cerebrospinal fluid (CSF); there may be an elevation in CSF pressure and the fluid can appear cloudy or milky (Figure 26.2). The specimen will be sent to the laboratory for analysis, the offending organism determined and the appropriate antibiotic commenced. There are contraindications to lumbar puncture, for example, if there are signs of raised intracranial pressure, such as abnormal posturing, dilated or poorly reactive pupils.

Chest and skull X-rays may be ordered and a computed tomography (CT) scan may be undertaken to rule out cerebral haematoma, haemorrhage or trauma.

Those who present with a CNS infection such as meningitis are often very ill. The person may be predisposed to seizures as a result of the combination of pyrexia, dehydration and cerebral oedema. Neurological deterioration, airway obstruction, respiratory arrest or cardiac dysrhythmias may occur. Nursing care associated with altered level of consciousness, increased intracranial pressure and seizures may be required for the person with meningitis.

Antibiotics can be given in the first instance when the cause of the meningitis is not known but antibiotics are stopped if the cause is found to be viral as antibiotics are ineffective against viruses.

In the primary care setting, those with suspected bacterial meningitis or suspected meningococcal septicaemia should be transferred to secondary care as an emergency by calling 999. Those with suspected bacterial meningitis without non-blanching rash should be directly transferred to secondary care, without the administration of antibiotics.

If urgent transfer to hospital is not possible or when the setting is in a remote location or during adverse weather conditions, the administration of antibiotics is required. In cases of suspected meningococcal disease (meningitis with non-blanching rash or meningococcal septicaemia), the person should be given parenteral antibiotics (intramuscular or intravenous benzylpenicillin) at the earliest opportunity. There should be no delay in urgently transferring the person to hospital to give the parenteral antibiotics, but the antibiotic may be given in the GP surgery or by a paramedic.

Admission to hospital usually requires intensive care. Whilst intensive care is required often to save life, the nurse must not forget the intensive care that the person's family may require. Clear and precise explanations need to be given to the family.

Oxygen therapy and in some cases ventilation are required. Intravenous fluid may be needed to correct shock and steroids given in an attempt to reduce inflammation. Anticonvulsant therapy helps control seizures along with sedatives to reduce restlessness and analgesia to control headache and fever. There may be a need to isolate the person; adhere to local policy and procedure. The person should be cared for in a quiet darkened room to reduce the impact of photophobia and irritability.

Antiemetics should be administered. An intravenous infusion is required to administer prescribed medication. Neurological observations will be required to detect any improvement or deterioration in neurological status. Skilled, competent and confident care is required for both the patient and the family.

27 Subarachnoid Haemorrhage

Figure 27.1 Subarachnoid haemorrhage

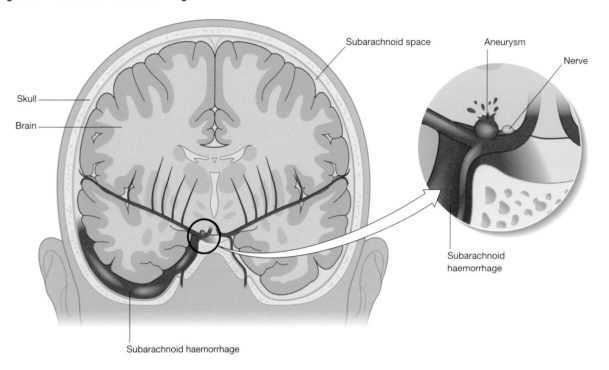

Skull

Brain

Subarachnoid space

Aneurysm

Nerve

Subarachnoid haemorrhage

Subarachnoid haemorrhage

Table 27.1 Some neurological deficits associated with brain injury

Neurological deficit		Manifestations
Visual field deficits	*Hemianopsia* *Loss of peripheral vision* *Diplopia*	• Unaware of people or objects on side of visual loss • Neglecting one side of the body • Difficulty judging distance • Difficulty with night vision • Unaware of objects or the boarder of objects • Double vision
Motor deficits	*Hemiparesis* *Ataxia* *Dysarthria* *Dysphagia*	• Weakness of the face, arm, leg on the same side • Unstable gait • Unable to keep feet together • Difficulty in forming words • Difficulty in swallowing
Sensory deficits	*Paraesthesia* *(opposite side of lesion)*	• Sensation of numbness or tingling • Difficulty with proprioception
Verbal deficits	*Expressive aphasia* *Receptive aphasia* *Global aphasia*	• Unable to form words that are understandable, uses sign word responses • Unable to comprehend the spoken word, may not make sense when speaking • Receptive and expressive aphasia
Cognitive deficits		• Short and long term memory loss • Decreased attention span • Impaired ability to concentrate • Poor abstract reasoning • Altered judgment
Emotional deficits		• Loss of self-control • Emotional labiality • Depression • Withdrawal • Fear, anger • Feelings of isolation

Medical-Surgical Nursing at a Glance, First Edition. Ian Peate. © John Wiley & Sons, Ltd. Published 2016 by John Wiley & Sons, Ltd.
Companion website: www.ataglanceseries.com/nursing/medsurg

Most cases of subarachnoid haemorrhage (SAH) (a haemorrhage in the subarachnoid space) occur where there is a ruptured intracranial haemorrhage (Figure 27.1). SAH is sometimes known as a haemorrhagic stroke.

Subarachnoid haemorrhage

The condition may occur as a result of an arteriovenous malformation, intracranial aneurysm, trauma or hypertension. Commonly, there is a leaking aneurysm in the area of the circle of Willis along with a congenital arteriovenous malformation of the brain.

Risk factors associated with subarachnoid haemorrhage

The larger the aneurysm, the more prone it is to bleed. The incidence increases with age and the average age is 50 years. Hypertension, smoking and excessive alcohol intake (all modifiable risk factors) double the risk. Genetic factors have a role to play in risk, although no single gene has been isolated. Those with a positive family history often have their first SAH at a younger age and are more likely to have large and multiple aneurysms.

Signs and symptoms

The person with SAH presents with a variety of neurological deficits. In the conscious patient, the most commonly reported symptom is severe headache; this may last seconds or even just a fraction of a second but the pain is so severe that the individual may think that somebody has hit them on the back of the head. A SAH should be considered in any patient who presents with sudden and severe onset headache with or without an alteration in consciousness.

The headache is often diffused and the main feature is the severity, as opposed to the suddenness of the headache; often this is described as the most severe ever experienced. It generally lasts for a week or two. The other features include vomiting and seizures, there may be neck stiffness and some people experience tinnitus. An overview of some neurological deficits associated with brain injury is outlined in Table 27.1.

Investigations and diagnosis

Rapid diagnosis and treatment of stroke are essential to reduce the likelihood of a subsequent disability. If the person is conscious, a full health history should be obtained. A depressed level of consciousness affects most people admitted to hospital, and coma is a predominant feature.

On examination, the person may have a stiff neck due to meningeal irritation. In some people ophthalmoscopic examination demonstrates intraocular haemorrhage which is more pronounced in those with a depressed level of consciousness. There can be focal neurological signs that may suggest a stroke. A marked rise in blood pressure may occur as a reflex following haemorrhage.

Assessment of arterial blood gases should be undertaken to exclude hypoxia.

A CT scan will be performed at the earliest opportunity if SAH is suspected – immediately if the person presents with sudden severe headache and as soon as possible in all other cases. CT angiography should follow immediately if there is confirmation of SAH. A lumbar puncture should be undertaken if the CT scan is negative. Spectrophotometry can allow detection of small amounts of xanthochromia (yellow discolouration of the spinal fluid).

Care and management

In early management, the aim is to avert further bleeding and reduce the rate of secondary complications, for example, cerebral ischaemia.

Calcium antagonists (for example, nimodipine) should be given to every patient as they help to reduce spasm and cerebral ischaemia.

In order to prevent seizure (or the spread of seizure activity), phenytoin may be given. A potent vasodilator such as nitroprusside along with labetolol is used to treat hypertension; the dose must be titrated in order to provide low enough levels to avert a rebleed whilst being high enough to sustain cerebral perfusion.

Referral to a specialist unit (often a neurosurgery centre) is required, within 24 hours if appropriate. Further investigations are undertaken (if CT angiogram has not been performed, this should be done, and imaging of all cerebral arteries is needed) and, if appropriate, definitive treatment.

An aneurysm that is associated with the haemorrhage is usually treated by surgical clipping or endovascular embolisation. Surgical interventions should be carried out earlier rather than later.

There may be contraindications to surgical intervention; each patient must be assessed individually.

Surviving patients should be offered advice on secondary prevention, particularly on treatment for hypertension and the need to stop smoking.

Those with residual impairment after investigation and treatment should be referred to an appropriate specialist rehabilitation service. Some patients may develop epilepsy after discharge.

As hypertension, smoking and excessive alcohol consumption are risk factors, the nurse needs to help individuals address such issues in order to prevent recurrence.

The care and management of people with SAH require a number of important decisions to be made; the patient's wishes must be considered and the role of the nurse is to provide support and act as patient advocate. Providing information so that the person understands it and permitting time for questions can help the person make an informed decision.

Specific aspects of nursing care include problems with airway maintenance, nutrition, mobility and specific hygiene requirements. The unconscious patient is at risk of ineffective airway clearance and aspiration, imbalanced nutrition and damage to the integrity of skin and related structures.

Nursing care for an unconscious person who has had a SAH is both general and specific. The nurse needs to ensure that all necessary supportive care is provided. Total patient care is required if the person has lost consciousness. An initial and ongoing assessment of care needs is essential if care is to be safe and effective. The patient and family must be given an explanation of investigations and all care that is being provided.

Maintaining a positive fluid balance and avoiding hypovolaemia will reduce the risk of vasospasm. Constipation, straining to pass stools and the administration of enemas will increase intra-abdominal pressure, which can in turn increase intracranial pressure and hasten a rebleed.

28 Epilepsy

Table 28.1 Generalised seizures: descriptions

Seizure	Characteristic
Generalised tonic–clonic seizures	Also known as the *'grand mal'* seizures' the most common type of seizure activity. Followed by a typical sequence: • ***Aura***. A warning may precede generalised seizure activity - a vague sense of uneasiness or an abnormal gustatory, visual, auditory or visceral sensation • ***Tonic phase***. Sudden loss of consciousness and sharp tonic muscle contractions. The person may cry out as air is forced out of the lungs, the person falls to the floor, muscles are rigid, arms and legs extended, jaw clenched. Urinary incontinence is common; bowel incontinence can occur. Breathing ceases and cyanosis, pupils are fixed and dilated. Lasts an average of 15 seconds, may persist for up to a minute • ***Clonic phase***. Follows the tonic phase and is characterised by alternating contraction and relaxation of the muscles in all the extremities with hyperventilation, eyes roll back, may froth at the mouth. Varies in duration, gradually subsides • ***Post-ictal period or phase***. Following the clonic phase, person remains unconscious and unresponsive to stimuli. Gradually regains consciousness, may be confused and disoriented. Headache, muscle aches and fatigue often follow, may sleep for several hours. Amnesia of the seizure is usual and amnesia of the events just prior to the seizure activity may occur
Tonic seizures	Involve sudden onset of stiffening of the muscles resulting in increased muscle tone, often leads to a fall.
Clonic seizures	Rapidly alternating contraction and relaxation of a muscle (repeated jerking) of the arms and legs (uncommon).
Myoclonic seizures	Brief, arrhythmic, jerking, motor movements, lasting less than a second, often occur in clusters
Atonic seizures	Consist of brief loss of postural tone, often resulting in falls and injuries.
Absence seizures	Often called 'petit mal' seizures, characterised by a sudden brief cessation of all motor activity accompanied by a blank stare and unresponsiveness. Classically last only 5–10 seconds but, some may last for 30 seconds or more

Medical-Surgical Nursing at a Glance, First Edition. Ian Peate. © John Wiley & Sons, Ltd. Published 2016 by John Wiley & Sons, Ltd.
Companion website: www.ataglanceseries.com/nursing/medsurg

Epilepsy is one of the most common neurological disorders and is also known as seizure disorder. This is a chronic disorder characterised by abnormal recurring, excessive and self-terminating electrical discharge from the neurones. This abnormal neuronal activity can involve all or part of the brain; it interrupts skeletal motor function, sensation, autonomic function of the viscera, and behaviour and may also impact on the person's level of consciousness.

Epilepsy

Epilepsy can be classed as idiopathic, with multiple episodes that are diagnosed as a seizure disorder, or it can be secondary to a number of conditions that affect the brain or other organs, for example, birth injury and toxaemia of pregnancy, drug and alcohol overdose and withdrawal, systemic metabolic conditions (e.g. hypoglycaemia, hypoxia, uraemia and electrolyte imbalances), pathologies of the brain, for example meningitis, cerebral haemorrhage, cerebral oedema, infection, trauma or tumours. Seizures can be provoked or unprovoked.

Signs and symptoms

The signs and symptoms of seizures depend on the brain location of the electrical discharges and the amount and pattern of the discharge in the brain. Characteristic symptoms include temporary changes in mental status and loss of consciousness, abnormal sensory changes and abnormal movements.

Classification of epilepsy

Focal or partial seizures

Abnormal neuronal activity can remain localised, which causes a partial or focal seizure, often involving a limited aspect of one cerebral hemisphere at the onset. Partial seizures can be further subdivided into simple partial seizure (without impaired consciousness), complex partial seizure (with impaired consciousness) and partial seizures developing into secondary generalised seizures.

Both types of seizures can spread, resulting in secondarily generalised tonic-clonic seizures; the signs and symptoms depend on the area of brain involved. Usually this is a portion of the motor cortex, resulting in recurrent muscle contractions. This may stay confined to one area or spread sequentially, known as Jacksonian march or Jacksonian seizure. In complex partial seizures, consciousness is compromised; the person may engage in repetitive, non-purposeful activity such as aimless walking or picking at clothing. Complex partial seizures may be heralded by an aura, such as an unusual smell, a sense of déjà vu or a sudden intense emotion.

Generalised seizures

The two hemispheres of the brain are affected, including deeper brain structures. Consciousness is always impaired. Generalised seizures can be further subdivided into six major categories (Table 28.1).

Status epilepticus

Can develop during seizure activity. In status epilepticus the seizure activity becomes incessant and there are only very short periods of calm between strong and unrelenting seizures. There is a great danger that the person may develop hypoxia, acidosis, hypoglycaemia, hyperthermia and exhaustion if unrelenting seizure activity is not stopped. This condition is considered a life-threatening medical emergency and the person requires immediate treatment. The condition is distressing for the person and those who may be watching (and this can include the person's family).

Non-epileptic seizures

These events look like epileptic seizures. There are two main types: psychogenic non-epileptic seizures (episodes of altered movement, sensation or experience, caused by a psychological process, not related to abnormal electrical discharges in the brain) and physiological non-epileptic seizures caused by physiological dysfunction, such as cardiac arrhythmias or hypotensive episodes. May result in loss of consciousness with or without associated motor signs.

If the cause is cardiac, these seizures can be life-threatening. An accurate diagnosis is needed to ensure appropriate treatment and improvement in quality of life.

Investigations and diagnosis

In order to make an accurate diagnosis, a detailed medical history is needed, which may be taken from the person and/or eyewitnesses. Diagnostic testing to confirm the seizure diagnosis and to ascertain any treatable causes and trigger factors often includes magnetic resonance imaging (MRI) or computed tomography (CT) scan and a skull X-ray to identify any bony abnormalities. An electroencephalograph helps localise any brain lesions and confirms diagnosis. Lumbar puncture is undertaken to assess spinal fluid for central nervous system infections, and a full blood count is assessed. A specialist in the field of epilepsy confirms diagnosis. Other causes of loss of consciousness will need to be established.

Treatment and care

The initial aspects of treatment focus on controlling the seizure; long term, the aim is to ascertain the cause and prevent impending seizures. A multidisciplinary approach is advocated, and diagnostic testing, medications and in some cases surgery will be indicated.

Nurses will focus on providing care during and immediately after the seizure has occurred for the person and the family.

The nurse is required to provide teaching to promote safety and reduce the incidence of seizure activity. Assisting the person (and if appropriate the family) to adjust to a diagnosis and providing relevant information are critical. Education includes interventions to maintain a patent airway: cushion the head, loosen anything tight around the neck, turn on the side, do not force anything into the mouth and if available administer oxygen. If the seizure lasts for more than 5 minutes, there is slow recovery, a second seizure or difficulty breathing after the seizure and if there are signs of injury, call for an ambulance. The person must be advised about the importance of follow-up care, attending medical appointments and continuing to take antiepileptic medications as prescribed. Information must also be given about relevant legislation, for example driving a motor vehicle; awareness of drug interactions with other prescribed, over-the-counter and recreational drugs and alcohol; identifying factors that precipitate a seizure; abrupt withdrawal from medication; fatigue, excessive stress, sights and sounds such as television, flashing video and computer screens.

29 Gastro-oesophageal Reflux Disease

Figure 29.1   Signs and symptoms of GORD

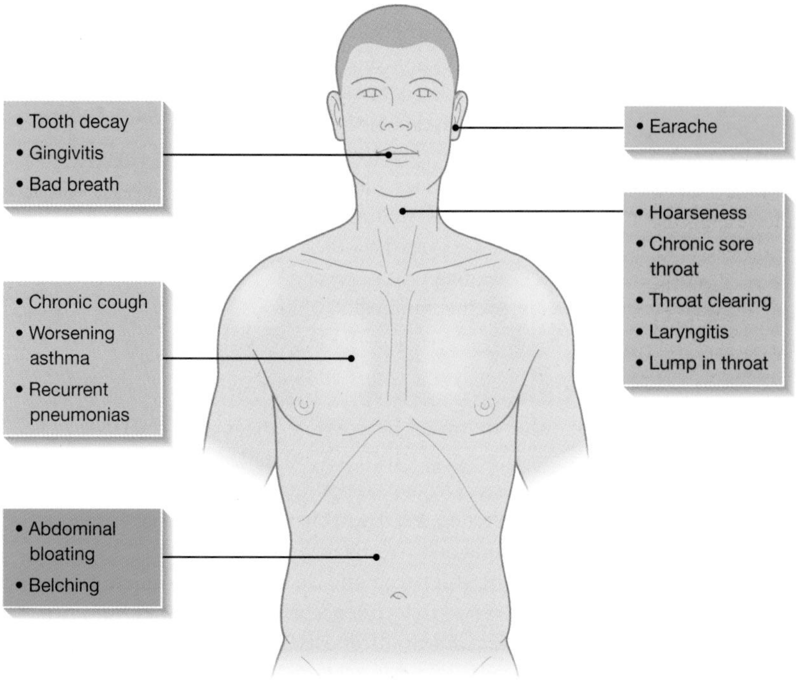

- Tooth decay
- Gingivitis
- Bad breath

- Chronic cough
- Worsening asthma
- Recurrent pneumonias

- Abdominal bloating
- Belching

- Earache

- Hoarseness
- Chronic sore throat
- Throat clearing
- Laryngitis
- Lump in throat

Table 29.1   Recommended lifestyle changes

- Reduce weight
- Stop smoking
- Reduce alcohol intake
- Elevate the head of the bed at night
- Eat small, regular meals
- Avoid hot drinks, alcohol
- Avoid eating during the three hours before going to bed
- Avoid drugs that alter oesophageal motility (nitrates, anticholinergics, tricyclic antidepressants) or damage the mucosa (NSAIDs, alendronate)

Figure 29.2   Gastroscopy

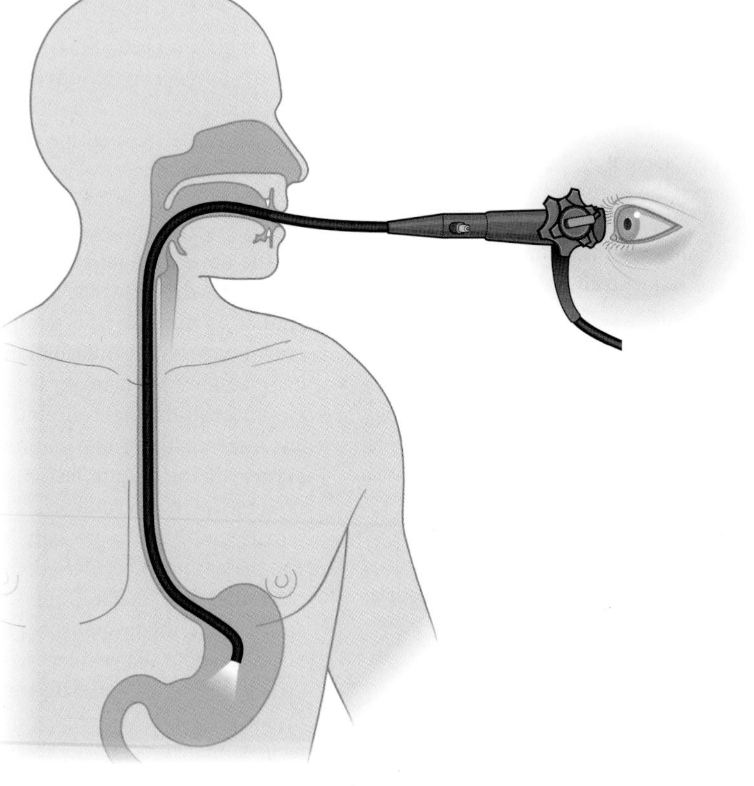

Gastro-oesophageal reflux disease (GORD) is sometimes called gastroesophageal reflux disease (GERD) or reflux oesophagitis.

Gastro-oesophageal reflux disease

A certain amount of gastro-oesophageal reflux of acid is normal. The lower aspect of the oesophagus has a natural protective mechanism. If reflux is protracted, however, or extreme it can result in a breakdown of this protective structure, causing oesophagitis (inflammation of the oesophagus).

GORD is 2–3 times more common in men than in women. This condition covers a spectrum of disorders ranging from the most common – endoscopy-negative GORD (no abnormal findings on endoscopic examination) – to oesophageal mucosal damage, which can progress to ulceration along with stricture formation.

Excessive reflux of gastric contents including acid and occasionally bile from the stomach can enter the oesophagus due to malfunction of the lower oesophageal sphincter.

Reflux of duodenal contents (bile) is more problematic than reflux of gastric contents alone as bile is very caustic.

On occasion, medications that have not been taken with a sufficient amount of water can lodge in the oesophagus where they are slowly released, causing oesophagitis. Non-steroidal anti-inflammatory drugs (NSAIDs) and doxycycline can cause the condition, and must be taken with adequate water. It is important to note that oesophageal reflux is considered a risk factor for cancer of the oesophagus.

Signs and symptoms

The key or typical symptom is heartburn. Heartburn is a burning feeling, starting from the stomach or lower chest and moving up towards the neck. Very often this is associated with eating a meal, lying down, stooping and straining; taking antacids alleviates it. There is retrosternal discomfort, acid brash (regurgitation of acid or bile) and excessive salivation (water brash). Odynophagia (pain on swallowing) can occur and this may be due to severe oesophagitis or stricture.

Atypical symptoms can include chest pain, epigastric pain and bloating. Respiratory symptoms include chronic hoarseness, chronic cough and symptoms associated with asthma, for example, wheezing and shortness of breath. See Figure 29.1 for an overview of the signs and symptoms associated with GORD.

Investigations and diagnosis

The investigation of choice is gastroscopy (Figure 29.2). A full blood count is performed to exclude the presence of anaemia. A barium swallow may show that the person has a hiatus hernia. Monitoring of oseophageal pH can help to determine if symptoms coincide with the presence of acid in the oesophagus. There are several ways in which this can be achieved.

- The introduction of a naso-oesophageal pH catheter (this is a 24-hour study).
- The insertion of a wireless pH capsule.
- Oesophageal impedance and pH through a nasal catheter (can provide quantitative information concerning the amount of fluid that has been refluxed).

Treatment and care

The role of the nurse in caring for people with GORD is multifaceted. The nurse:

- provides comfort
- prevents complications
- acts as an educational resource.

The various investigations and tests required to make a diagnosis of GORD can be invasive and as such the nurse is required to assist the patient before, during and after the procedure. In order to provide care that is safe, effective and patient centred, the nurse must understand the condition and various treatment options available.

National guidance has been produced concerning the management of dyspepsia (including reflux symptoms) that will guide and inform clinical practice.

The initial pharmacological treatment for patients with reflux symptoms includes administration of full-dose proton pump inhibitors (PPIs) for 1 month.

In instances of uninvestigated dyspepsia, consideration should be given to eradication therapy for *H. pylori* if infection is evident. Where there is known GORD (for example, after a positive gastroscopy), then the eradication of *H. pylori* is not recommended.

If after treatment symptoms return and long-term acid suppression is needed, a step-down strategy to the lowest dose of PPI that provides effective relief of symptoms is required (as opposed to a step-up approach). Start acid suppression at a healing dose for 1–2 months. All patients should have a treatment plan and should be told that if they are symptom free they can stop treatment.

Referral for endoscopy

Referral to an endoscopic specialist for a second opinion may be appropriate for some patients who have an inadequate response to therapy, or where there are new symptoms.

The patient's medications should be reviewed for possible causes of dyspepsia. There are some calcium antagonists, nitrates, theophyllines, bisphosphonates, steroids and NSAIDs, for example, that may cause and exacerbate dyspepsia. The patient who requires endoscopy should be free from medication with either a PPI or an H2-receptor antagonist for a minimum of 2 weeks.

If endoscopy is performed and oesophagitis is seen, a healing dose of PPI should be prescribed for 2 months. Usually in these patients symptoms relapse when treatment is withdrawn, so maintenance PPI therapy is usually required.

The majority of patients are treated with lifestyle interventions and medication. However, surgical intervention may be needed. Laparoscopic fundoplication surgery is more effective than medical management for the treatment of GORD in the short to medium term.

Lifestyle

Most patients unfortunately do not respond to lifestyle advice and require further therapy. However, the lifestyle changes in Table 29.1 are recommended.

30 Diverticular Disease

Figure 30.1 Diverticular disease

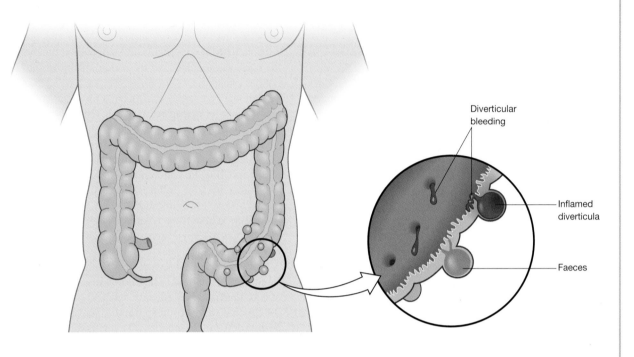

Diverticular bleeding

Inflamed diverticula

Faeces

Figure 30.2 Colonoscopy

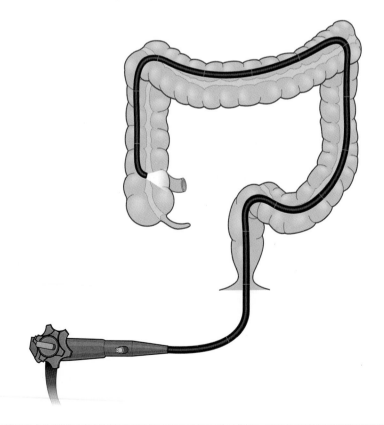

Diverticular disease consists of three conditions involving the development of small sacs or pockets in the wall of the colon: diverticulosis, diverticular bleeding and diverticulitis.

Diverticulosis

Diverticula vary from solitary findings to many hundreds. They are usually 5–10 mm in diameter but they can exceed 2 cm. Diverticula can range from very small pea size to much larger sizes; they are formed by increased pressure on weakened areas of the intestinal walls by flatus or faeces. Diverticula can form whilst straining during a bowel movement. They are most common in the sigmoid colon and the descending colon.

Complications can occur; one of these complications is rectal bleeding, called diverticular bleeding, and another is diverticular infection known as diverticulitis (Figure 30.1).

Diverticular bleeding

Diverticular bleeding occurs with chronic injury to the small blood vessels that are located next to the diverticula.

Diverticulitis

Diverticulitis occurs when there is inflammation and infection in one or more diverticula. This typically happens when the outpouchings become blocked with faecal matter, permitting bacteria to accumulate and resulting in infection.

Risk factors associated with diverticular disease

The main risk factors are age over 50 years and low dietary fibre. In young people obesity is a significant risk factor. In complicated diverticular disease, an increased frequency occurs in those who smoke, use non-steroidal anti-inflammatory drugs (NSAIDs) and paracetamol, those who are obese and those who have low-fibre diets.

Signs and symptoms

Uncomplicated diverticular disease is often an incidental finding occurring during assessment of the patient for another reason, for example, during routine screening for colon cancer. Patients can present with non-specific abdominal complaints, such as lower abdominal pain that is usually left-sided. There may be pyrexia or an increase in white blood cells (signs of inflammation) which may indicate diverticulitis.

Pain is often aggravated by eating and reduces when the person defaecates or passes flatus; bloating, constipation or rectal bleeding can also occur. Physical examination can uncover fullness or mild tenderness in the left lower quadrant.

In diverticulitis, often the patient will present with left lower quadrant pain. Some Asian patients have predominantly right-sided diverticula, presenting with right lower quadrant pain. The pain can be sporadic or constant and may be linked to a change in bowel habits. Pyrexia and tachycardia are present in most patients, hypotension and shock are uncommon. The person may be anorexic and nauseous and vomiting can occur.

Localised tenderness is apparent on examination and sometimes there is a palpable mass. Bowel sounds are often reduced but in mild cases they may be normal or increased in obstruction. A rectal examination may reveal tenderness; there may be a mass, particularly if there is a low-lying pelvic abscess.

Further complications can develop and include perforation, abscess, fistula, stricture and/or obstruction.

A common cause of lower gastrointestinal haemorrhage is related to diverticular bleeding. Often presentation is abrupt with painless bleeding. The patient may have mild lower abdominal cramps or experience the urge to defaecate, followed by passage of a large amount of red or maroon blood or clots. It is uncommon for melaena to occur. In the majority of patients haemorrhage will stop spontaneously. There may be a rebleed.

Investigations and diagnosis

There is a need to undertake a thorough investigation, including a colonoscopy (Figure 30.2), for patients with symptomatic disease to confirm the diagnosis and exclude other possible diagnoses, in particular bowel cancer.

A full blood count is required. In the initial stage blood haematology should be normal in those with uncomplicated diverticular disease. The white cell count is often elevated with diverticulitis or abscess. Bleeding can cause a raised platelet count and anaemia.

In uncomplicated diverticular disease, a barium enema offers information on the number and location of colonic diverticula. If there is diverticulitis a chest X-ray with the patient upright can aid detection of pneumoperitoneum. Abdominal X-rays may show small or large bowel dilation or ileus, pneumoperitoneum, bowel obstruction or lesion suggestive of soft tissue abscesses. When an abscess is suspected, computed tomography (CT) scanning is the best tool for making the diagnosis and following its course.

Flexible sigmoidoscopy is an appropriate initial approach to rule out an obvious rectosigmoid lesion if there is haemorrhage.

Care and management

People who have diverticulosis without symptoms or complications do not need specific treatment, but it is important to adopt a high-fibre diet to prevent the further formation of diverticula.

No treatment or follow-up is needed for those who are asymptomatic or have no complications but a high-fibre diet may help. The risk of perforation may be increased by the use of NSAIDs and long-term use of opioids so medications need to be reviewed.

With significant blood loss, a blood transfusion may be required. Advise a high-fibre diet along with adequate fluid intake. If required paracetamol should be used for pain.

The patient should be admitted to hospital with diverticulitis when pain cannot be managed with paracetamol, there is a risk of dehydration or oral antibiotics cannot be tolerated, perforation and peritonitis occur. Admit if symptoms persist after 48 hours in spite of conservative management at home.

If cared for at home, broad-spectrum antibiotics should be prescribed; treatment should last for at least 7 days and paracetamol should be used for pain. Advise clear liquids only; gradually reintroduce solid food as symptoms improve over 2–3 days. After 48 hours, or sooner if symptoms deteriorate, arrange for hospital admission.

If the patient does not respond to conservative treatment, surgery may be needed.

31 Constipation

Figure 31.1 Constipation

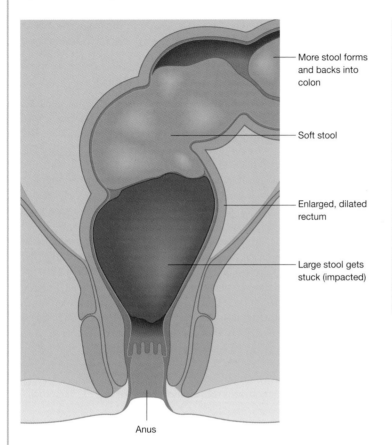

- More stool forms and backs into colon
- Soft stool
- Enlarged, dilated rectum
- Large stool gets stuck (impacted)
- Anus

Table 31.1 Some causes of constipation

- Lack of exercise, bed rest
- Inadequate fluid intake
- Low-fibre diet
- Certain medications:
  – some types of antacids, opioids, anticholinergics, antidepressants, tranquilisers and sedatives, antihypertensives, iron preparations
- Large bowel conditions:
  – diverticular disease, inflammatory disease, tumour, obstruction, changes in rectal or anal structure or function
- Certain psychogenic conditions:
  – voluntary suppression of urge, perceived need to defaecate at certain times, depression
- Systemic issues:
  – advanced age, pregnancy, neurological conditions endocrine and metabolic disorders
- Chronic laxative or enema use

Table 31.2 Some drugs used in the treatment of constipation

Drug	Example
Bulk producers	• Bran powder • Ispaghula husk • Methylcellulose
Stool softener	• Aracis oil enema • Liquid paraffin enema
Stimulants	• Bisccodyl, senna • Docusate sodium • Glycerol suppositories • Sodium picosulfate, lactulose
Osmotic agents	• Magnesium salts • Macrogols • Sodium phosphate enemas and glycerin suppositories • Sodium salts (such as micolette and micralax enemas)

Medical-Surgical Nursing at a Glance, First Edition. Ian Peate. © John Wiley & Sons, Ltd. Published 2016 by John Wiley & Sons, Ltd.
Companion website: www.ataglanceseries.com/nursing/medsurg

Globally, chronic constipation is a common problem. The term chronic constipation is used for those patients who have had symptoms for more than 6 months.

Constipation

A person's quality of life can be affected by constipation and it may be associated with haemorrhoids and anal fissures as well as serious underlying causes, for example, colorectal cancer.

Constipation is not a diagnosis, it is a symptom, meaning different things to different people. The nurse should always ask patients what exactly they mean by the term constipation.

Although the transit of faeces in the large intestine slows with ageing, the increased incidence in this condition may be related more to impaired general health status, an increased medication use and a decrease in physical activity in the older person (Figure 31.1).

Some causes of constipation are outlined in Table 31.1.

Signs and symptoms

There are various formal definitions of constipation. It is defined as defaecation that is unsatisfactory because of infrequent stools (passing a stool less than three times weekly), difficult stool passage (passing of the stool is accompanied with straining or discomfort), or apparently inadequate or incomplete defaecation. With constipation, stools are frequently dry and hard, and they may be abnormally large or abnormally small. Some patients may mean that:

- faeces are too hard
- they do not defaecate often enough
- defaecation hurts.

Investigations and diagnosis

There are several causes of constipation. Taking a careful and detailed history can help to ascertain the probable cause. The nurse must always consider the possibility of a serious underlying cause. When taking the history, be sure to ask particularly about weight loss or rectal bleeding which are 'red flags' alerting the nurse to potential serious underlying causes.

As part of the history taking, enquire about frequency, nature and consistency of the stool. Ask 'Is there blood or any mucus in/on the stools? Is there any diarrhoea that alternates with constipation? Have there been any recent changes in bowel habit?' Enquire about the person's diet and any medications they are taking.

As well as the oral history of the condition, a thorough examination of the abdomen must be performed; this will also include a rectal examination.

In most cases of constipation, there is no need for any investigations, particularly in the young and those who are mildly affected. If there is a need for any investigations these are usually indicated in:

- those aged over 40 years
- people reporting a recent change in their bowel habit
- those presenting with associated symptoms, such as weight loss, rectal bleeding, mucous discharge or tenesmus.

Other investigations may include the following.

- A full blood count, estimation of urea and electrolytes, calcium levels, thyroid function tests.
- Sigmoidoscopy and biopsy of abnormal and normal mucosa.
- If there is suspected colorectal malignancy, a barium enema should be performed.
- Occasionally a range of special investigations may be indicated. In certain cases these include transit studies and anorectal physiology.

Care and treatment

Laxative (milder preparations) and cathartic preparations (these have a stronger effect) are used to encourage stool evacuation. The majority of laxatives are usually only appropriate for short-term use. These preparations interfere with normal bowel reflexes and should be avoided when the person complains of simple constipation. If a person has an undiagnosed intestinal obstruction, abdominal pain, impacted faeces, rectal fissures, ulcerated haemorrhoids, Crohn's disease, ulcerative colitis or chronic inflammatory bowel disease then they should not be given laxative or cathartics. Dangerous mechanical damage can occur and perforate the bowel when laxatives or cathartics are given if there is bowel obstruction.

The cause of the constipation (if known) should be treated. The nurse should encourage and assist the person to mobilise. If safe to do so, fluid intake should be increased, as should the intake of high-fibre foods, such as fruits, vegetables, whole wheat and bran.

Laxatives and cathartics should only be considered if the above actions fail. Drugs should be used for short periods only. Drug therapy is outlined in Table 31.2. It is essential that each person is assessed individually and treatment plans are tailored to meet the person's needs in a holistic way. Caution must be exercised with some types of medication.

Bulk-producing agents increase faecal mass and this then stimulates peristalsis. They must, however, be taken with plenty of fluid. Contraindications include difficulty in swallowing, intestinal obstruction, colonic atony and faecal impaction.

Side effects associated with the use of stool softeners include anal seepage, lipoid pneumonia and malabsorption of fat-soluble vitamins.

Stimulants work by increasing intestinal motility; they should not be used in intestinal obstruction. Prolonged use should be avoided, as this can result in colonic atony and hypokalaemia.

Promoting health

Providing education can prevent constipation. Explain the importance of maintaining a diet high in natural fibre; foods such as fresh fruits, vegetables, wholegrain products and bran provide natural fibre. Reducing consumption of meats and refined foods, which are low in fibre, can prevent constipation. It is important to emphasise the need to ensure a high fluid intake daily, particularly during hot weather, and exercise. Explain the association between exercise and bowel regularity. Encourage the person to engage in some form of exercise, such as walking daily. Discuss normal bowel habits, explaining that a daily bowel movement is not the norm for everyone. Encourage the person to respond to the need to defaecate when it occurs. Advise setting aside a time, usually after a meal, for elimination.

32 Osteoporosis

Table 32.1 Causes of osteoporosis

- Advancing age
- Reduced bone mineral density
- Parental history of hip fracture
- Consumption of 4 or more units of alcohol per day
- Rheumatoid arthritis
- Gender (female)
- Corticosteroid therapy
- Cushing's syndrome
- Ankylosing spondylitis
- Crohn's disease
- Untreated premature menopause or prolonged secondary amenhorrhoea
- Low body mass (less than 19 kg/m2)
- Anorexia nervosa
- Poor diet (calcium-deficient)
- Malabsorption syndromes (such as coeliac disease)
- Lengthy periods of immobilisation
- Smoking
- Primary hypogonadism
- Primary hyperparathyroidism
- Hyperthyroidism
- Osteogenesis imperfecta
- Caucasian or Asian origin
- Post organ transplantation
- Chronic renal failure

Figure 32.1 Normal and osteoporotic spine

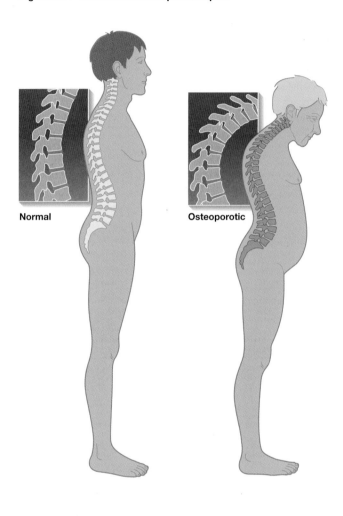

Normal   Osteoporotic

Table 32.2 Some investigations used to diagnose osteoporosis

- A full blood count, erythrocyte sedimentation rate or C-reactive protein, serum calcium, albumin, creatinine, phosphate, alkaline phosphatase and liver function tests
- Thyroid function tests (including parathyroid hormone)
- Bone densitometry (DXA)
- Various radiographs (for example, thoracico-lumbar spine)
- Protein immunoelectrophoresis and urinary Bence-Jones protiens
- 25-hydroxyvitamin D (a pre hormone)
- Serum testosterone, sex hormone binging globulin, follicle stimulating hormone, luteinising hormone (in men)
- Serum prolactin
- 24 hour urinary cortisol/dexamethasone suppression test
- Isotope bone scan

Medical-Surgical Nursing at a Glance, First Edition. Ian Peate. © John Wiley & Sons, Ltd. Published 2016 by John Wiley & Sons, Ltd.
Companion website: www.ataglanceseries.com/nursing/medsurg

Over the age of 30 years, more bone cells are lost than replaced; this is referred to as bone thinning. Women are more affected by this than men, probably because the bones of men are denser than those of women. The condition is the most prevalent bone condition globally.

Osteoporosis

This is a metabolic bone disorder. It has been estimated that around 250,000 fractures occur annually as a result of osteoporosis; this has an impact on an individual's health and well-being, their family and the nation. Many people who sustain a fracture due to osteoporosis will lose their mobility and independence. People die each year as a result of sustaining a hip fracture.

The definition of osteoporosis is based on bone mineral density (BMD) measurements in white women. The definition applies to postmenopausal women and men aged 50 years or older. Bone formation initially exceeds bone resorption, but by the time the person reaches 30 years, this has reversed and there is a net loss of bone mass causing increased bone fragility and fracture susceptibility.

Osteoporotic (fragility) fractures arise from mechanical forces that would not usually result in a fracture. Osteoporotic fractures are defined as fractures associated with a low BMD, for example, spine, wrist, hip and shoulder fractures.

Risk features for osteoporosis

The following hormone-related problems influence osteoporosis.

- Hyperthyroidism
- Cushing's syndrome
- Diabetes mellitus
- Coeliac disease

Other factors include:

- low calcium and vitamin D levels in the diet
- consumption of alcohol
- smoking.

See also Table 32.1. Having risk factors means the person is more prone to developing bone modelling and maintenance problems.

Signs and symptoms

The process that leads to recognised osteoporosis is asymptomatic; often the condition presents only after bone fracture. 'Fragility fractures' (a fracture caused by a force equivalent to the force of a fall from the height of an ordinary chair or less) most commonly occur in the spine (vertebrae), hip (proximal femur) and wrist (distal radius). They can also occur in the arm (humerus), pelvis, ribs and other bones. The signs will differ depending on the fracture site. See Figure 32.1 for an illustration of a normal and an osteoporotic spine.

As bone loss continues to decrease and the density of the bones reaches a severely low level, osteoporosis symptoms can manifest through various means, including bone and joint pain. The bone and joint pain will be felt throughout the body; many people often assume the pain is part of the ageing process. The pain can be felt in the lower back due to spinal bone fractures. The person may experience neck pain due to fractures in the spinal bones. There are a number of things that can cause bone and joint pain and osteoporosis is one of them. Bone and joint pain due to osteoporosis occurs as the bones get to such a weakened state that it becomes an effort for them to hold the person's body weight.

Investigations and diagnosis

The diagnosis of osteoporosis relies on the quantitative assessment of BMD, usually by central dual energy X-ray absorptiometry (DXA). The BMD is calculated using the femoral neck as the reference site.

A detailed history is taken and physical examination is carried out. The aims of the history, physical examination and investigations are to exclude diseases akin to osteoporosis such as osteomalacia and myeloma, to identify the cause of osteoporosis and contributory factors, assess the risk of subsequent fractures and select the most appropriate type of treatment. Table 32.2 notes some of the procedures that may be appropriate when investigating osteoporosis.

Care and treatment

National guidance exists for the treatment of osteoporosis. General management will include an assessment for the risk of falls and their prevention (the nurse should consider suggesting hip protectors). Ensuring mobility and correction of nutritional deficiencies, particularly of calcium, vitamin D and protein, should be advised; calcium and vitamin D supplementation may be needed. The person's drug regimen should be reassessed and medications such as sedatives should be reconsidered.

The key pharmacological interventions are the bisphosphonates, denosumab, strontium ranelate, raloxifene and parathyroid hormone peptides. All these interventions have the ability to reduce the risk of vertebral fracture when given with calcium and vitamin D supplements. Some have demonstrated the ability to reduce the risk of non-vertebral fractures, in some cases particularly at the hip.

Generic bisphosphonates have a broad spectrum of anti-fracture efficacy and are the first-line treatment for most people.

For those who are unable to tolerate generic bisphosphonates or in whom they are contraindicated, other bisphosphonates, denosumab or raloxifene may provide treatment options. Strontium ranelate is restricted to people with severe osteoporosis for whom treatment with other approved drugs is not possible. Other approved pharmacological interventions for postmenopausal women include calcitriol, etidronate and hormone replacement therapy.

The relief of pain is a key nursing consideration and the nurse should administer and record the outcome of any prescribed pain relief. Working with the patient, the nurse can suggest that lying on the side or the back in bed for short periods may help to relieve pain; the trunk should be moved as a whole unit as opposed to twisting. Local heat and back rubs may also ease the pain.

Constipation is a problem related to immobility and some of the medications prescribed for osteoporosis may contribute to constipation. A high-fibre diet with increased fluids could help to avoid constipation. Prescribed stool softeners may help to prevent or minimise constipation.

A multidisciplinary approach to care, with the patient at the centre of all that is done, is advocated, working with physiotherapists, occupational therapists and dieticians.

33 Gout

Figure 33.1 Gout

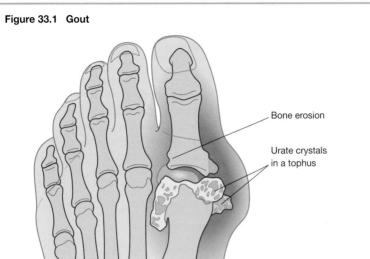

Bone erosion

Urate crystals in a tophus

Table 33.1 Risk factors for gout

- Gender (male)
- Meat eaters
- People who eat seafood
- Consumption of alcohol
- The use of diuretics
- Obesity
- Hypertension
- Coronary heart disease
- Diabetes mellitus
- Chronic renal failure
- High triglycerides

Figure 33.2 Risk foods and joints affected

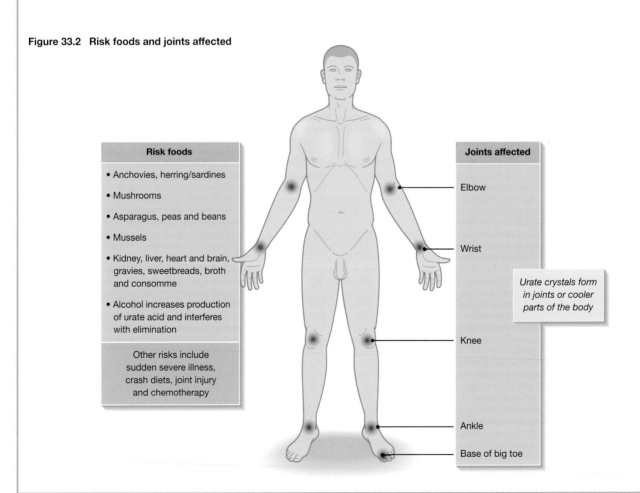

Risk foods

- Anchovies, herring/sardines
- Mushrooms
- Asparagus, peas and beans
- Mussels
- Kidney, liver, heart and brain, gravies, sweetbreads, broth and consomme
- Alcohol increases production of urate acid and interferes with elimination

Other risks include sudden severe illness, crash diets, joint injury and chemotherapy

Joints affected

Elbow

Wrist

Knee

Ankle

Base of big toe

Urate crystals form in joints or cooler parts of the body

Medical-Surgical Nursing at a Glance, First Edition. Ian Peate. © John Wiley & Sons, Ltd. Published 2016 by John Wiley & Sons, Ltd.
Companion website: www.ataglanceseries.com/nursing/medsurg

Gout (a type of arthritis) is an extremely painful condition; it is the most common form of inflammatory arthritis. It arises from inflammation caused by accumulation of serum uric acid (hyperuricaemia), which precipitates as sodium monourate crystals in the joints, resulting in an erosion of cartilage and bone (Figure 33.1). This is a metabolic disease as it results from the byproducts of metabolism of alcohol, in particular beer and foods that are rich in purine such as meat, full-fat dairy products and seafood. In response to high levels of metabolites from the digestion of red meats and alcohol, the liver produces uric acid and suppresses the production of insulin. The kidneys fail to excrete all the uric acid, and this causes higher levels of serum uric acid. Renal calculi may develop due to the high levels of sodium monourate crystals.

Classification and risk factors

Gout can be classed as primary or secondary depending on the cause of hyperuricaemia. Primary gout occurs mainly in men aged 30–60 years who present with acute attacks. Secondary gout is usually due to long-term diuretic therapy. It occurs in older people and is often related to osteoarthritis. The hallux valgus (big toe) is most often affected by the condition, but it can occur elsewhere (see figure 33.1). Gout affects the upper and lower limbs with acute attacks. It can present with painful, tophaceous deposits (there may be discharge) in Heberden's and Bouchard's nodes.

There are four types of gout:

- asymptomatic
- hyperuricaemic
- acute gout (sometimes called acute gouty arthritis)
- intercritical gout and chronic tophaceous gout.

Risk factors for gout can be seen in Table 33.1 and Figure 33.2.

Signs and symptoms

The development of acute pain in a joint which becomes swollen, tender and erythematous and which reaches its crescendo over a 6–12-hour period is highly suggestive of crystal arthropathy, but this may not necessarily be gout.

The first metatarsophalangeal joint is the joint most commonly affected; other sites include the knee, midtarsal joints, wrists, ankles, small joints in the hand, and elbows.

Within 24 hours the inflammation reaches its peak (crescendos), often accompanied by a pyrexia and malaise. There is a clear synovitis and swelling and severe tenderness with overlying erythema. The attack will resolve spontaneously over 5–15 days if untreated, often with itching and desquamation of overlying skin. Atypical attacks may occur with tenosynovitis, bursitis and cellulitis, accompanied by a mild discomfort without swelling, which lasts for 1–2 days.

In chronic tophaceous gout, there are large crystal deposits producing irregular firm nodules predominantly around extensor surfaces of the fingers, hands, forearms, elbows, Achilles tendons and ears. Characteristically, tophi are asymmetrical with a chalky appearance underneath the skin. Injury is usually located in the first metatarsophalangeal joints, midfoot, small finger joint and wrist; there is restricted movement, crepitus and deformity.

Investigations and diagnosis

A detailed history is undertaken and physical examination performed. Where there is typical presentation such as inflammation of the first metatarsophalangeal joint (the podagra) with hyperuricaemia, a clinical diagnosis can be made with a degree of accuracy but this is not definitive until the presence of uric acid crystals can be demonstrated by polarised light microscopy of the synovial fluid or the finding of tophi confirms the diagnosis of gout. Culture of synovial fluid should be arranged as gout and sepsis can co-exist.

A 24-hour urine specimen can determine renal uric acid secretion; this may be helpful in diagnosis. Radiographs may be useful in chronic gout, when punched-out lesions, areas of sclerosis and, in the later stages, tophi may be seen. Computed tomography (CT) scanning may be helpful in less accessible areas. In early attacks of gout or an acute attack, radiography may be less helpful.

Care and treatment

The aim of treatment is to decrease the amount of sodium urate in order to prevent deposits forming. In acute cases pain must be managed. Rest, elevation of an affected limb and the application of ice pack may provide some relief from the severe pain. Accidental trauma to the limb should be avoided. A bed cradle should be placed over the affected limb. reducing the pressure from bedlinen.

Colchicine (given orally or parenterally) is useful in suppressing inflammation; indomethacin (a non-steroidal anti-inflammatory) or a corticosteroid are also helpful in managing pain and inflammation. The choice of medication for a particular patient will depend on contraindications, the time lapse between onset of symptoms and the start of treatment and risks versus benefits.

Care and management are based on assessing and responding to individual needs. The patient should be advised to inform the nurse if they are experiencing any gastrointestinal symptoms (the person may complain of diarrhoea).

Uric acid-lowering medications are required after the acute phase has passed; allopurinol can significantly reduce the occurrence of gout flare-up.

Gout cannot be cured but the attacks can usually be controlled. Lifestyle changes should be discussed with the person covering issues such as:

- avoiding purine-rich foods (such as meat and fish)
- overweight or obese patients are encouraged to lose weight
- a high fluid intake (unless contraindicated) encourages the excretion of uric acid
- alcohol should be reduced or avoided altogether.

Prior to discharge, the nurse will need to explain to the person about long-term drug and diet therapy and the need to attend for follow-up and monitoring of the condition.

Provide information in a way that the person will understand; this may be supplemented by written instruction. The person should be given detailed information concerning the various medical regimens, such as the importance of increasing fluid intake in order to reduce the risk of renal calculi forming.

34 Rheumatoid Arthritis

Figure 34.1 Rheumatoid arthritis: joints affected

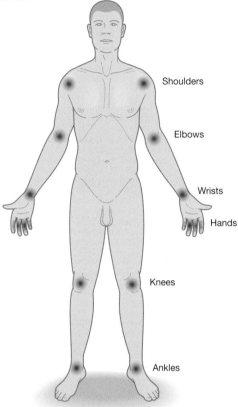

Shoulders

Elbows

Wrists

Hands

Knees

Ankles

Table 34.1 Some localised symptoms

- Joint pain (arthralgia)
- Swelling
- Warmth
- Erythema
- Limitations of mobility/stiffness
- On palpation tissue feels spongy
- There may be excessive collection of fluid in the joints

Table 34.2 Other features of the condition

- Anaemia
- Pyrexia
- Vasculitis
- Neuropathy
- Scleritis
- Pericarditis
- Splenomegaly
- Dry eyes and mucous membranes (Sjögen's syndrome)

Table 34.3 Some treatment options

- Disease-modifying anti-rheumatic drugs (DMARDs), prescribed soon after diagnosis to slow down the disease process
- Non-steroidal anti-inflammatory drugs (NSAIDs), may be given with DMARDs to reduce inflammation and pain
- Biologics, including anti-TNFs (tumour necrosis factors), these also reduce inflammation
- Steroids are used to reduce severe inflammation quickly
- Joint replacement surgery is only be considered if the joint is extremely painful or if there is a risk that loss of overall function will be lost

Medical-Surgical Nursing at a Glance, First Edition. Ian Peate. © John Wiley & Sons, Ltd. Published 2016 by John Wiley & Sons, Ltd.
Companion website: www.ataglanceseries.com/nursing/medsurg

Arthritis is a disorder of the musculoskeletal system and can impact on the person's ability to perform the activities of living independently. Most people with arthritic conditions are cared for in their own homes or in a community setting but some may require hospital admission and the nurse may be required to assist the patient to carry out some of the activities of living.

Arthritis is a general condition that is typified by inflammation and degeneration of the joint.

Rheumatoid arthritis

There are over 100 different types of recognised rheumatic disorders (inflammatory disorders). This condition is described as a chronic progressive inflammatory autoimmune disease of connective tissue and/or joints that is characterised by chronicity, remissions and exacerbations. It is also classified as an immune disorder of unknown origin.

Rheumatoid arthritis (RA) can affect anyone irrespective of where they live and what climate they live in; however, it is less widespread in Asian communities and in certain parts of Africa it is unheard of. It is considered a systemic disease as it affects the whole body, producing flu-like symptoms, anaemia and general malaise. In contrast to osteoarthritis where only one joint may be affected, rheumatoid arthritis is a symmetrical disease, occurring on both sides of the body, affecting the synovial membranes covering the joints in the hands, wrists, feet, ankles, knees and shoulders (Figure 34.1).

Signs and symptoms

For many people the onset of symptoms is acute. Localised symptoms are highlighted in Table 34.1.

As the condition progresses and over several weeks, more joints will become involved, the swelling and pain may come and go, the person may be anorexic, easily fatigued, and experience weight loss. Other features of this condition can be seen in Table 34.2.

Investigations and diagnosis

A detailed health history and physical examination are often all that are needed to make a diagnosis (this is a clinical diagnosis). However, in order to make a definitive diagnosis and exclude other potential diagnoses, undertaking a range of investigations can help. The nurse may be required to assist with the investigations. Pain, stiffness and deformity all severely restrict use of the affected joint, along with muscle wasting. The patient may need assistance prior to the investigations, during the investigations and after they have been performed. The nurse should bear in mind that the person may have restricted mobility and that mobilisation and manipulation of position for some investigations such as X-rays may cause pain and discomfort.

There are national guidelines available to guide the most appropriate investigations. Specifically, blood is taken to determine the presence of rheumatoid factor; if rheumatoid factor is negative then anticyclic citrullinated peptide antibodies are assessed. With regard to imaging, radiography is first choice, with X-ray of the hands and feet. Non-specific investigations include a full blood count, C-reactive protein and plasma viscosity, liver function tests and uric acid/synovial fluid analysis.

Care and treatment

The nurse must work with the patient in providing patient-centred care.

Drug management intends to relieve symptoms, as pain relief is the priority for people with RA as well as modifying the progression of the disease. Disease modification slows or stops radiological progression. Where there is radiological progression, this is linked to a reduction in mobility. There are a variety of medications available for RA. Some are used for pain relief and some reduce inflammation whilst others attempt to try and slow the course of the disease. Treatment options are highlighted in Table 34.3.

People with rheumatoid arthritis should have access to a named member of the multidisciplinary team, often a specialist nurse. The nurse should ensure that patients have the opportunity to make informed decisions concerning their care and treatment, in partnership with healthcare professionals.

Nursing priorities will include pain relief, increase and continuation of mobility, promotion of positive self-concept, encouraging and supporting independence and providing information concerning the condition, how it progresses, prognosis and treatment needs. Regular review of the patient's condition is needed; other specialists will include podiatrists, orthotists, dieticians, pharmacists and neurologists.

Referral to a pain clinic or pain specialists can help with non-drug management options, such as transcutaneous electrical nerve stimulation and behavioural approaches. Issues that are non-clinical in nature may need the assistance of social workers, voluntary organisations and wheelchair services.

Analgesics (paracetamol, codeine) should be offered, to potentially reduce the person's need for long-term treatment with NSAIDs or cyclo-oxygenase-2 (COX-2) inhibitors. NSAIDs (ibuprofen, diclofenac, naproxen) should be prescribed with a suitable proton pump inhibitor (PPI). NSAIDs are highly effective but they do not slow progression or prevent long-term disability. They have a rapid onset of action, but beneficial effects are offset by toxicity. The nurse needs to note that NSAIDs can interact with diuretics, warfarin, lithium and methotrexate.

COX-2 drugs (such as celecoxib, etoricoxib) should also be prescribed with a suitable PPI. These drugs have a very similar effect to the standard NSAIDs. COX-2s should not be used for patients with established ischaemic heart disease, heart failure or cerebrovascular disease. Care should be taken with those patients with any cardiovascular disease risk factors; the drugs should be used at the lowest effective dose for the shortest period possible.

Oral corticosteroids in low dose can be used in combination with DMARDs (for example, azathioprine, ciclosporin, methotrexate, sulfasalazine) for short-term relief of signs and symptoms and in the medium to long term to minimise radiological damage. Intra-articular corticosteroid injections can provide symptomatic relief and alleviate symptoms in particularly troublesome joints.

Biological therapies (cytokine modulators) have been shown to be effective in the treatment of RA, including those resistant to methotrexate. These include adalimumab, rituximab and infliximab.

35 Diabetes Mellitus

Table 35.1 Some of the types of diabetes mellitus

- **Type 1 diabetes mellitus:** the body's failure to produce sufficient insulin

- **Type 2 diabetes mellitus:** results from resistance to the insulin, often initially with normal or increased levels of circulating insulin

- **Gestational diabetes** – pregnant women who have never had diabetes before but who have high blood glucose levels during pregnancy have gestational diabetes

- **Maturity-onset diabetes of the young**

- **Secondary diabetes**. Causes include, pancreatic disease, endocrine disorders (e.g. Cushing's syndrome), genetic

- **Drug-induced diabetes**

Table 35.2 Risk factors for diabetes

- Obesity

- Lack of physical activity

- Ethnicity

- History of gestational diabetes

- Impaired glucose tolerance

- Impaired fasting glucose

- Some forms of drug therapy

- Low-fibre, high-glycaemic index diet

- Metabolic syndrome

- Polycystic ovarian syndrome

- Family history

- Those born with low birth weight for gestational age

Table 35.3. Components of a plan of care

- A structured approach concerning diabetes education should be provided at diagnosis, reviewed regularly and reinforced with the aim of encouraging self-management and to promote awareness

- If the person is overweight, diet and lifestyle will need to be addressed; this includes smoking cessation, regular physical exercise, healthy diet and weight loss

- Maximise glucose control whilst at the same time reducing adverse effects of treatment, for example, hypoglycaemia

- Reduction of risk factors for complications of diabetes, for example, early detection and management of hypertension, drug treatment to modify lipid levels and consideration of aspirin as antiplatelet therapy

- Monitoring and early intervention for complications, this includes cardiovascular disease, problems with the feet, ophthalmic problems, renal problems and neuropathy

Medical-Surgical Nursing at a Glance, First Edition. Ian Peate. © John Wiley & Sons, Ltd. Published 2016 by John Wiley & Sons, Ltd.
Companion website: www.ataglanceseries.com/nursing/medsurg

Diabetes mellitus is a disease caused by deficiency or diminished effectiveness of endogenous insulin and is characterised by hyperglycaemia, disturbed metabolism and sequelae that mainly affect the vasculature. Some of the types of diabetes mellitus are shown in Table 35.1.

Type 1 diabetes mellitus

Type 1 diabetes mellitus is based on a combination of genetic predisposition with an autoimmune process, resulting in gradual destruction of the pancreatic beta cells, causing an absolute deficiency of insulin. Likely triggers for the process include viruses, dietary factors, environmental toxins and emotional or physical stress. The most at-risk population is Caucasian of northern European ancestry. Highest incidence is in Scandinavian people.

Type 2 diabetes mellitus

The majority of people with diabetes are usually older at presentation (over 30 years of age) but increasingly it is diagnosed in children and adolescents. This type of diabetes is associated with excess body weight and inactivity. There is increased prevalence in people of South Asian, African, African-Caribbean, Polynesian, Middle Eastern and American-Indian ancestry but all racial groups are affected. Impaired insulin secretion and insulin resistance with a gradual onset cause the condition. Eventually those with type 2 diabetes may need insulin treatment.

Risk factors for diabetes can be found in Table 35.2.

Signs and symptoms

In all types of diabetes mellitus, patients can experience polyuria, polydipsia, lethargy, boils, pruritus vulvae or frequent, recurrent or prolonged infections. In type 1 diabetes there may also be weight loss, dehydration, ketonuria and hyperventilation. Presentation of type 1 diabetes is often acute with a short duration of symptoms whereas with type 2 diabetes symptoms are usually subacute and are of longer duration. There may be acute or chronic complications associated with diabetes such as diabetic ketoacidosis and hyperosmolar hyperglycaemic state, cardiovascular disease, diabetic neuropathy. diabetic retinopathy, diabetic foot and diabetic leg ulcers. Repeated, recurrent and persistent infections can also occur.

Investigations and diagnosis

Making an early diagnosis is beneficial as treatment can then commence with the aim of reducing any complications. Diabetes is a serious condition that can lead to heart disease, stroke, blindness and renal failure if left untreated.

A diagnosis of diabetes is based on a urine specimen (a dipstick test) for the presence of glucose (urine does not usually contain glucose). A definitive diagnosis is based on a blood test that reveals an abnormal plasma glucose (random greater than 11.1 mmol/L or fasting greater than 7 mmol/L) in the presence of a range of diabetic symptoms, for example, thirst, polyuria, recurrent infections, weight loss, drowsiness and coma.

The fasting blood glucose test is the preferred test for diagnosing diabetes. It is more reliable when done in the morning.

In those who are asymptomatic with an abnormal random plasma glucose, two fasting venous plasma glucose samples in the abnormal range (greater than 7 mmol/L) are recommended for diagnosis. Venous plasma glucose concentration greater than 11.1 mmol/L 2 hours after 75 g anhydrous glucose is an oral glucose tolerance test.

Glycated haemoglobin (HbA1c) can be used as a diagnostic test for diabetes. An HbA1c of 48 mmol/mol (6.5%) is recommended as the cut-off point for diagnosing diabetes; less than 48 mmol/mol does not exclude diabetes diagnosed using glucose tests. HbA1c indicates the average blood sugar level for the past 2–3 months.

Treatment and care

The care and treatment of the person with diabetes demand a tailored approach that will meet their individual physical and psychological needs. Table 35.3 provides an overview of the components of a care plan for a person with diabetes.

Treatment for type 1 diabetes requires the injection of insulin (or the use of an insulin pump), frequent checking of blood sugar levels and carbohydrate counting. Type 2 diabetes is predominantly managed by monitoring blood sugar, along with diabetes medications, insulin or both.

Depending on the person's plan of care, blood sugar may be checked and recorded several times a week or up to three or more times daily.

Careful monitoring is the only way to ensure that blood sugar levels remain within the target range; to do this, the person should aim for preprandial blood glucose 4.0–7.0 mmol/L, postprandial less than 9.00 mmol/L. Those receiving insulin therapy may choose to monitor blood sugar with a continuous glucose monitor but more generally the glucose meter is used, providing information about trends in blood sugar levels.

The amount of sugar in the blood can change unpredictably even when the person is on a controlled diet. Blood sugar levels change in response to food, physical activity, medications, illness, alcohol, stress and variations in hormone levels.

As well as daily blood glucose assessments, regular HbA1c testing may also be needed as this better indicates how well the diabetes treatment plan is working overall. An elevated HbA1c may signal the need for a change in the person's insulin regimen or meal plan. Target HbA1c can vary depending on age and other factors.

Most people with type 1 diabetes need insulin therapy although some with type 2 diabetes can also require insulin therapy. Insulin is injected using a fine needle and syringe or an insulin pen; insulin pumps may be an option. Insulin is available in many types, including rapid-acting, long-acting and intermediate options. The type of insulin prescribed depends on individual needs; a mixture of insulin types can be used throughout the day and night.

Oral or injected medications are also prescribed. Some diabetes medications stimulate the pancreas to produce and release more insulin, whilst others inhibit the production and release of glucose from the liver. Some medications block the action of stomach or intestinal enzymes that break down carbohydrates or make tissues more sensitive to insulin.

A pancreas transplant may be an option. With a successful pancreas transplant, insulin therapy will no longer be needed. Transplantation is usually reserved for those whose diabetes cannot be controlled or for those who have serious complications.

36 Thyrotoxicosis

Figure 36.1 Signs and symptoms of thyrotoxicosis

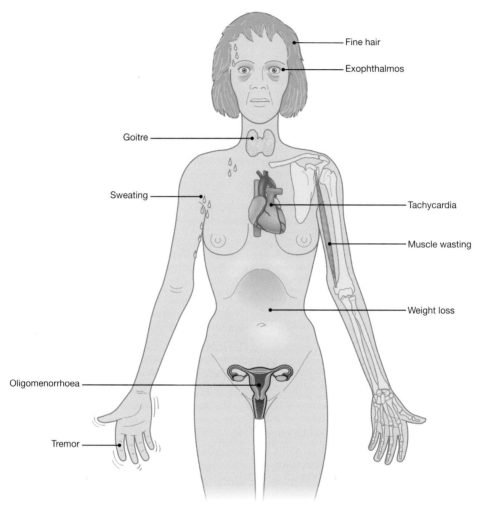

- Fine hair
- Exophthalmos
- Goitre
- Sweating
- Tachycardia
- Muscle wasting
- Weight loss
- Oligomenorrhoea
- Tremor

Table 36.1 Classic signs and symptoms of thyrotoxicosis

- Excessive sweating
- Heat intolerance
- Increased bowel movements
- Tremor (usually fine shaking)
- Nervousness; agitation
- Tachycardia
- Tachypnoea
- Weight loss
- Fatigue
- Decreased ability to concentrate
- Irregular and scant menstrual flow

Thyrotoxicosis is also called hyperthyroidism or an overactive thyroid. The condition is more common in women than men. Thyrotoxicosis can be the result of Graves' disease or toxic nodular goitre and most commonly develops between 20 and 40 years. Toxic nodular goitre increases with age.

Hyperthyroidism refers to overactivity of the thyroid gland; this results in a number of signs and symptoms. The condition can significantly accelerate the body's metabolism.

Thyroid gland

The thyroid gland produces two chief hormones, thyroxine (T_4) and tri-iodothyronine (T_3). These hormones influence every cell in the body, maintaining the rate at which the body metabolises fats and carbohydrates, helping to control body temperature, influencing heart rate and helping regulate the production of protein. The thyroid also produces the hormone calcitonin, which assists with the amount of calcium in the blood.

Risk factors

These include family history, high iodine intake, smoking (particularly for thyroid-associated ophthalmopathy), trauma to the thyroid gland (including surgery), toxic multinodular goitre, childbirth and the use of highly active antiretroviral therapy (HAART). There is a genetic susceptibility associated with Graves' disease. Other potential triggers include smoking, stress, pollutants, allergy, iatrogenic causes and selenium intake.

Signs and symptoms

Several signs and symptoms suggest hyperthyroidism (Figure 36.1); however, those people with mild disease will usually experience no symptoms. In patients older than 70 years, the typical signs and symptoms can also be absent. Usually the symptoms become more obvious as the degree of hyperthyroidism increases. The symptoms are often related to an increase in the body's metabolic rate. Common symptoms are identified in Table 36.1.

In older patients, dysrhythmia and heart failure can occur. In the most severe form, if left untreated hyperthyroidism can result in thyroid storm, a condition involving pyrexia and heart failure. Changes to cognition such as confusion and delirium may also occur.

Investigations and diagnosis

A medical history is taken and a physical examination performed. During the examination a tremor may be detected as the fingers are extended; overactive reflexes, eye changes and warm, moist skin can indicate thyroid disease. The thyroid gland is palpated as the person swallows.

A range of blood tests will be taken. A diagnosis can be confirmed with blood tests measuring the levels of thyroxine and thyroid-stimulating hormone (TSH) in the blood. High levels of thyroxine and low or even non-existent amounts of TSH signify an overactive thyroid. These tests are particularly important for the older adult, who may not have the classic symptoms of hyperthyroidism. If blood tests demonstrate hyperthyroidism, other tests are required to help determine why the thyroid gland is overactive.

The radioactive iodine uptake test requires the person to take a small, oral dose of radioactive iodine (radioiodine), which accumulates in the thyroid gland. Assessment is made after 2,

6 or 24 hours, and in some cases after all three time periods, to determine how much iodine has been absorbed by the thyroid gland. A high uptake of radioiodine indicates that the thyroid gland is producing too much thyroxine. The most likely cause is either Graves' disease or hyperfunctioning nodules. If there is hyperthyroidism and the radioiodine uptake is low, this may indicate thyroiditis.

A thyroid scan requires the injection of a radioactive isotope; images of the thyroid gland are produced on a computer screen.

Care and treatment

There are a number of options for treating hyperthyroidism: treating the symptoms, administration of antithyroid drugs, provision of radioactive iodine or surgery that treats symptoms.

Medications

Medications used to treat the symptoms caused by excessive thyroid hormones, for example tachycardia, are from the beta-blocker class of drugs and they include propranolol, atenolol and metoprolol; they are used for rapid symptom control whilst waiting for thyroid function to normalise. These medicines counteract the effect of thyroid hormone in increasing metabolism but they do not alter the levels of thyroid hormones in the blood.

Methimazole (carbimazole) and propylthiouracil are two types of antithyroid drugs. They act quickly and accumulate in the thyroid tissue, blocking the production of thyroid hormones; it may take 2–3 weeks for the full benefit to become apparent. Caution must be exercised to prevent drug-induced hypothyroidism from occurring.

The major risk of these medications is the potential suppression of production of white blood cells by the bone marrow, resulting in agranulocytosis. The nurse needs to inform the patient that if they develop a fever, a sore throat or any signs of infection, they should see a doctor immediately. The patient usually commences with methimazole which is adjusted depending on response and the outcome of thyroid function tests. The dose is adjusted (titrated) to maintain the patient in as close to a normal thyroid state as possible (euthyroid). Once stable, the patient takes the lowest amount. If a patient's condition relapses, antithyroid drug therapy can be restarted, or radioactive iodine or surgery may be considered.

Radioactive iodine

Radioactive iodine is given orally on a one-time basis to ablate (destroy) a hyperactive gland. It can take 3–4 months to take effect (some people may need a second treatment). Radioactive iodine is cleared via the urine and can be passed on so patients are advised to avoid close contact with children and pregnant women; patients should also sleep alone for a week. This form of therapy is the treatment of choice for recurring Graves' disease, those with severe cardiac involvement, multinodular goitre or toxic adenomas and people who cannot tolerate antithyroid drugs.

Surgery

Surgery partially removes the thyroid gland. The aim is to remove the thyroid tissue that was producing the excessive thyroid hormone. With the introduction of radioactive iodine therapy and antithyroid drugs, surgery for hyperthyroidism is not as common as it used to be.

37 Erectile Dysfunction

Table 37.1 Some causes of ED

Organic	• Cardiovascular diseases • Atherosclerosis • Hypertension • Diabetes mellitus • Hyperlipidaemia • Smoking • Pelvic surgery or radiotherapy to the pelvis/retroperineum • Trauma
Neurological	• Parkinson's disease • Cerebrovascular accident • Multiple sclerosis • Tumour • Traumatic brain injury • Intervertebral disc disease • Spinal cord disease or injury • Polyneuropathy • Peripheral neuropathy • Alcoholism • Uraemia
Hormonal	• Hypogonadism • Hyperprolactinaemia • Thyroid disesae • Cushing's disease
Anatomical	• Peyronies's disease • Micro penis and other penile anomalies
Drug related	• Anti hypertensives • Beta blockers • Diuretics • Anti depressants • Antipsychotics • Hormonal agents • Anticonvulsants • Antihistamines • Recreational drugs • H_2 antagonists
Psychogenic/ other	• Disorders of sexual intimacy • Lack of arousability • Partner, performance or stress (situational) • Generalised anxiety • Depression • Psychosis

Table 37.2 Investigations for ED

• Testosterone
• Prolactin
• Glucose
• LH/FSH
• T_4
• TSH
• Liver and renal function
• Neurological tests
• Vascular imaging

Table 37.3 Psychogenic and organic causes of ED

Psychogenic causes	Organic causes
• Sudden onset	• Gradual onset
• Early collapse of erection	• Normal ejaculation
• Self-stimulated or waking erections	• Normal libido (except hypogonadal men)
• Premature ejaculation or inability to ejaculate	• Risk factor in medical history (cardiovascular, endocrine or neurological)
• Problems or changes in relationship	• Operations, radiotherapy, or trauma to pelvis or scrotum
• Major life events	• Current drug recognised as associated with erectile dysfunction
• Psychological problems	• Smoking, high alcohol consumption, use of recreational or body-building drugs

Figure 37.1 Model of vascular events controlling erection

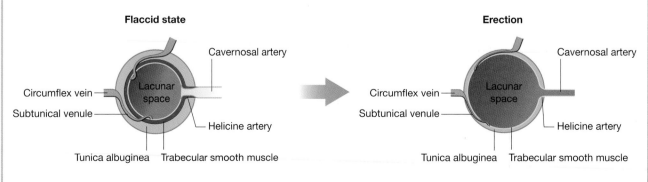

Medical-Surgical Nursing at a Glance, First Edition. Ian Peate. © John Wiley & Sons, Ltd. Published 2016 by John Wiley & Sons, Ltd.
Companion website: www.ataglanceseries.com/nursing/medsurg

Erectile dysfunction (ED), previously known as impotence, concerns the inability to achieve and maintain an erection that is sufficient for satisfactory sexual intercourse. ED can affect men at any age. It is a psychophysiological condition impacting on sexual arousal. ED is strongly associated with cardiovascular disease, and any newly presenting patient should be thoroughly evaluated for cardiovascular and also endocrine risk factors.

Erectile dysfunction

Erectile dysfunction is one of a number of male sexual dysfunctions. It is no longer discussed in a hushed voice behind closed doors, and the taboo that was associated with it has almost disappeared. Treatments have become easier to obtain and are provided in a more patient-acceptable way. However, the condition is still disturbing for men and their partners who suffer as a result of the problem despite the understanding. It is important that patients are appropriately assessed and investigated prior to commencing treatment.

Erection

The penis contains two cylindrical, sponge-like structures called the corpus cavernosa. When the man becomes sexually aroused, nerve impulses increase blood flow to both corpus cavernosa. The penis becomes erect due to the dilation of blood vessels entering the corpora cavernosa and corpus spongiosum. The increased flow of blood into the cavernous spaces increases tissue pressure, restricting venous drainage and resulting in a further build-up of pressure. making the penis fully erect. The parasympathetic nerves cause vasodilation releasing acetylcholine, vasoactive intestinal peptide and, primarily, nitric oxide (NO). NO increases the production of cyclic guanosine monophosphate (cGMP) in blood vessel smooth muscle cells to cause them to relax. Figure 37.1 depicts the vascular events controlling erection.

Risk factors and causes of erectile dysfunction

Erectile dysfunction is often multifactorial; the causes may be organic and/or inorganic disorders (a combination of both factors). Organic causes are related to physiological disorders; inorganic causes are psychological in nature and may be more common in the younger person. See Table 37.1 for some of the causes of ED. Psychogenic factors are involved in the majority of cases, in spite of the fact that in the majority of men with ED, the dominant pathophysiology is organic. Risk factors also associated with cardiovascular disease are shared with ED:

- inactivity
- obesity
- smoking
- hypercholesterolaemia
- hypertension
- metabolic syndrome
- diabetes mellitus.

Vasculopathy has come to be recognised as the most common cause of ED; this means that ED is a sentinel marker for cardiovascular disease. Identification of cardiovascular risk factors should be a routine part of the evaluation for ED.

Signs and symptoms

The predominant symptom is the man's inability to achieve and maintain an erection for satisfactory intercourse; this can be extended to other aspects of sexual activity, for example, the inability to maintain an erection for fellatio and masturbation. There are instances when ED only occurs in specific situations; for example, the man may be able to get an erection when he masturbates, or he may sometimes experience nocturnal erections but he is unable to get an erection with his sexual partner.

Erectile dysfunction should not be confused with other ejaculatory problems such as premature ejaculation; in these situations the underlying cause of ED is likely to be primarily psychological. If, however, the man cannot achieve erection under any circumstances, then the underlying cause is usually physical.

Investigations and diagnosis

History taking, physical examination and clinical investigations help to make a diagnosis. Investigations differ, depending on the findings from the history and physical examination. Clinical investigations can be divided into three: essential, possible and specialised. Table 37.2 outlines the investigations for ED. Other investigations can include nocturnal penile tumescence and rigidity (NPTR) monitoring. This can differentiate between psychogenic and organic causes and the number and quality of erections occurring during REM sleep can be assessed. Cavernosometry and cavernosography measure pressure and outline radiographically if there are any difficulties within the penile chambers; the aim is to assess arterial inflow and venous outflow of penile blood.

A diagnosis will need to be made prior to offering treatment and providing the man with a choice of treatment options.

Care and treatment

Treatment options are based upon the underlying cause. Table 37.3 outlines psychogenic and organic origins of ED. Treatments are provided after individual assessment and can include the increasingly popular oral pharmacological therapies. Other treatments are also available:

- hormonal treatment
- mechanical/physical devices, e.g. vacuum devices
- surgical treatment
- natural/homeopathic remedies.

The use of intercavernosal and transurethral medications, vacuum and ring devices have the potential to cause harm and discomfort and may be seen as unpleasant by some men and their partners. The surgical insertion of penile implants can also lead to complications such as infection.

Some men with ED may not be aware of the cause; not knowing the cause can increase anxiety. The man may believe himself to be less than a man and the cause may be blamed on unrelated factors, such as age, medications, illness or sexual partner. The nurse must adopt a non-judgemental approach.

Panbiological approaches (including gene therapies) may fail to include the humanistic aspects of sexuality. Other therapeutic interventions such as psychological and behavioural interventions should be considered.

38 Chlamydia

Figure 38.1 The impact of chlamydia on the female reproductive system

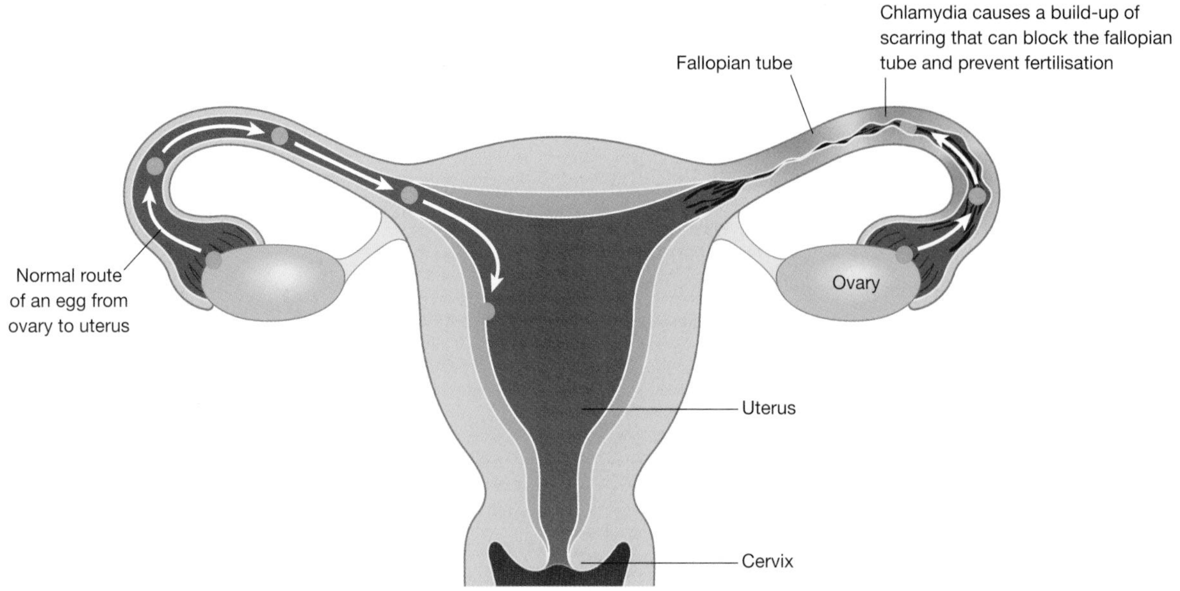

Fallopian tube

Chlamydia causes a build-up of scarring that can block the fallopian tube and prevent fertilisation

Normal route of an egg from ovary to uterus

Ovary

Uterus

Cervix

Table 38.1 Female and male symptoms

Female symptoms	Male symptoms
• Vaginal discharge	• Dysuria
• Dysuria	• Urethral discharge
• Lower abdominal pain	• Epididymo-orchitis (presents as testicular pain and/or swelling)
• Pyrexia	• Pyrexia
• Inter menstrual bleeding (this is vaginal bleeding at any time during the menstrual cycle other than during normal menstruation)	
• Bleeding after sex (postcoital)	
• Dyspareunia (pain during sexual intercourse)	

Table 38.2 Other symptoms that may be suggestive of chlamyidal infection in both sexes

• Reactive arthritis also called Reiter's syndrome especially in younger people (this is a triad of urethritis, arthritis and conjunctivitis)
• Upper abdominal pain as a result of perihepatitis (also known Fitz-Hugh-Curtis syndrome)
• Proctitis (inflammation of the rectum) with mucopurulent discharge this can be due to rectal chlamydia following anal intercourse
• Throat infection

Table 38.3 Female and male signs

Signs in the female may include:	Signs in men may include:
• A friable (the cervix easily prone to bleeding), inflamed cervix	• Epididymal tenderness
• Mucopurulent endocervical discharge	• Mucoid or mucopurulent discharge
• Abdominal tenderness	
• Pelvic adnexal tenderness on bimanual palpation	
• Cervical excitation (a tender and painful cervix on examination)	

Medical-Surgical Nursing at a Glance, First Edition. Ian Peate. © John Wiley & Sons, Ltd. Published 2016 by John Wiley & Sons, Ltd.
Companion website: www.ataglanceseries.com/nursing/medsurg

The most commonly diagnosed sexually transmitted infection (STI) in the western world is chlamydia. Chlamydia diagnosis rates are higher in females than males. It is the most common preventable cause of infertility globally. In approximately 50% of men and 80% of women, it is asymptomatic but sequelae can include pelvic inflammatory disease, ectopic pregnancy, tubal infertility in women (Figure 38.1) and epididymitis and epididymo-orchitis in men. Raising awareness of chlamydia is key to preventing the disease. People requiring care come from all walks of life. This infection is highest in sexually active people under the age of 25.

Untreated or repeated chlamydial infection can result in serious complications for a person's health and well-being and has a specific impact on the reproductive system.

Chlamydia

The bacterium *Chlamydia trachomatis* is an intracellular pathogen; this pathogen cannot reproduce outside its host cell, its reproduction is entirely dependent on resources within the cell. Chlamydia was originally thought to be a virus because of the way it was able to develop. The ways in which chlamydia develops (the pathogenesis) are not fully understood. This bacterium is found in the semen and vaginal fluid of those who have the infection; it infects human columnar and transitional epithelium tissues that line parts of the urinary and reproductive tracts.

Risk factors

There are a number of risk factors associated with chlamydia. The most consistent risk factor is younger age; in women the highest prevalence occurs between 16 and 19 years and in men between 20 and 24 years. Other factors include:

- two or more sexual partners in the preceding year
- a recent change in sexual partner
- non-barrier contraception
- co-infection with another STI
- poor socioeconomic status
- genetic predisposition.

Signs and symptoms

In most cases this infection is asymptomatic (it causes no symptoms) and is usually only detected through screening or during investigations for other genitourinary conditions. Approximately 50% of men and 80% of women are asymptomatic. Female and male symptoms are outlined in Table 38.1.

There are other symptoms, in both sexes, that may be suggestive of chlamydial infection (Table 38.2). Table 38.3 outlines male and female signs.

Investigations and diagnosis

There are a number of new tests being developed for detecting chlamydia. It is important, however, to always obtain a sexual health history, either at the time of testing or when managing a positive chlamydia test result. Gaining a sexual health history means that time must be set aside for this important activity and the person must be put at ease; a non-judgemental approach is

essential. Many of the skills required to undertake a sexual health history are already used by nurses when making an assessment of a person's general health, such as asking open-ended questions and refraining from making any assumptions.

As well as the sexual history, a number of laboratory tests are needed in order to make a definitive diagnosis. The nurse may be required to assist in obtaining a sample of fluid from the cervix or vagina using a speculum or occasionally, in the case of a vaginal swab, by inserting a swab into the vagina. The patient may also perform the vulvo-vaginal swab herself. Specimens taken from the cervix and the vagina can have similar reliability. A swab may be taken from the penis, although a urine test for chlamydia is just as reliable and more acceptable to patients.

Self-taken vulvo-vaginal swabs need to be performed using the swabs and transport medium specifically required by the laboratory. The nurse should be familiar with local arrangements. A specific technique is required, and this must be fully discussed with the patient. It is good practice to check their understanding of what is being asked of them prior to them taking the swab themselves. These specimens are sent for analysis in the laboratory, looking for the causative organism (the bacteria causing chlamydia). Rectal, pharyngeal or conjunctival tests may be required; if this is the case, local policy and procedure must be followed.

Another test used is one that looks for the *Chlamydia* bacterium in a urine sample. This does not require a pelvic examination or swabbing of the penis. Results are available quickly (within 24 hours) and often the person can do this themselves but the nurse must carefully explain the correct technique. This test is less reliable for women than those tests discussed above. The person should not have passed urine for at least 2 hours before the sample being collected; a first-catch specimen (between 10 and 30 mL) is passed into a sterile container.

Testing kits are available at some pharmacies, GP practices and genitourinary medicine clinics and are also available by post where the envelope is delivered unmarked, containing full instructions for use.

Care and treatment

Treatment should be provided in such a way that it is effective, easy to take, has limited side effects and has the least impact on a person's lifestyle. Advice should be offered about the impact chlamydia can have on the person's health and well-being, the implications for their partner(s) and the long-term complications.

Those people with suspected or confirmed diagnosis of chlamydia should be offered screening for other STIs and an HIV test. Hepatitis screening and, if appropriate, vaccination should be provided. National advice is available regarding treatment regimens. Treatment should be commenced prior to outcome of test results in those with signs or symptoms that would strongly suggest they have chlamydia.

In order to ensure that the person receiving the treatment has the best chance of treating the infection effectively, the nurse should reinforce safer sex practices as chlamydia is an STI; for example, correct and consistent use of condoms. Provide clear written advice and instructions for taking the prescribed medications. Reinforce the fact that it is important that sexual partner(s) are also tested. The person should abstain from sexual intercourse (including oral, anal and vaginal sex and mutual masturbation) even with a condom, until they and their partner(s) have completed their therapy.

39 Dysmenorrhoea

Figure 39.1 Typical sites of pain associated with dysmenorrhoea

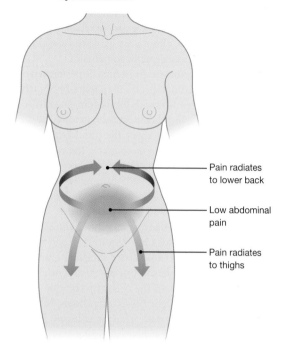

Pain radiates to lower back

Low abdominal pain

Pain radiates to thighs

Table 39.1 Some menstrual terms and conditions

Term	Explanation
Amenorrhoea	Absence of menses (typically 6 months or more)
Dysmenorrhoea	Painful menstrual bleeding prior to or during the period
Hypermenorrhoea (or flooding)	Episodes of heavy menstrual bleeding
Menarche	Age when periods commenced
Menorrhagia	Heavy menstrual bleeding at regular intervals
Metrorrhagia	Irregularly timed menstrual bleeding
Oligomenorrhoea	Periods occurring at intervals longer than 35 days and/or being particularly light
Perimenopause	Period around menopause when periods become unpredictable with menopausal symptoms
Postmenopausal bleeding	Spontaneous vaginal bleeding occurring more than one year after last menstrual period

Table 39.2 Medical conditions associated with increased risk

- Early age of menarche
- Nulliparous
- Obesity
- Smoking
- Alcohol consumption
- Family history of dysmenorrhoea
- Pelvic infection (i.e. pelvic inflammatory disease)
- History of (or current) sexually transmitted infection
- Endometriosis
- Leiomyomas
- Use of an intrauterine device

Table 39.3 Details of comprehensive history

- Age at menarche
- Length of menstrual cycle
- If the cycle is regular
- Extent of bleeding
- Timing of pain in relation to period
- History of smoking
- If the woman is sexually active
- Obstetric history
- History of contraceptive use

Medical-Surgical Nursing at a Glance, First Edition. Ian Peate. © John Wiley & Sons, Ltd. Published 2016 by John Wiley & Sons, Ltd.
Companion website: www.ataglanceseries.com/nursing/medsurg

ysmenorrhoea is a term used to describe low anterior pelvic pain that occurs in association with periods.

Dysmenorrhoea

Dysmenorrhoea is very common but the exact incidence is not known, as often it goes unreported by women. The most commonly given reason for absence from school amongst adolescent girls is primary dysmenorrhoea.

Classification

This condition can be thought of as either primary or secondary.

Primary dysmenorrhoea

Primary dysmenorrhoea usually occurs in young women who do not have a pelvic pathology. Often it begins with the onset of ovulatory cycles 6 months to 1 year after the menarche. The pain commences with the onset of the period and can last for 24–72 hours.

Secondary dysmenorrhoea

Secondary dysmenorrhoea occurs alongside some form of pelvic abnormality (pathology). The pain typically comes before the start of the period by several days and can last the duration of the period. There may be associated dyspareunia (painful sexual intercourse). Secondary dysmenorrhoea may occur as a result of a number of conditions including fibroids, endometriosis and pelvic inflammatory disease.

Some menstrual terms and conditions can be found in Table 39.1.

Risk factors

There is increased risk in those in the younger age group and if they have any of the medical conditions listed in Table 39.2.

Signs and symptoms

Dysmenorrhoea is thought to be due to a release of prostaglandins and leukotrienes (inflammatory mediators) in the menstrual fluid; this then produces vasoconstriction in the uterine vessels, causing the uterine contractions that cause the pain. The prostaglandin release may also be responsible for gastrointestinal disturbance that can also occur in association with dysmenorrhoea. The reason why some women produce excessive prostaglandin is unknown.

Symptoms of dysmenorrhoea can include throbbing or cramping pain in the lower abdomen that can be intense (Figure 39.1). The pain may be described as a dull, constant ache that radiates to the lower back and thighs. Some women can also experience nausea, loose stools, headache and dizziness.

Investigations and diagnosis

In order to make the diagnosis, a comprehensive history is taken from the woman (Table 39.3). The nurse should pay particular attention to the type of pain that the woman is describing, the duration and what (if any) remedies she is using in order to alleviate the pain.

A detailed physical examination should be undertaken. A pelvic examination is essential for eliminating uterine irregularities and includes inspection of the external genitalia, the vaginal vault and the cervix, and bimanual examination.

There are no tests specific to the diagnosis of primary dysmenorrhoea. Laboratory studies may be undertaken to identify or exclude organic causes of secondary dysmenorrhoea. Diagnosis may be confirmed by ultrasound, hysterosalpingogram, laparoscopy, laparotomy, and dilation and curettage.

Care and treatment

Many women never seek medical help for dysmenorrhoea. Women often self-medicate using analgesics and non-steroidal anti-inflammatory drugs (NSAIDs) as well as applying direct heat (hot water bottle).

The treatment of dysmenorrhoea is aimed at providing symptomatic relief as well as addressing the underlying processes that cause symptoms. Controlling the pain associated with dysmenorrhoea is a primary nursing intervention. Medications used may include NSAIDs such as ibuprofen, and mefenamic acid and naproxen are very effective in the treatment of pain associated with dysmenorrhoea. In addition to pain relief, mainstays of treatment include the provision of physical and psychological support along with education.

Non-steroidal anti-inflammatory drugs are able to inhibit the synthesis of prostaglandin. The nurse must be aware that some patients are unable to take NSAIDs as they can cause gastrointestinal bleeding, nephrotoxicity, nausea, vomiting, dyspepsia and headache. NSAIDs are contraindicated in those with aspirin-induced asthma, peptic ulcer, renal disease and clotting disorders.

It should be suggested to the woman that she takes the NSAID as soon as she knows that the period is imminent or as soon as the bleeding begins; the medication should be taken on a regular basis for the first 1–3 days of the period as it prevents pain.

The oral contraceptive pill is an effective first-line agent for the treatment of primary dysmenorrhoea when NSAIDs have failed. In those women in whom the oral contraceptive pill or NSAIDs do not work, transdermal glyceryl trinitrate patches may be of benefit as they can cause relaxation of uterine contractions.

Second-line treatment such as oral contraceptives may be effective in treating primary dysmenorrhoea; they block ovulation, thus reducing blood flow to the uterus. Vitamin E is another prostaglandin inhibitor.

In secondary dysmenorrhoea, the aim of treatment is to identify and correct the underlying organic cause; options include surgical intervention and/or pharmacological intervention.

Pelvic inflammatory disease (PID) is a cause of secondary dysmenorrhoea; this should be treated to relieve the associated symptoms.

Transcutaneous electrical nerve stimulation (TENS) can help with or without pharmacological analgesics. Acupuncture may be of value but there is insufficient evidence to determine its effectiveness in reducing pain.

In rare cases surgical intervention may be required for some women. Hysterectomy can help to relieve the presenting symptoms; this is usually performed once childbearing is complete.

Exercise can cause the release of endogenous endorphins, which are the body's own analgesics.

40 Eczema

Figure 40.1 Eczema

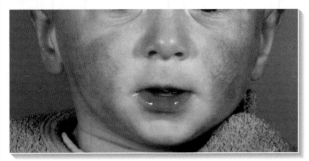

Table 40.2. Signs and symptoms of atopic eczema

- The skin often feels dry
- Some areas of skin become red and inflamed (next to skin creases, for example, wrists, cubital and popliteal fossae and around the neck). Any areas of skin may be affected
- Inflamed skin is itchy
- Scratching can cause patches of skin to become thickened
- Inflamed areas of skin may become blistered and ooze
- Inflamed areas of skin can become infected

Table 40.1 Eczema triggers

Environmental irritants and allergens:

- Irritants, such as soaps and detergents, shampoos, bubble baths, shower gels and washing-up liquids
- Skin infections Staphylococcus aureus is an important exacerbating factor in atopic eczema
- Contact allergens
- Extremes of temperature and humidity. The condition improves in the summer and worsens in winter
- Abrasive fabrics, such as wool
- Dietary factors aggravate atopic eczema more in children less frequently in adults
- Inhaled allergens, for example, house dust mites, pollens, pet dander and moulds

Endogenous factors:

- Stress can exacerbate atopic eczema, which can then become a cause of psychological distress
- Hormonal changes in women – premenstrual flare-ups, deterioration in pregnancy

Table 40.3 A guide to the severity of eczema

Clear	Normal skin, no evidence of active atopic eczema
Mild	Areas of dry skin, infrequent itching (with or without small areas of redness)
Moderate	Areas of dry skin, frequent itching, redness (with or without excoriation and localised skin thickening)
Severe	Widespread areas of dry skin, incessant itching, redness (with or without excoriation, extensive skin thickening, bleeding, oozing, cracking and alteration of skin pigmentation)

Medical-Surgical Nursing at a Glance, First Edition. Ian Peate. © John Wiley & Sons, Ltd. Published 2016 by John Wiley & Sons, Ltd.
Companion website: www.ataglanceseries.com/nursing/medsurg

Skin disorders are the most common diseases seen by health professionals; there are thousands of skin disorders. They are also the most common group of occupational health problems causing an absence from work; this leads to lost working time with an economic impact on individuals, their family and society.

Eczema is divided into a small number of subgroups; it is a chronic, widespread, non-infective inflammatory condition that results in severe pruritus, erythema and scaling. This condition can occur at any age; usually it arises during infancy or early childhood (Figure 40.1). This chapter focuses upon atopic eczema.

Some people with eczema have to cope with ill-informed remarks and incorrect anxieties that this condition is contagious. Understanding and education can help reduce the damaging effects that skin conditions such as eczema can have on the person and their family.

Causes of atopic eczema

The cause of atopic eczema is complex and as yet not fully understood. Genetic and environmental factors are likely to contribute, together with defects in epithelial barrier function as a result of abnormalities in structural proteins, causing the skin to become extremely permeable and more liable to damage from environmental irritants and allergens. Trigger factors can be found in Table 40.1.

Impact of eczema

As with the majority of visible skin conditions, eczema can have a intense effect on a person's self-esteem. The patient may also experience disturbed sleep as a result of the clinical manifestations. For younger patients, there may be a significant impact on their behaviour and their development as a result of disturbed sleep, lowered self-esteem and social isolation. Repeated visits to the general practice, the need to apply messy topical skin applications and the use of special clothing can add to the burden of the disease. Eczema can have a profound effect not only on the patient but also on their family.

Signs and symptoms

Stage of illness causes the signs and symptoms of atopic eczema to differ. Early in the acute phase of eczema, the rash can be inflamed, weeping and blistering, in the subacute phase dry, scaly and burning, and in the chronic phase the skin becomes dry, thickened, fissured and excoriated. Atopic eczema can start as early as 4 months of age and can commence as a dry scaly rash on the face that may spread to the rest of the body.

National guidance is available to help with the diagnosing of atopic eczema. The patient may present with three of the following in conjunction with a dry, itchy rash:

- previous history of rashes to the back of the knees and elbows
- family history or medical history of asthma and/or hay fever
- tendency to dry skin
- onset under 2 years of age.

Acute eczema is characterised by pruritus, erythema and vesiculation, and chronic eczema by pruritus, xerosis, lichenification, hyperkeratosis and fissure formation (rare). See Table 40.2 for the signs and symptoms of atopic eczema.

Investigations and diagnosis

Investigations are not often needed to make the diagnosis, which is made on clinical examination; referral to a dermatologist may be required. Diagnosis is based on visual assessment as well as a patient history. A guide to visual assessment of eczema severity has been developed (Table 40.3). Other diagnostic tests include blood tests, a patch test and allergy tests.

Care and treatment

There is no cure for eczema, so treatment aims to control or ease symptoms. It is usual for the treatment plan to be made up of three parts (avoidance of irritants and triggers, the use of emollients and application of topical steroids).

In atopic eczema, one main complication is infection due to a break in the skin. When skin is infected, it contains pustules that are green or yellow in colour, with large blisters; the patient may feel unwell and have a raised temperature. Prevention of infection is paramount; this can be achieved by providing information to the patient, explaining how the infection may be caused and that it can spread by scratching.

Establishing what causes or makes the eczema worse can lead the nurse to request a patch test. If an allergen or irritant has been identified, this should, if possible, be avoided. Approaches to care should be tailored to meet individual needs. If possible, remove the irritant or allergen causing the antibody-antigen reaction. Offer support to the patient and their family to empower, educate and motivate; this may raise self-esteem and self-awareness.

Creams, ointments and oils can be used as emollients to reduce the drying and itching effects of the disease. Aqueous cream may be used as opposed to soap. Perfumed products should be avoided. If infection occurs then antibiotics or antifungal medication may be required. These can be given systematically or applied topically. In some cases, topical steroid preparations can be used to reduce inflammation; these preparations should be used with caution and should not be used for longer than is necessary. Topical preparations containing antibiotics and steroids are available; these should only be used for the short term. Antihistamines may be prescribed.

There are other issues that the nurse will need to consider. Encourage rest as sleeping may be difficult for some patients. Dietary advice may be required if the allergen is a food product; refer to a dietician. Complementary therapies may help some patients. Complementary therapies are complementary, not a substitute for conventional medicine, but the patient's wishes must be respected.

If the nurse is applying topical medications, at all times wear gloves not only to combat the risk of cross-infection but also to prevent absorbing the medications.

41 Psoriasis

Figure 41.1 Psoriasis

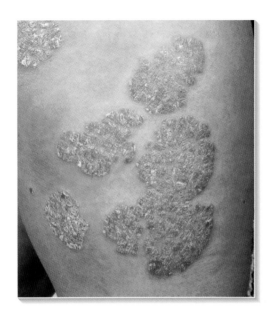

Figure 41.3 Penetration of UVA and UVB radiation

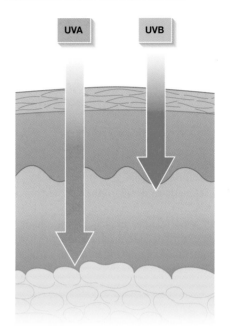

Figure 41.2 Common sites of psoriasis

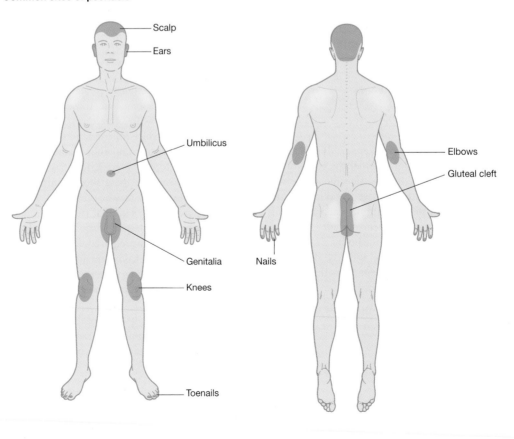

There are some skin conditions that have the potential to cause stigma, such as eczema and psoriasis. As advocate, the nurse can be instrumental in dispelling any misunderstanding regarding contagion and in so doing enhance the individual's social well-being. Appearance and image are often associated with success and achievement and the blemish-free individual usually portrayed in the media in most western societies is the image to which many aspire; for those who have skin problems this can become increasingly challenging. People with a skin problem can experience difficulties in other aspects of their lives, for example, forming relationships and also regarding issues concerning self-esteem and self-concept. Altered body image can have a negative impact on the individual, their partner and their family. Patients may report feeling stigmatised and isolated.

Psoriasis

Psoriasis a common, chronic, relapsing, inflammatory skin disorder which has a strong genetic basis. It is a T cell-mediated autoimmune disorder that results from the interaction between multiple genetic and environmental factors. T cells are provoked to produce cytokines; these stimulate keratinocyte proliferation and the production of dermal antigenic adhesion molecules in the local blood vessels, stimulating further the T cell cytokine response.

Males and females are equally affected by psoriasis and the condition can occur at any age but most cases first present before the age of 35 years. It is uncommon in children. Plaque psoriasis accounts for the majority of all cases of psoriasis.

There are several forms of psoriasis; this non-infectious, inflammatory disorder can appear as a red raised demarcation of skin patches with silvery whitish scales, and the condition varies from mild to severe. The aetiology is unknown. The condition brings with it many challenges for the patient and the nurse because of its unpredictable periods of exacerbation and remission.

Risk factors

There are several risk factors associated with the condition. There is a pattern of inheritance associated with psoriasis, about a third of patients with psoriasis having a family history. Environmental factors may trigger or exacerbate plaque psoriasis, including sunlight; there is usually a decrease in severity during periods of increased sun exposure (the condition often improves in the summer and is worse in the winter). Streptococcal infection is strongly related with the development of psoriasis. The presence of an immune disorder such as HIV plays a role in psoriasis. It is widely believed that psychological stress also plays a role but evidence for a causal relationship is scarce. There is a range of drugs that may be considered as risk factors, including some antidepressants, NSAIDs, angiotensin-converting enzyme inhibitors and certain antibiotics (tetracycline, for example), Smoking and alcohol are also risk factors.

Signs and symptoms

Erythematous plaques appear in plaque-type psoriasis with silvery scales and symmetrical involvement. This can be pruritic and painful, and often appears at areas of epidermal injury (Figure 41.1). Guttate psoriasis appears as individual red drop-like patterns on the trunk, arms or legs; these are not as thick as plaque psoriasis. Inverse, bright red patches that are smooth and shiny affect flexural areas such as the axilla and groin (Figure 41.2). Erythrodermic redness over most of the body has a scalded look with a relentless pruritus along with signs of systemic illness.

Pustular psoriasis, mainly seen in adults, is exacerbated by the sun; blisters form containing non-infective material surrounded by red skin on the palms and the soles or on widespread areas. Psoriatic arthritis is associated with joint pain and accompanying skin involvement.

Investigations and diagnosis

A diagnosis is made on clinical findings.

Care and treatment

Treatment should include both physical and psychological care. Treatment for psoriasis should be tailored to meet the individual needs of the person and is based on the severity of the skin disorder.

Topical treatment is prescribed for mild to moderate disease, phototherapy is used in moderate disease and in severe cases along with systemic treatment. Often, however, patients may be given a combination of treatments.

Topical treatments include the use of emollients, which aim to lubricate the skin and ease scaling as well as providing patient comfort, and vitamin D analogues such as calcipotriol, tacalcitol and calcitriol which inhibit cell proliferation. Coal tar preparations have an antipruritic and anti-inflammatory effect (but they can stain clothing); dithranol is used to suppress cell proliferation and topical steroids are used to reduce inflammation but should only be used for short periods. Retinoids are preparations that influence the activity of the epidermis and methotrexate is often used in the treatment of cancer; it causes inhibition of cell division.

Often patients find topical treatments messy with an offensive smell. Spending time with the patient discussing treatment options and offering support may help those who are undergoing this level of treatment. The nurse has a role to play in motivating and encouraging the patient to apply the therapies meticulously and adhere to the treatment regimen.

If there is poor response to topical treatments, phototherapy and photochemotherapy are considered; these can be used to inhibit cell division for some forms of psoriasis. Phototherapy involves irradiation using UVB, whereas photochemotherapy necessitates the use of a photoactive drug (psoralen) along with UVA irradiation (Figure 41.3). During treatment, patients will be required to attend hospital 2–3 times per week for 6 weeks. It is essential that during this type of therapy, the nurse documents the patient's lifetime exposure, as there is a risk of cutaneous malignancy.

Those patients who require systemic treatment include those with pustular psoriasis and extensive disease.

It should be noted that regardless of the treatment chosen, this is not a cure for the condition. There is no single treatment that will suit everyone and individual assessment is absolutely essential.

42 Skin Cancer

Table 42.1 The ABCDE of melanoma

A = **Asymmetry** – the two halves of melanoma may not look the same

B = **Border** – the edges of a melanoma can be irregular, blurred or jagged

C = **Colour** – the colour of a melanoma may be uneven with more than one shade

D = **Diameter** – the majority of menaonmas are at least 6mm in diameter

E = **Evolving** – any change in size, shape, colour, elevation or any new symptom,
e.g. bleeding, itching or crusting may be due to a melanoma

Table 42.2 Assessing changes in moles (lesions)

Characteristic	Points
Change in size*	2
Change in colour (becoming darker, becoming patchy or multi-shaded)*	2
Change in shape*	2
7 mm or more across in any direction	1
Inflammation	1
Oozing or bleeding	1
Change in sensation (such as, itching or pain)	1
*Represents the major features	

Medical-Surgical Nursing at a Glance, First Edition. Ian Peate. © John Wiley & Sons, Ltd. Published 2016 by John Wiley & Sons, Ltd.
Companion website: www.ataglanceseries.com/nursing/medsurg

Skin cancer is the most common cancer in the UK. Skin cancers are divided into melanoma (malignant melanoma), developing from melanocytes, and non-melanoma skin cancers which are around 20 times more common than melanomas and are divided into basal cell carcinoma (BCC), developing from basal cells, and squamous cell carcinoma (SCC), developing from keratinocytes. There are other types of skin cancer which are rare.

Melanoma is the most serious type of skin cancer, affecting young adults as well as older people. If this cancer is diagnosed at an early stage, then treatment offered is likely to be curative. The outlook is poor if the melanoma has spread prior to being treated.

Malignant melanoma

The most dangerous form of skin cancer is malignant melanoma. Melanocytes are the cells that produce the pigment melanin located in the basal layer of the skin, where melanomas occur, a third of them originating in pre-existing moles.

Melanoma usually develops in a naevus (also known as a mole); it can metastasise rapidly via the circulatory and lymphatic systems. This type of skin cancer spreads quickly, which makes it the most dangerous type. These cancers are more common in young people and are closely related to sunburn and overexposure.

Risk factors

There is one key risk factor for melanoma, i.e. sun or sunbed exposure (ultraviolet light). However, some people are more at risk than others. More women than men get melanoma; it is the seventh most common cancer in women. In those aged under 14 years, this disease is rare; in those aged over 15 years, the incidence steadily rises with age and the highest incidence is in those aged 80 years and over. Risk grows the more moles a person has.

Those who are fair skinned are more at risk than those who are dark skinned but people with dark skin can and do get malignant melanoma. Those with fair skin and a tendency to freckle when in the sun are most at risk, as are people who do not tan at all; these people usually peel before getting a tan.

People with melanoma are twice as likely to have been badly sunburned at least once in their lives; sunburn as a child is even more harmful than sunburn as an adult because during childhood the skin is at its most vulnerable. Risk is also associated with geographical location and where the person was born. Those who are fair skinned and were born in a hot country, for example Australia, have an increased risk of melanoma for life, in contrast to those people who went to live there as a teenager or compared to those with a similar skin colour who live in cooler climates. Whilst the person was young, their skin would have been exposed to the damaging effects of the sun, when the skin was at its most delicate. A family history of skin cancer, i.e. a family member who has had melanoma, puts a person more at risk.

Signs and symptoms

The characteristics of a melanoma are a slowly developing, symmetrical, flat lesion, more than 6 mm in diameter. Initially, they are classified as malignant melanoma *in situ*. These are considered benign but have the potential to infiltrate the dermis and metastasise by spreading through the blood and lymph network. The melanoma's characteristics change to a raised nodular appearance with satellite lesions around the margins (Table 42.1).

Investigations and diagnosis

Patient history and a full physical examination are required in order to make a diagnosis. The whole of the person's body should be examined and closely observed. Lentigo maligna (also known as Hutchinson's freckle) is a premalignant melanoma condition that can be seen on the face or other areas of the person's body that has been exposed to the sun; in some people, the lesion has been slowly enlarging for a number of years.

The only definitive method of confirming a diagnosis of malignant melanoma is to take a biopsy of the lesion and expose it to histological testing (histology). Diagnosis should be based on a full-thickness excisional biopsy. Typically, the specimen is taken under a local anaesthetic but this depends on the aspect of the body where the lesion is located. If the lesion is suspected to be cancerous then urgent referral must be made. The lesion must be measured; a photograph is usually taken in order to make comparisons at a later stage.

National guidance suggests that a seven-point scale is used in order to help make the decision to refer to a specialist service (Table 42.2). In the scale, there are three major features and four minor ones. Two points are allocated for any of the major features and one for the minor features; if the mole (lesion) scores three points or above then urgent referral is required. However, if there is any cause for concern, irrespective of the score, then the patient should be referred to a specialist.

Dermatoscopy may be performed in order to examine the lesion. This is a painless test that has the ability to magnify the area up to ten times, distinguishing benign from malignant pigmented lesions in a more accurate manner.

Sentinel lymph node biopsy (SLNB) identifies and removes the lymph node(s) immediately draining the area of the primary tumour for histological analysis; this provides prognostic information.

Further investigations may be needed and include chest X-ray and liver ultrasound, or computed tomography (CT) scan of the chest, abdomen and pelvis. Blood tests will include a full blood count, liver function tests and lactate dehydrogenase (LDH). Bone scans are performed only if there is an indication of bone disease.

Care and treatment

Treatment depends on whether the skin cancer is diagnosed at an early, medium or advanced stage. Early stage requires a wide local excision of the lesion under anaesthetic, with or without sentinel lymph node biopsy. If the results are positive, other lymph nodes are removed at a later date. Medium stage requires the same surgery as the early stage, with adjuvant treatment such as chemotherapy, radiotherapy and biological therapy (the use of interferon). At the advanced stage, the treatment and management depend on metastasis, symptoms currently experienced and prior treatments. Surgery and adjuvant therapies may be offered, but palliation may be the only option, with symptom control. Plans for end-of-life care may need to be discussed, with support for the family and significant others.

43 Lung Cancer

Figure 43.1 Types of cancer caused by smoking

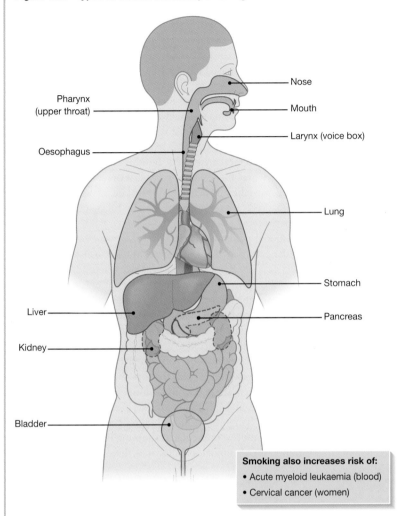

Nose

Pharynx (upper throat)

Mouth

Larynx (voice box)

Oesophagus

Lung

Stomach

Liver

Pancreas

Kidney

Bladder

Smoking also increases risk of:
- Acute myeloid leukaemia (blood)
- Cervical cancer (women)

Table 43.1 Benign and malignant tumours

Benign tumours
• Non-cancerous
• May grow large and compress adjoining tissue/organs
• Slow spreading
• Does not grow abnormally
• Usually encapsulated
• Differentiated
• Usually non-life threatening (has the potential to become malignant)

Malignant tumours
• Cancerous
• Potential to destroy nearby tissue
• Fast rate of spread
• Grows abnormally
• Non encapsulated
• Undifferentiated
• Can be life threatening

Table 43.2 Classification

Tumour	• **T-1** denotes that the primary tumour is contained within the lung
	• **T-2** tumour is between 3–7 cm across
	• **T-3** the tumour is larger than 7 cm
	• **T-4** the tumour has invaded nearby structures, for example, the mediastinum, the trachea, a major blood vessels
Nodes	• **N-0** means there has been no spread to the lymph nodes
	• **N-1** signifies that some of the local lymph nodes have been affected
	• **N-2** suggests that there has been a more extensive spread to local lymph nodes
	• **N-3** there is lymph node involvement on the opposite side of the chest
Metastases	• **M-0** signifies that there are no metastases
	• **M-1** means there are metastases to some other area of the body, e.g. the lungs or the pleural fluid
	• **M-1b** there is cancer in distant sites – liver or bones

Medical-Surgical Nursing at a Glance, First Edition. Ian Peate. © John Wiley & Sons, Ltd. Published 2016 by John Wiley & Sons, Ltd.
Companion website: www.ataglanceseries.com/nursing/medsurg

Lung cancer has the highest rate of all known cancers in the western world. In the UK, the most common cancers are lung, prostate, breast and bowel. The most significant risk factor is smoking; lung cancer is rare in those who have never smoked. The majority of primary lung tumours are malignant. Table 43.1 differentiates between malignant and benign cancers.

Other risk factors include passive smoking, occupational exposure to asbestos, silica and nickel as well as pulmonary fibrosis. Genetic factors also play a part.

Lung cancers

Nearly all lung cancers develop in bronchial tissue. There are two main types of bronchial carcinoma: non-small cell and small cell. Non-small cell carcinomas are responsible for 70% of all lung cancers. Non-small cell carcinomas can be subdivided into squamous cell carcinomas and adenocarcinomas or large cell carcinomas. Squamous cell carcinomas often develop within the larger bronchi, although other non-small cell carcinomas are located in the smaller airways, which makes them much harder to detect. Small cell carcinomas usually grow close to the large bronchi; these are the most aggressive bronchial carcinomas.

Smoking or other irritants such as asbestos can damage the pseudostratified epithelium in lung tissue; this makes the tissue more susceptible to inflammation. Inhalation of asbestos dust can cause cancer of the lining of the lungs (mesothelioma).

Some chemicals present within cigarette smoke are carcinogenic; these chemicals promote the development of tumours within the lung. Risk factors for cancer of the lung are, therefore, smoking, passive smoking and exposure to pollutants. Other types of cancer caused by smoking can be found in Figure 43.1.

Signs and symptoms

The following signs and symptoms are associated with cancer of the lung in those people who smoke tobacco: cough, haemoptysis, dyspnoea, chest pain, wheeze and stridor, clubbing of the fingers, bone pain, lethargy, dysphagia and hoarseness (if there is recurrent laryngeal nerve involvement).

Investigations and diagnosis

A comprehensive history is undertaken as well as a detailed physical examination. Cytological examination of sputum, chest X-ray, lung function tests, computed tomography and a range of blood tests will be required to confirm a diagnosis.

When a diagnosis of cancer has been made, the person is usually told what stage the cancer is, which helps to determine how much it has grown and spread. Usually, the earlier the stage and the lower the grade of the cancer, the better the prognosis.

Staging helps decide upon the most appropriate management of the disease and how well it might respond to treatment. If a person has malignant lung cancer it is essential to determine if the cancer has spread, as this can help them make an informed decision concerning care needs.

The most commonly used system for staging solid tumours is the TNM system (Table 43.2).

- T for tumour – how far the primary tumour has grown locally (tumour extension)

- N for nodes – if there is spread to the local lymph nodes (lymph node dissemination)
- M for metastases – if there is spread to other parts of the body (distant tumour spread)

After staging occurs, a number is given for the three features. As soon as possible after initial diagnosis, the stage of cancer should be told to the patient. Investigations (including pathology, radiography and bronchoscopy) determine the stage. During this time the nurse offers support to the patient and family, making referrals to organisations such as Macmillan.

Care and treatment

When a person is diagnosed with cancer, this is likely to be a traumatic event, not only for the individual receiving the diagnosis but also for their family and friends. The nurse is required to provide care that reflects a person's individual needs (consideration should be given to physical and psychological health and well-being), using a sound evidence base. It is essential that whatever the person's circumstances, the nurse does not make assumptions or prejudge the individual.

The success of treatment depends on early detection of the disease, careful staging and grading in order to assess the extent of the cancer, intervening quickly and offering appropriate support as well as advances in technology and medicine.

There are a number of ways in which cancer can be treated, depending on the type of cancer and whether it has spread. Cancer treatment aims to cure, control the disease process or provide palliation of symptoms. People are sometimes given more than one type of treatment such as surgery, chemotherapy, radiotherapy, percutaneous radiofrequency ablation and biotherapy. The goals of treatment are to eradicate the tumour or malignant cells, prevent metastatic spread, reduce the growth of cells and promote independence and functional abilities. The nurse provides pain relief as required.

There are side effects with all forms of treatment. Surgical intervention can cause nerve destruction. If diseased regional lymph nodes are removed, this can cause long-term lymphoedema, impacting on the person's quality of life. If the tumour is inoperable or widespread metastases exist, surgery may only be palliative.

Chemotherapy is the treatment of cancer using cytotoxic drugs. These drugs can cause side effects, as they affect some of the healthy cells in the body; damage is usually temporary and most side effects will disappear once treatment ends. Side effects vary depending on the drug used and duration of treatment.

Many patients with cancer receive radiotherapy (and some receive combination therapy) as part of their treatment. The nurse should offer psychological and physical support. The site to be treated is usually marked with a semi-permeable marker, which should not be washed off, otherwise all the measurements for positioning of the radiotherapy beam will need to be recalculated.

The nurse should also advise the patient not to wash the treated area with soap or to apply creams, talcum powder or other topical preparations, as this can cause skin damage. They should avoid rubbing, scratching, shaving or exposing the area to sunlight, and hot or cold packs should not be applied to the area. The skin should be checked daily and any changes reported.

44 Cervical Cancer

Table 44.1 Stages of cervical cancer

Stage 1	Cancer cells within the cervix only
Stage 2	Cancer spreads into surrounding structures, e.g. upper part of the vagina or tissues adjacent to the cervix
Stage 3	Cancer has spread to areas such as lower aspect of the vagina, or tissues at the sides of the pelvic area
Stage 4	Cancer has spread to the bladder or bowel or beyond the pelvic area

Table 44.2 Signs and symptom of cervical cancer

- Intermittent or continuous vaginal discharge
- Bleeding – may be spontaneous, post-coital, during micturition or whilst defaecating
- Vaginal bleeding can be severe
- Vaginal discomfort/urinary symptoms
- On examination there maybe white or red patches on the cervix

Later symptoms can include:

- Painless haematuria
- Chronic urinary frequency
- Painless fresh rectal bleeding
- A change in bowel habit
- Leg oedema, pain and hydronephrosis
- Pelvic pain or discomfort
- There may be a rectal mass or bleeding due to erosion
- Bimanual palpation may reveal pelvic bulkiness/masses as a result of pelvic spread
- Leg oedema may cause lymphatic or vascular obstruction
- Hepatomegaly may indicate liver metastases
- Pulmonary metastases can cause pleural effusion or bronchial obstruction
- On examination due to erosion, ulcer or tumour cervix and vagina, may appear abnormal

Medical-Surgical Nursing at a Glance, First Edition. Ian Peate. © John Wiley & Sons, Ltd. Published 2016 by John Wiley & Sons, Ltd.
Companion website: www.ataglanceseries.com/nursing/medsurg

Carcinogens (chemicals or environmental factors) can cause cells to become abnormal and cancerous. They cause damage and can initiate mutation of a cell's genetic material – the DNA and RNA. Smoking increases a person's risk of lung cancer, overexposure to ultraviolet sunlight increases the possibility of melanoma and the breathing of asbestos dust can cause mesothelioma. There are some viruses that are known to be carcinogenic, such as the human papilloma virus (HPV), which is associated with cancer of the cervix. Some strains of HPV are responsible for genital and anal warts and others are responsible for the majority of cervical and anal cancers.

Vaccination

The HPV vaccine is offered routinely to girls aged 12 and 13 years with the aim of reducing the risk of cervical cancer. Currently HPV vaccines cover four types of HPV (HPV 6 and 11, responsible for causing warts, and HPV 16 and 18, the two most common cancer-causing strains of the virus). The vaccine given to young women in the UK only offers protection against HPV 16 and 18. However, this vaccine may also offer protection against throat, penile and anal cancers. HPV vaccines are very successful at preventing the infection of susceptible women with the HPV types that are covered by the vaccine. In young women with no evidence of previous infection, vaccines are over 99% effective at preventing precancerous lesions associated with HPV types 16 or 18.

There are around 100 types of HPV; approximately 40 of these cause infections of the genital tract. Most infections are asymptomatic and self-limiting; infection of the genitalia by HPV is related to genital warts and anogenital cancers in males and females. Depending on their association with the development of cancer, HPV viruses are classed as 'high-risk' or 'low-risk' types.

Risk factors

Genital HPVs are transmitted by sexual contact; this is mainly through sexual intercourse. As a result, risk factors are associated with the number of sexual partners, the introduction of a new sexual partner and the sexual history of any partner.

Other risk factors for cervical cancer include being heterosexual, smoking and the woman's socioeconomic status (women living in the most deprived areas have cervical cancer rates more than three times higher than women living in least deprived areas), co-infection with HIV (and immunosuppression).

Cervical cancers are preventable, by avoiding infection with HPV; HPV is present in all cervical cancers. Smoking plays a part in causing some cervical cancer; it increases the possibility of HPV infection or causes HPV infection to be more persistent.

Grading/staging cervical cancer

There are four systems of grading (four stages are used in cervical cancer) used to determine the extent of dysplastic changes in the cervix – cervical intraepithelial neoplasia (CIN). An awareness of the stage of the cancer helps determine treatment options. Grading/staging incorporates the size of the cancer and if it has spread beyond its original site. The four main stages can be found in Table 44.1.

Squamous cell cancers spread by direct invasion of accessory structures and include the vaginal wall, pelvic wall, bladder and rectum. Usually metastatic spread is limited to the pelvic area; distant metastasis may occur via the lymphatic system.

Signs and symptoms

Most cervical cancers are detected by screening. When carcinoma of the cervix is established, the signs and symptoms in Table 44.2 may be present.

Investigations and diagnosis

The nurse will be expected to assist the woman before, during and after procedures and investigations. The woman should be provided with information in such a way that she understands it and is able to make an informed decision.

Colposcopy allows the nurse or doctor to visualise the surface of the cervix and a cone biopsy may be undertaken if any abnormal tissue has been identified, providing a sample for histology. A pelvic examination under general anaesthetic shows through examination that there may be a need for sigmoidoscopy and cystoscopy. Radiological investigations include magnetic resonance imaging (MRI) or computed tomography (CT) scan, positron emission tomography (PET)-CT scan, chest X-ray and a variety of blood tests.

Care and treatment

If precancerous changes are identified (mild to severe) then it is advised that treatment commences. All types of treatments aim to remove or destroy the abnormal cells. Laser ablation, cold coagulation and cryotherapy just treat the part of the cervix containing abnormal cells. This will permit normal cells to grow back. Depending on the outcome of colposcopy, the cone biopsy and the woman's individual needs, hysterectomy may be required.

Carcinoma *in situ* is treated, according to the stage, with surgery, radiotherapy or chemotherapy or a combination of these treatments. Some women may decide to have treatment to control symptoms.

Surgical intervention can range from hysterectomy for early-stage cervical cancer to surgery for advanced cervical cancer. Advanced cervical cancer includes both cancer that has spread at the time of diagnosis and cancer that returns after previous treatment; advanced cancer involves structures within the pelvis. Removal of the uterus, cervix, top aspect of the vagina and lymph nodes and other organs is known as pelvic exenteration (there are three types: anterior, posterior and total exenteration), the aim being to cure the cancer.

If the woman is pregnant then treatment may be delayed until a viable fetus can be delivered, with the proviso that the delay is only for a few weeks; a therapeutic abortion may be necessary. In all instances, the wishes of the woman in discussions with the multidisciplinary team are respected.

Follow-up is required for some years after treatment; initially this will usually be every few months, gradually becoming less frequent if the woman's condition continues to progress well. The frequency of appointments varies according to the guidelines used by the doctor. One example of follow-up is 3–4-month check-ups to start with.

45 Prostate Cancer

Table 45.1   Signs and symptoms of local, locally invasive and metastatic prostate disease

Local disease	Locally invasive disease	Metastatic disease
• Raised PSA on screening	• Haematuria	• Bone pain or sciatica
• Weak stream, hesitancy, sensation of incomplete emptying of the bladder, urinary frequency, urgency, urge incontinence	• Dysuria	• Paraplegia as a result of spinal cord compression
• Urinary tract infection	• Urinary incontinence	• Lymphadenopathy
	• Haematospermia	• Loin pain or anuria due to ureteric obstruction by lymph nodes
	• Perineal and suprapubic pain	• Lethargy
	• Obstruction of ureters, causing loin pain, anuria, symptoms of acute kidney injury or chronic kidney disease	• Anaemia
	• Erectile dysfunction	• Uraemia
	• Rectal symptoms – e.g. tenesmus	• Weight loss, cachexia
		• The most common sites for metastases are bone and lymph nodes

Table 45.2   Treatment options for prostate cancer

Option	Comment
Watchful waiting/active surveillance	This involves regular check-ups (follow up) to determine if and how the cancer is developing, as opposed to radical treatment
Radical prostatectomy	There are a number of surgical procedures and approaches that can be used to perform prostatectomy and if needed lymphadenectomy
Radiation therapy	This includes external beam radiation therapy and brachytherapy
Hormonal treatment	Bilateral orchidectomy, oestrogen therapy, luteinizing hormone – releasing hormone, anti-androgen therapy, androgen depravation therapy
Chemotherapy	Chemotherapy will not eradicate prostate cancer, but can help to control or delay symptoms, and it may help some men to live longer
Cryosurgery, proton beam therapy and other treatment options	These treatment options are under clinical evaluation

Medical-Surgical Nursing at a Glance, First Edition. Ian Peate. © John Wiley & Sons, Ltd. Published 2016 by John Wiley & Sons, Ltd.
Companion website: www.ataglanceseries.com/nursing/medsurg

Prostate cancer arises in the prostate gland, a small, walnut-sized structure which is part of the male reproductive system. The gland wraps around the urethra and when it enlarges, this can have an impact on the man's ability to void urine. Prostate cancer is the most common cancer in men in the UK; it is the second most common cause of cancer death after lung cancer.

Epidemiology

Globally, it is estimated that more than 1.11 million men were diagnosed with prostate cancer in 2012. Incidence rates across the world vary.

In 2011 in the UK, 41,736 men were diagnosed with prostate cancer, with 10,793 deaths. In England, 81.4% of adult prostate cancer patients survived their cancer for 5 years or more in 2005–2009.

This cancer accounts for approximately 25% of all new cases of cancer diagnosed in men in the UK. Prostate cancer rates in the UK have tripled over the last 35 years. It is suggested that this is the result of higher detection rates through the increased use of the prostate specific antigen (PSA) test.

Whilst cancer of the prostate gland is often associated with age (more than a third of prostate cancer cases are diagnosed in men aged 75 years or over), men under 65 years are also affected, accounting for approximately 25% of all cases.

Risk factors

The greatest risk factor for prostate cancer is age; there is a very low risk in men under the age of 50 but the risk increases with age. Black men have a higher risk of prostate cancer than white men and Asian men have a lower risk of prostate cancer than white men.

Those men with one or more first-degree relatives (a father, brother or son) diagnosed with prostate cancer have an increased risk, particularly if the relative was diagnosed at an early age. Mutations in the BRCA2 gene increase the risk of developing prostate cancer.

Signs and symptoms

Cancer of the prostate is usually slow growing and there may be no immediate symptoms. Symptoms often occur as the prostate enlarges, irritating and compressing the urethra and resulting in an obstruction to urinary flow. Local advanced prostate cancer can cause lower urinary tract symptoms. See Table 45.1 for an overview of the signs and symptoms of prostate cancer related to local, locally invasive and metastatic disease.

Investigations and diagnosis

A detailed medical history and clinical examination is undertaken. There are several tests used to diagnose prostate cancer. Digital rectal examination (DRE) is usually undertaken, to determine if there is an enlarged or irregular prostate gland. Blood is taken to measure levels of PSA in the bloodstream (this is a protein produced by the prostate gland); the PSA test alone will not confirm a diagnosis of prostate cancer but it is a useful method of monitoring the cancer and the effects of treatment.

The removal of a small amount of prostatic tissue (transrectal ultrasonography, TRUS) is taken for examination under the microscope. This can determine if there are any cancer cells present.

A urinary flow test assesses the rate of flow and ascertains if there are any outflow/obstruction difficulties. Radiological investigations can include a computed tomography (CT) scan, magnetic resonance imaging (MRI) scan or bone scan.

Staging

Staging of the cancer is an important step in deciding on the most appropriate treatment option as well as determining prognosis. The stage is based on the prostate biopsy results, the PSA level and any other examinations or investigations that have been undertaken to determine if and how far the cancer has spread. Prostate cancer can be divided into non-metastatic and metastatic.

The Tumour, Node, Metastasis (TNM) staging system is used along with the histological result of the TRUS biopsy from which a Gleason score can be obtained (histological grading, sometimes called pathological stage). This approach estimates the grade of cancer according to its differentiation. The higher the score, the worse the prognosis; a score of 2 demonstrates a well-differentiated tumour and 10 is the most poorly differentiated with a 75% 10-year risk of local progression.

Care and treatment

There have been a number of significant improvements concerning the ways in which men with advanced prostate cancer are treated. Table 45.2 summarises a number of available treatment options. The option chosen will depend on whether the man's cancer is localized (contained within the prostate gland), locally advanced (has spread just outside the prostate) or advanced, whereby the cancer has metastasized.

The decision to move from an active surveillance regimen to radical treatment has to be taken in conjunction with the man and by considering his individual and personal needs, co-morbidities and also his life expectancy. The nurse has a duty to act as the patient's advocate, offering him support physically and psychologically during this important time when decisions concerning treatment options need to be considered.

Some of the treatment options, for example, chemotherapy, may be given alongside other treatments such as hormone therapy, steroids and radiotherapy; if there is advanced cancer, bisphosphonates may be administered.

National guidelines have been issued by NICE concerning the treatment of prostate cancer. New hormone treatments, such as abiraterone (Zytiga) and enzalutamide (Xtandi; also known as MDV3100), have been recommended. The rationale underpinning the NICE guidance is to provide an assurance that the treatment offered is evidence based and that it is to be given to those men who will gain from it.

Men should be offered support by healthcare providers who can explain the various treatment options and advice on the support services available. Providing information, offering support and knowing how to make appropriate referrals are key aspects of the role and function of the nurse, especially if men are to make the treatment choices that are right for them.

46 Glaucoma

Figure 46.1 Glaucoma

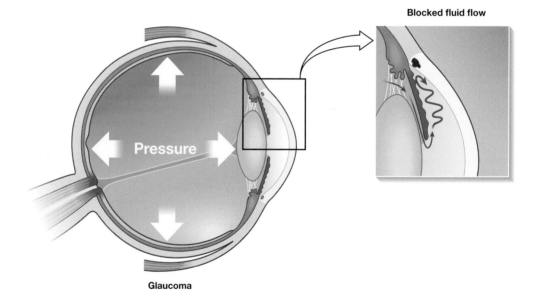

Drainage channel

Normal fluid flow

Cornea

Retina

Lens

Optic nerve

Normal eye

Blocked fluid flow

Pressure

Glaucoma

Table 46.1 Some ophthalmological examinations

Examination	Tests
Tonometry	The inner eye pressure
Perimetry (visual field test)	The complete field of vision
Ophthalmoscopy (dilated eye exam)	The shape and colour of the optic nerve
Gonioscopy	The angle in the eye where the iris meets the cornea
Pachymetry	Thickness of the cornea

Medical-Surgical Nursing at a Glance, First Edition. Ian Peate. © John Wiley & Sons, Ltd. Published 2016 by John Wiley & Sons, Ltd.
Companion website: www.ataglanceseries.com/nursing/medsurg

Sight

The eye is the organ of vision; it has a complex structure. Vision occurs when light is processed by the eye and interpreted by the brain. Light passes through the transparent eye surface, the cornea. The pupil is an opening to the inner aspects of the eye. It can dilate and constrict, regulating the amount of light entering the eye. The iris is a muscle that controls the size of the pupil. Most of the eye's interior is filled with vitreous, a gel-like substance helping the eye maintain a round shape. There is a flexible, transparent lens that focuses light which hits the retina (the back of the eye). The retina converts light energy into a nerve impulse carried to the brain and it is then interpreted. See Figure 46.1.

Glaucoma

Glaucoma is known colloquially as the sneak thief of sight. The leading cause of irreversible blindness globally is glaucoma. First-degree relatives of glaucoma patients have an eight-fold increased risk of developing this condition. Black ethnicity, raised intraocular pressure, myopia and diabetes mellitus are also risk factors. Risk increases with age. A significant proportion of people with glaucoma (around 50%) are undiagnosed.

Glaucoma is the name given to a group of eye diseases in which the optic nerve is slowly destroyed. In most people, this damage is usually (but not always) due to increased pressure inside the eye, the result of a blockage of the circulation of aqueous, or its drainage. In some people, the damage may be caused by poor or reduced supply of blood to the optic nerve fibres, there may be a weakness in the structure of the nerve and/or a problem with the nerve fibres themselves.

Glaucoma is classified as congenital or acquired and is further subdivided into open-angle or closed-angle glaucoma, depending on how the aqueous outflow is impaired. Primary or secondary types of the condition are identified depending on the existence of any underlying contributory factors.

Signs and symptoms

Symptoms of open-angle glaucoma

Usually there are no early warning signs or symptoms associated with open-angle glaucoma. This type of glaucoma develops slowly and occasionally without noticeable sight loss for a number of years. Generally most people who have open-angle glaucoma are well and do not notice a change in their vision; this is because the initial loss is of side or peripheral vision and the visual acuity or sharpness of vision is maintained until late in the disease. When a patient becomes aware of vision loss, the disease is often relatively advanced.

Loss of vision caused by glaucoma cannot be reversed with treatment, even with surgery. As open-angle glaucoma has few warning signs or symptoms before damage has happened, regular eye examinations are important.

Symptoms of closed-angle glaucoma

- Misty or blurred vision
- The appearance of rainbow-coloured circles around bright lights
- Severe eye and head pain
- Nausea or vomiting (accompanying severe eye pain)
- Sudden sight loss

Blocked drainage canals in the eye cause this type of glaucoma; this then results in a sudden rise in intraocular pressure. The condition develops very quickly and demands immediate medical attention (this is a much more rare form of glaucoma). Compared to open-angle glaucoma, symptoms of acute angle-closure glaucoma are very noticeable and damage occurs quickly. Anyone experiencing any of these symptoms should seek immediate care.

Investigations and diagnosis

Regular, detailed and comprehensive eye examination is the key to protecting vision from damage caused by glaucoma. A detailed medical history and examination are essential in order to make the diagnosis. See Table 46.1.

Care and treatment

A number of medications (a combination may be prescribed) can be used to treat glaucoma. Medications are intended to reduce raised intraocular pressure and prevent optic nerve damage. Eye drops work by decreasing eye pressure by helping the fluid of the eye to drain more effectively and/or decreasing the amount of fluid produced by the eye. The drugs used to treat glaucoma are classified by their active ingredient.

- Prostaglandin analogs (increase the outflow of intraocular fluid from the eye)
- Beta-blockers (decrease production of intraocular fluid)
- Alpha-agonists (decrease production of fluid and increase drainage)
- Carbonic anhydrase inhibitors (reduce eye pressure by decreasing the production of intraocular fluid, available as eye drops and in tablets)

Combination drugs are available for those who require more than one type of medication. The nurse must explain to the patient how the drops are to be used, for how long and how to store them.

There is no cure for glaucoma but it can usually be controlled and further loss of sight can be prevented or at least slowed down. Treatment can save the remaining vision but it does not improve eye sight. Treatments include the following.

- Eye drops: this is the most common form of treatment and must be used regularly. In some cases tablets may be prescribed. The drops are varied in order to best suit the patient and the type of glaucoma.
- Laser trabeculoplasty: this is undertaken when eye drops do not stop deterioration in the field of vision. In most cases eye drops will need to be continued after trabeculoplasty. This procedure can usually be performed as a day case.
- Trabeculectomy: this is performed after eye drops and laser have failed to control the pressure in the eye. A new channel is created in order for the fluid to leave the eye.

47 Conjunctivitis

Figure 47.1 Conjunctivitis

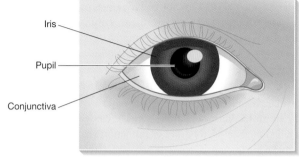

Iris
Pupil
Conjunctiva

Normal eye

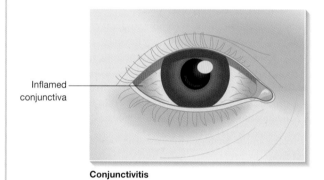

Inflamed conjunctiva

Conjunctivitis

Figure 47.2 Test for visual acuity

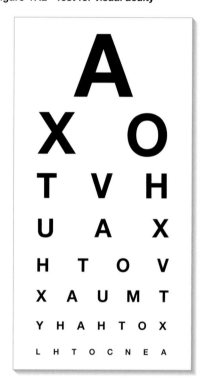

Figure 47.3 Instillation of eye ointment

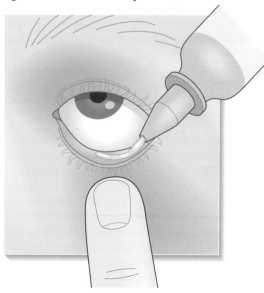

How to administer an ophthalmic ointment

- Wash hands

- Hold the ointment tube in the hand for a few minutes to warm and soften the ointment

- Gently cleanse the affected eyelid with warm water and a soft cloth before applying the ointment

- With the affected eye looking upward, gently pull the lower eyelid downward with the index finger to form a pouch.

- Squeeze a thin line (approximately ¼ – ½ inch) of the ointment along the pouch. **DO NOT** allow the tip of the ointment tube to touch the eyelid, the eyeball, finger, or any surface

- Close the eye gently and rotate the eyeball to distribute the ointment. Blink several times to evenly spread the ointment.

- Replace the cap on the ointment tube

- After applying the ointment, vision may be blurred temporarily. This will clear up in a short while, do not drive a car or operate machinery until vision has cleared

Medical-Surgical Nursing at a Glance, First Edition. Ian Peate. © John Wiley & Sons, Ltd. Published 2016 by John Wiley & Sons, Ltd.
Companion website: www.ataglanceseries.com/nursing/medsurg

The conjunctiva

The conjunctiva is the thin, transparent tissue covering the outer surface of the eye. It begins at the outer edge of the cornea, covering the visible aspect of the sclera, and it lines the inside of the eyelids. The conjunctiva is nourished by many very small blood vessels that are nearly invisible to the naked eye. The conjunctiva also secretes oils and mucus that provide moisture and lubricate the eye, permitting it to move freely in its socket. The conjunctiva is composed of three sections or regions.

- The palpebral: lines the undersurface of the eyelids
- The bulbar: covers the front, external eyeball
- The fornix: this forms the junction located between the eyelid and eyeball

The palpebral is moderately thick, although the bulbar is very thin and movable and easily slides back and forth over the front of the eyeball that it covers. As the bulbar is clear, it is easy to see the underlying blood vessels. Within the bulbar, conjunctivae are 'goblet cells' which secrete an important part of the precorneal tear layer, that protects and nourishes the cornea. The fornix is a loose pocket of conjunctiva between the upper eyelid and the eyeball, permitting the eyeball to rotate freely.

Conjunctivitis

The term conjunctivitis covers any form of conjunctival inflammation (Figure 47.1). When the eye is irritated or injured, or if it is infected, these tiny blood vessels dilate and this makes the white part of the eye look red. Bacteria and viruses can cause an inflammation of the conjunctiva and this can lead to conjunctivitis. Whilst the conjunctiva is usually a tough, resilient tissue, it may be lacerated with sharp or pointed objects such as a fingernail, tree branches or the edge of a piece of paper. Infections, inflammatory conditions and trauma can all potentially extend from one structure to the other. Conjunctivitis is usually accompanied by blepheritis and this will also need treatment.

A number of micro-organisms can infect the conjunctiva; bacterial infections include:

- *Staphylococcus aureus*
- *Staphylococcus epidermidis*
- *Streptococcus pneumoniae*
- *Haemophilus influenzae*
- *Neisseria gonorrhoeae*
- *Chlamydia trachomatis*.

The common viral infections causing conjunctivitis include:

- adenoviruses
- herpes virus.

Systemic childhood viral infection such as measles or chicken pox can also result in conjunctival involvement.

Non-infective conjunctivitis (allergic conjunctivitis) typically occurs after exposure to pollen or some other form of allergen.

Signs and symptoms

Bacterial conjunctivitis is usually seen as a sticky red eye with an acute onset, often accompanied by itching, a burning sensation or a feeling of grit in the eye (grittiness). There is little or no impact on the person's vision. Onset is usually unilateral but bilateral involvement usually occurs soon after.

The eyelid swells, there is conjunctival hyperaemia and a purulent discharge is present. This discharge can cause mild blurring of vision; if visual acuity is reduced then further investigation concerning the cause is needed. The conjunctival papillae have the appearance of velvet.

Bacterial and viral conjunctivitis are symptomatically similar but the discharge with viral conjunctivitis is watery as opposed to purulent. Discharge at night will cause the eyelids to become sticky when waking. As with bacterial infection, this is unilateral but then progresses to both eyes with the typical itching and grittiness. Where the papillae in bacterial conjunctivitis have a velvet appearance, in viral conjunctivitis they resemble grains of rice. There may be concomitant systemic symptoms such as pyrexia and respiratory tract infection. There may be preauricular lymphadenopathy and eyelid swelling that can result in eye closure. If the infection is due to herpes simplex virus, there may be a vesicular rash.

Non-infective conjunctivitis (allergic conjunctivitis) is rapid in onset and causes itching, lid swelling, eye watering and conjunctival oedema, which usually settle spontaneously after a few hours.

Investigations and diagnosis

The initial eye examination includes measurement of visual acuity (Figure 47.2) along with an external and internal eye examination using an ophthalmoscope. The person may report that they have had recent contact with conjunctivitis.

Clinical examination and the taking of a history are usually sufficient to make a diagnosis of conjunctivitis in the majority of cases. There are some cases where further diagnostic tests would be helpful. In all cases of suspected infectious neonatal conjunctivitis, cultures of the conjunctiva are required. Bacterial cultures may also be of value for recurrent or severe purulent conjunctivitis when the condition has failed to respond to medication.

Laboratory advice should be obtained concerning viral cultures, as these are not routinely used to establish a diagnosis. If adult and neonatal chlamydial conjunctivitis is suspected, this can be confirmed by laboratory testing. Immunologically based diagnostic tests are available.

A conjunctival biopsy can be helpful where conjunctivitis is unresponsive to therapy. Directed biopsy may be a vision- and life-saving investigation if a neoplasm is suspected.

Care and treatment

The majority of cases of bacterial conjunctivitis are self-limiting and do not require treatment. A broad-spectrum antibiotic (for example, chloramphenicol) is often prescribed (Figure 47.3). If the infection does not respond to this treatment then a swab will be taken and sent for microscopy and culture. The patient may be referred to an ophthalmologist if there are atypical features or the infection persists.

Viral conjunctivitis without treatment will often settle within around 2 weeks but the stickiness (usually after waking), irritation and redness can continue for months. Aciclovir (an antiviral medication) administered topically may be effective against herpes simplex virus.

Symptom control (i.e. itchiness) can include the administration of antihistamine. Artificial tears can promote comfort and soothe the eyes and prophylactic administration of topical antibiotics may be advised.

48 Age-Related Macular Degeneration

Figure 48.1 The eye showing the position of the macula

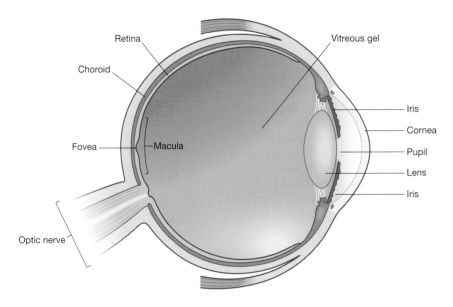

- Retina
- Choroid
- Fovea
- Macula
- Optic nerve
- Vitreous gel
- Iris
- Cornea
- Pupil
- Lens
- Iris

Figure 48.2 Normal macula and degenerated

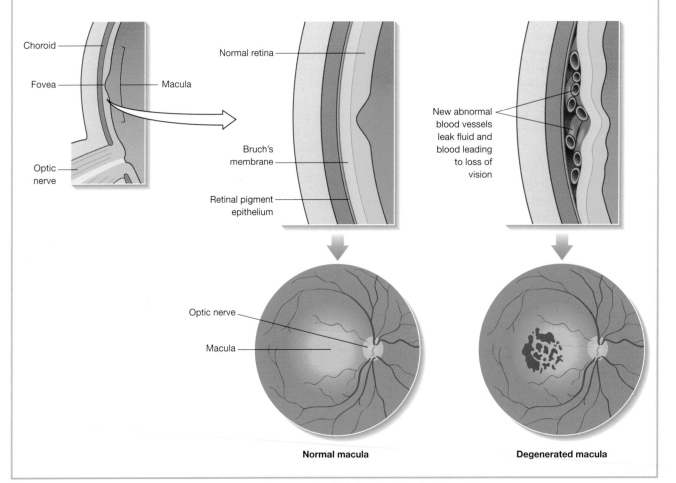

- Choroid
- Fovea
- Macula
- Optic nerve
- Normal retina
- Bruch's membrane
- Retinal pigment epithelium
- New abnormal blood vessels leak fluid and blood leading to loss of vision
- Optic nerve
- Macula

Normal macula

Degenerated macula

Medical-Surgical Nursing at a Glance, First Edition. Ian Peate. © John Wiley & Sons, Ltd. Published 2016 by John Wiley & Sons, Ltd.
Companion website: www.ataglanceseries.com/nursing/medsurg

There are a number of age-related conditions that can affect the eyes; these are more pronounced after the age of 40 years. By the time they reach 70 years, the majority of people will need some type of visual aid as the elasticity of the eye decreases with age, focusing becomes affected, tear film is reduced, leading to tears being evaporated more quickly, and dryness and irritation ensue. However, some older people complain of excess watering of the eyes as a result of muscle weakness and malposition of the eyelids.

Age-related macular degeneration (AMD)

This condition is the major cause of blindness in the developed world. Primarily AMD affects the central and colour vision (Figures 48.1, 48.2). The person notices that they are having difficulty with some activity such as reading or sewing; they may also have some problems in recognising faces and identifying coins. Distorted and burred vision can occur when new blood vessels have developed, lifting the central retina, but peripheral vision is maintained.

Classification

There are two types of AMD – wet and dry. These can also appear with other eye conditions (co-morbidities) such as cataract or glaucoma. This can lead to complications concerning the diagnosis and the treatment to be offered.

Ageing (as the name of the condition suggests) and smoking are the most common risk factors associated with the development of AMD. The condition may be hereditary; if a family member has or had the condition, the risk for developing macular degeneration may be higher. Hypertension, high cholesterol, obesity and being light-skinned are also risk factors for macular degeneration. AMD is more common among Caucasians.

Dry AMD

In the majority of people it is usual for AMD to begin with the dry type, which develops slowly and in most cases the symptoms it causes are mild. There can, however, be marked visual loss with advanced dry AMD. If dry AMD occurs unilaterally there is an increased risk of this occurring in the other unaffected eye.

Wet AMD

This is a chronic condition. This type of AMD can very quickly damage the macula and cause rapid and severe visual loss. Wet AMD is generally caused by abnormal blood vessels that leak fluid or blood into the region of the macula.

Signs and symptoms

In the early stages of AMD the person may be asymptomatic and the condition can go unrecognised until it progresses or affects both eyes. AMD may also be an incidental finding during an eye examination. Often, the first sign of macular degeneration is distortion of straight lines (straight lines that appear crooked). The centre of vision becomes distorted. Dark, blurry areas or white-out appears in the centre of vision. There may also be diminished or changed colour perception.

This can then progress to a gradual loss of central vision.

A common presentation is difficulty with reading, initially with the smallest sizes of print and then later with larger print. Patients also report difficulty in performing tasks that require visual discrimination, for example, driving, reading and recognising faces.

Investigations and diagnosis

Only a comprehensive dilated eye examination can detect AMD. A detailed patient history should be taken. The eye exam may include a visual acuity test and dilated eye examination, in which drops are placed into the eyes to dilate the pupils, which provides a better view of the back of the eye. The retina and optic nerve are looked at using a special magnifying lens for signs of AMD and for any other eye problems. As changes in central vision may occur, an Asler grid can be used; central vision changes will cause the lines in the grid to disappear or appear wavy which is a sign of AMD. Retinal imaging is an essential aspect of patient management and is required for making a diagnosis and monitoring any response to therapy.

A fluorescein angiogram may be performed; an intravenous fluorescent dye is injected into the arm whilst images are taken as the dye passes through the blood vessels in the eye. This provides an opportunity to identify if there are any leaking blood vessels. Optical coherence tomography (OCT) uses light waves, and can achieve very high-resolution images of any tissues that can be penetrated by light, such as the eyes. OCT is used to support the initial diagnosis and help assess the severity of the disease.

Care and treatment

Whilst AMD is rarely a totally blinding condition, it can be a source of significant visual disability. The nurse will need to give consideration to the needs of the visually impaired person. The person will require physical and also psychosocial support. Care should be planned using a systematic approach and the nurse has to be aware of the degree of assistance the visually impaired person may need. This must be undertaken with respect and compassion by ensuring the individual remains as independent as possible.

There is no cure for AMD but treatments can prevent severe vision loss or slow disease progression considerably. A number of treatment options are available, and these include antiangiogenic drugs that are injected into the eye to prevent or block the development of new blood vessels and leakage from the abnormal vessels that cause wet macular degeneration. The patient may require follow-up treatments.

High-energy laser light therapy can be used to destroy any growing abnormal blood vessels that occur. Photodynamic laser therapy is a two-step treatment, in which photoreactive chemicals are injected into the patient and irradiated with light that is strong enough to activate the chemicals, causing them to emit free radicals and destroy the targeted abnormal cells.

Radiation therapy, other medicines and surgery to the retina (such as submacular surgery and retinal translocation) are being investigated. Research in this area is ongoing.

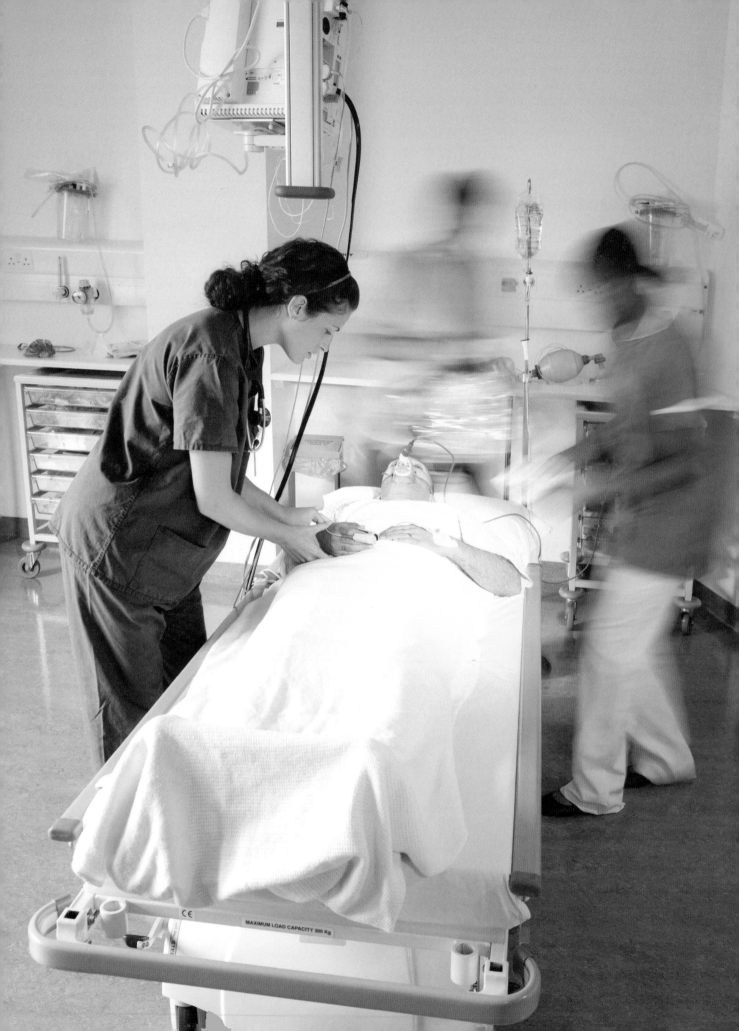

Surgical nursing

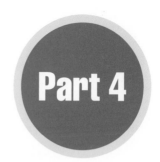

Part 4

Chapters

49 Preoperative Care

Table 49.1 Types of surgery

Classification	Description
Diagnostic	Surgery that is undertaken to confirm or make a diagnosis
Palliative	This type of surgery aims to relieve pain or to reduce the symptoms caused by a disease
Ablative	Surgery carried out in order to remove diseased body parts
Constructive	This type of surgery restores function or appearance that has been lost or reduced
Transplant	The aim here is to replace (to transplant) malfunctioning structures

Table 49.2 Types of surgery and degree of urgency along with the perceived degree of risk

Type of surgery	Description
Emergency surgery	Needs to be performed immediately to save life, limb to preserve function
Urgent surgery	Usually undertaken within hours of the decision to operate for events that may possibly threaten life, limb or function or for the relief of pain
Expedited surgery	Surgery undertaken within days of the decision to operate and where the condition is not an immediate threat to life, limb or function
Elective surgery	Performed when surgery is the preferred treatment the aim is to achieve the required outcome for the patient. This type of surgery is planned and booked in advance
Surgery may also be categorised according to risk	
Major surgery	This is associated with a high degree of risk it may be a complex procedure and prolonged operation. There may be a large loss of blood and vital organs may be involved
Minor surgery	Minor surgery brings with it little risk; there may be some potential complications. Generally this is performed as day or short stay surgery

Table 49.3 Information giving

- An outline of the procedure
- Preoperative preparation
- The operating theatre environment
- Postoperative expectations (including length of stay)
- Details of the anaesthesia

Medical-Surgical Nursing at a Glance, First Edition. Ian Peate. © John Wiley & Sons, Ltd. Published 2016 by John Wiley & Sons, Ltd.
Companion website: www.ataglanceseries.com/nursing/medsurg

The opening chapters of this text have provided the reader with principles of care from a general perspective and these can be applied to medical and surgical nursing. The remaining chapters are concerned with surgical nursing. Technology continues to make advances in the field of surgery. The introduction of robotics into the operating theatre has assisted surgeons in their quest to advance and make safer the care of the person who is undergoing surgery. The control, decision making and knowledge required, however, remain with the surgeon. Many surgical procedures are still carried out by direct hand of the surgeon. In some instances, appropriately prepared and educated nurses are also undertaking certain surgical procedures.

Surgery is usually categorised according to its purpose (Table 49.1) as well as degree of urgency and risk (Table 49.2).

Minimally invasive surgery, often called 'keyhole' surgery, includes laparoscopic procedures; the use of minimally invasive surgery continues to expand but it requires specific expertise and specialist equipment. This technique reduces wound size, decreases undesired inflammatory responses and pain and has the potential to reduce recovery time and prompt an earlier patient discharge. Preoperative assessment determines those patients who are suitable for this type of surgery as not all people are suitable, for example, those who are obese or who have undergone previous surgery to the proposed operative site.

Preoperative care

Often successful postoperative outcomes are dependent upon effective preoperative care. The preoperative phase begins when the patient makes the decision to undergo the recommended surgical procedure and culminates when the patient is transferred into the operating theatre. Whilst the decision to offer surgery rests with the surgeon, the decision to undergo surgery remains with the patient, unless the patient is deemed incompetent to make the decision.

As the patient enters the preoperative phase of the surgical journey, the impact of the decision to undergo surgery will vary from person to person – many will be nervous and anxious. The role of the nurse is multifaceted and will include caring for the person from a biopsychosocial perspective, educating, reassuring, preventing potential complications and alleviating anxiety.

Anxiety

Often patients are anxious about the anaesthetic and surgery, and feel fear of the unknown, of death and dying and of the treatment, and may have concerns about pain and safety. Anxiety causes a number of unwanted physical responses, such as tachycardia, hypertension, sweating and nausea as well as psychological responses including behavioural changes, increased tension, apprehension, aggression, nervousness and withdrawal.

Information giving

Addressing the psychological needs of the patient can reduce the risk of complications and improve postoperative outcomes. Providing information and giving the patient time to ask questions will reduce preoperative anxiety but this must be tailored to each person's unique needs. Other anxiety reduction strategies may include the use of medication to reduce preoperative anxiety, distraction techniques and relaxation techniques, for example, visualisation or deep breathing. Information provided preoperatively varies depending on the surgical procedure (Table 49.3).

Preoperative teaching

The type/content of preoperative teaching will depend on the person's individual needs; the aim is to aid the patient in their postoperative recovery. This includes deep breathing exercises in order to reduce the incidence of chest infection when the patient has reduced mobility and is not taking breaths deep enough to expand the lungs; an incentive spirometer aids deep breathing exercises. Leg exercises are taught in an attempt to diminish the effects of reduced mobility on the circulation. Usually, it is preferable for the patient to mobilise as soon as possible after surgery; this increases lung expansion and improves circulation. Reduced mobility leads to venous stasis and this may lead to the development of deep vein thrombosis and a pulmonary embolus.

Teaching splinting to support incisions when coughing is important, particularly in those who are to undergo abdominal or thoracic surgery, as they are less likely to cough post surgery; they may be frightened that the sudden pressure will damage the suture line as well as the fear of increased pain.

Preparing for surgery

The patient will be required to be nil by mouth for a set period. Those who are nil by mouth should be offered mouthcare. Only those medications deemed medically necessary should be administered. A premedication may be prescribed for a variety of reasons and may be taken with up to 60 mL of water. Time-critical premedication, for example eye drops or antibiotics, must be given as prescribed.

Rigorous skin decolonisation may be required for some types of surgery. Nail polish and make-up should be removed prior to surgery. If hair removal is required, it should be done on the day of surgery using depilatory cream or electric clippers with a single-use disposable head. Jewellery should be removed if possible; all metal jewellery increases the risk of burns where diathermy is used in theatre; local policy should be adhered to.

Antiembolic stockings and/or low molecular weight heparin injections may be required.

Details on the patient's wristband must be checked with the patient and against the medical notes, X-rays, test results and nursing documentation. Allergies should be documented and recorded on a suitable allergy wristband.

The operating surgeon should mark the site of surgery with an indelible marker prior to the patient receiving any medication that may cause drowsiness.

Checklists

At all times the nurse must adhere to local policy and procedures with regard to any checklists in use. Surgical checklists are used in the preoperative period throughout the UK. The checklist ensures that mandatory issues have not been omitted or forgotten with the intention of reducing risk and ensuring patient safety.

Maintaining a patient's dignity while they are waiting for surgery is important. They may be wearing a surgical gown (with the opening to the rear) and patients often complain that the gowns do not keep them covered. Wherever possible, the patient may keep on their underwear until the moment they are to be transferred. Those who have a dressing gown should be encouraged to wear it, those without should be given a second surgical gown to wear in place of a dressing gown.

50 Perioperative Care

Table 50.1 Sample of patient care plan

Preoperative patient checklist	Yes	No	N/A

Patient details
- Name, address, hospital number:
- Patient documents present:
- Consent form:
- Allergies:
- Operation site marked:
- Blood results:
- ECG results:
- Fasted as per policy:

Medication
- Premed:
- Medications taken:
- Anticoagulants:

Personal
- Contact lenses removed:
- Glasses removed:
- Dentures removed:
- Status of teeth:
  (caps, crowns, bridges, etc.)
- Make-up and nail varnish removed:
- Hearing aid:
- Prosthesis:
- Pacemaker:
- Patient is safe on trolley:
- Ward nurse name and signature:

Anaesthetic care

- Anaesthetic: General, spinal, epidural, regional, local

- Airway equipment:

- Monitoring sites: ECG, pulse oximeter, arterial line, CVP, other

- Peripheral IV access:

- Airway maintenance:

- Skin integrity:

- Nasogastric tube:

- Drugs used:

Intraoperative care plan – circle, tick or complete using text as appropriate

Position
- Supine
- Lithotomy
- Left lateral
- Right lateral
- Prone
- Knee/elbow
- Other:

Arm position
- At side
- On arm board
- Palm down
- Palm up
- Palm at side
- Concerns:

Aids used
- Arm boards
- Tissue support mattress
- Warming blanket
- Bair Hugger
- Other warming device:
- Arm retainer
- Heel support
- Lloyd Davies stirrups
- Lithotomy stirrups
- Head support
- Sacral wedge
- Lateral support
- Pillows
- Flowtron boots
- Other:

Concerns

Electrosurgery
- Monopolar Bipolar
- Patient plate site:
- Shaved:
- Concerns:

Skin preparation
- Chlorhexidine
- Betadine
- Other:

Skin closure
- Absorbable steristrips
- Clips Non-absorbable
- Other:

Dressings
  Adhesive   Melonin
  Velband   Backslab
  Crepe   Tegaderm
  Plaster of Paris
  Jelonet
- Other:

Specimens
- Specify:

  Histology   Microbiology
  Cytology   Frozen section
- Specimen sent:

Tourniquet
- Position: Left Right
- Arm
- Leg
- Finger
- Toe
- Time on:
- Time off:
- Pressure:
- Concerns:

Urinary catheter
- 2-way catheter
- 3-way catheter
- Suprapubic
- Bladder irrigation
- Balloon (mL)
- Catheter type and size:

Dressing packs
- Pack *in situ*:
- Site:

Wound drains
- Suction
- Site:
- Non-suction
- Site:
- Chest drain
- Site:
- Other:
  Specimens:
- Specify:

Postoperative inspection
- Airway status
- Skin integrity
- Diathermy site
- Tourniquet site
- Peripheral perfusion of limbs

Surgical procedure
- Final count correct: Register completed:
- Computer record completed:
- Final count incorrect (specify reasons):
- Surgeon informed: X ray taken: Incident form completed:

Comments, concerns and handover information

Medical-Surgical Nursing at a Glance, First Edition. Ian Peate. © John Wiley & Sons, Ltd. Published 2016 by John Wiley & Sons, Ltd.
Companion website: www.ataglanceseries.com/nursing/medsurg

Perioperative care or the intraoperative phase begins when the patient arrives in the operating theatre and concludes when transferred to the recovery area. However, for some, 'perioperative' can also refer to the entire surgical experience, including the pre-, intra- and postoperative phases of the person's surgical journey.

Preoperative visiting

In order to ensure that the person's perioperative journey is safe, it is essential to prepare them for their perioperative journey. Safe preparation will help to achieve the best possible results after surgery and anaesthesia. Preoperative visiting of the patient can be seen as the first step towards the provision of high-quality care. The anaesthetist, theatre nurse or operating department practitioner may undertake the preoperative visit.

Perioperative care planning

The provision of perioperative care throughout the perioperative journey is usually undertaken through the formulation of a perioperative care plan (Table 50.1). It should be noted that the perioperative care plan also includes aspects of care that are related to the preoperative phase of the patient journey. The plan of care must be focused on meeting the individual needs of the person. A holistic approach to care provision requires the nurse to consider the person's physical, psychosocial and spiritual needs.

Perioperative care plans are used to document the care that was provided. Most care plans contain elements of the following: preoperative checklist, surgical safety checklist, care received in the anaesthetic room, intraoperative care interventions and postoperative care.

Preoperative checks

There are several points along the patient's journey where the preoperative checklist is considered, for example, on the ward and then again when the person is admitted to the operating department. The various points at which the checks are made demonstrate the whole team's commitment to the health and safety of the person who is to undergo surgery.

Checks will be made on the completion and signing of the consent form, to determine if the person has any known allergies, to ascertain if any preoperative investigations were undertaken, the type of investigation(s) and the results, to learn about any medication the patient has taken, has been given or is currently using, to check for the presence of any jewellery, the use of any communication aids such as spectacles, contact lenses or a hearing aid, and if the person has any loose teeth, caps, crown or dentures (partial or full palate).

It is essential that all discussions and the checks undertaken concerning the patient's condition are documented and shared with the whole care team as well as any treatment that has been carried out. Perioperative practitioners may use a number of processes including sign in, time out and sign out procedures. There may also be a group meeting that takes place during the 'sign in' phase, the point of which is to ensure that team members are aware of their roles, responsibilities and duties associated with the intended plan of care (the person's treatment). The overarching aim of these checks and the 'sign in' meeting is to reduce the risk of errors occurring during surgery and during the initiation and continued administration of anaesthesia during surgery.

Communication between all healthcare staff, perioperative staff and the patient is paramount if the patient's specific needs are to be identified at an early stage. Preparation undertaken by perioperative staff can ensure that the patient's needs are met.

The perioperative environment

Preparation of the perioperative environment begins prior to the arrival of the patient. Of all clinical environments, it could be suggested that the perioperative environment is possibly one of the most hazardous.

The patient is escorted to the operating theatre by a registered nurse or staff who have been deemed competent. A number of checks are made such as checking the patient's identity and ensuring the operating consent form is signed and complete. Local policy and procedure will demand that the patient's notes and all relevant documentation are completed before the patient is transferred to theatre.

The patient may be anxious at this stage and perioperative healthcare staff must communicate effectively to ensure that the patient understands the actions being performed as well as giving them the opportunity to ask questions.

Assessment at this stage will form the basis for the delivery of high standards of patient care. Parents or other adults may escort a child or young patient to theatre and perioperative care therefore extends to the whole family.

The anaesthetic room

Care provided in the anaesthetic room usually includes recording and monitoring vital signs and identifying the type of anaesthetic required and whether there are any particular anaesthetic needs.

Intraoperative care

Patient and staff safety is key throughout the perioperative care stage, with proactive clinical risk management strategies in place. During the intraoperative phase, the patient is vulnerable and totally dependent on perioperative healthcare staff. Potential risks are associated with surgical access and positioning, risk of infection, danger of developing deep vein thrombosis, risk of hypothermia and risk to staff and patients from the use of equipment. For each risk, strategies should be in place to minimise harm to patients and staff.

All swabs, instruments, needles and other sharps are counted and must be accounted for at all times throughout the procedure; a 'swab board' is used to record these on. This is done whenever there are any invasive procedures where swabs, instruments or needles might accidentally be retained.

Ensuring that risks are managed or the impact of harm is minimised in the pre- and perioperative period can mean that in the postoperative period the patient will make a quicker, safer recovery.

When the procedure concludes, the perioperative care plan is completed. The patient is prepared for transfer to the recovery room or postanaesthetic unit; this may involve moving the patient to another bed or trolley. It is essential to preserve the patient's dignity and to ensure that their safety is maintained. After safe transfer of the patient, cleaning of the theatre can commence using an evidence-based approach and in accordance with hospital policy and procedure.

51 Postoperative Care

Table 51.1   Criteria to be met prior to a patient being discharged from the recovery room

- The patient is fully conscious, is responding to voice or light touch, can maintain a clear airway and has a normal cough reflex
- Respiration and oxygen saturation are satisfactory (10–20 breaths per minute and SpO_2 greater than 92%)
- The cardiovascular system is stable with no unexplained cardiac irregularity or persistent bleeding. The patient's pulse and blood pressure should approximate to normal preoperative values or should be at a level commensurate with the planned postoperative care
- Pain and emesis should be controlled and suitable analgesic and anti-emetic regimens should be prescribed
- Temperature should be within acceptable limits (greater than 36°C)
- Oxygen and fluid therapy should be prescribed when required

Table 51.2   The six physiological parameters associated with the National Early Warning Score (NEWS)

1.	Respiratory rate
2.	Oxygen saturation
3.	Temperature
4.	Systolic blood pressure
5.	Pulse rate
6.	Level of consciousness (patients who have had recent sedation or are receiving opioid analgesia, this will be impaired)

Table 51.3   Issues the nurse must take into consideration prior to discharging the patient from the recovery room to the ward

- Awake with their eyes open
- Extubated
- Maintaining satisfactory blood pressure and pulse
- Is able to lift their head from the pillow on command
- Not hypoxic
- Breathing quietly and comfortably
- Not persistently bleeding from wound sites or into drains
- Appropriate analgesia has been prescribed and is safely established

The handover must incorporate information on:

- The procedure undertaken
- Any complications
- Any changes in treatment from that planned
- A comment on medical and nursing observations

Handover from the recovery nurse to the ward nurse must include comprehensive orders for:

- Vital signs
- Pain control
- Rate and type of IV fluids
- Urine and gastrointestinal fluid output
- Other medications
- Laboratory investigations

Medical-Surgical Nursing at a Glance, First Edition. Ian Peate. © John Wiley & Sons, Ltd. Published 2016 by John Wiley & Sons, Ltd.
Companion website: www.ataglanceseries.com/nursing/medsurg

There are national guidelines concerning postoperative management. In order to ensure that the optimal management of patients occurs throughout the postoperative phase, appropriate clinical assessment and monitoring are necessary. Postoperative care requires preventive management. Regular assessment, appropriate monitoring and timely documentation are central to safe and effective postoperative care.

Postoperative care

The key aims of care provision in the recovery room are to critically evaluate and stabilise the patient postoperatively, to predict and prevent any probable complications and to safeguard the individual's health and well-being until they are able to do this for themselves.

The recovery room is located close to the operating theatre. Practitioners providing care in the recovery room must be skilled and knowledgeable concerning anaesthetic and operating theatre techniques. They must be confident and competent in being able to deal quickly and efficiently with any untoward changes in the patient's condition.

Immediate postoperative care

This aspect of the patient's journey is associated with immediate assessment of the person's condition when they enter the recovery area (sometimes called the recovery room or postanaesthetic unit), and then regular monitoring of vital signs until the patient has recovered enough to return to the ward. The most important aspects to be monitored include breathing, circulation, fluid and electrolyte balance and pain relief. The criteria noted in Table 51.1 must be satisfied prior to a patient being discharged from the recovery room.

In the recovery room, recorded observations will include blood pressure, respiration, condition of wound, type, patency and position of wound drains, central venous pressure, temperature and pulse. Prior to discharge, recovery staff should record in the notes that patients have met the criteria.

Healthcare staff should record the following items in the case notes: the anaesthetic, surgical or intraoperative complications, any specific postoperative instructions regarding potential problems, any particular treatment or prophylaxis needed (such as fluids, nutrition, antibiotics, analgesia, antiemetics, thromboprophylaxis).

National Early Warning Score

The National Early Warning Score (NEWS) provides a national standard for assessing, monitoring and tracking acutely and critically ill adults. The NEWS has six physiological parameters (Table 51.2).

As well as assessing the postoperative patient using NEWS, they must also be observed for signs of haemorrhage, shock and sepsis as well as the effects of any analgesia administered and their response to the anaesthetic. Those people who are receiving intravenous opiates must be closely observed for the side effects associated with this type of medication. There are a number of potential problems that could put the person at risk of deterioration in conscious levels.

Vital signs must be carried out with due regard to local policies or guidelines and a comparison should be made with the baseline observations obtained in the perioperative period, during surgery and the preoperative period and in the recovery room. An understanding of the parameters for these observations and what is normal for the patient is required. A holistic perspective should be adopted when carrying out observations on a patient who is recovering from anaesthesia and surgery; the nurse should look at the patient and physically touch them even if vital signs are performed using adjuncts.

If a patient's condition is deteriorating, the nurse must pass this information on verbally to an appropriate senior healthcare professional using the SBAR tool – citing the Situation, Background, Assessment and Recommendation.

Often if there is a change in cardiac or neurological status, the respiratory rate and function is usually the first vital sign affected. The nurse should observe and record the following:

• the person's airway, noting respiratory rate, rhythm and depth
• hypoventilation or bradypnoea: this can indicate respiratory depression and may be due to the use of opiates or anaesthetic gases. Oxygen therapy may be prescribed to help anaesthetic gases to be transported out of the body. The following should be recorded: the prescribed oxygen therapy, how the oxygen is administered and the rate. Continuous oxygen therapy should be humidified
• whether the person received an epidural, is receiving patient-controlled analgesia or is on a morphine infusion.

Acceptable oxygen saturation (pulse oximetry) should be above 95% on air, unless the patient has lung disease, and be maintained above 95% if oxygen therapy is prescribed to prevent hypoxia or hypoxaemia. The following should be checked and recorded: rate, rhythm and volume of pulse, blood pressure, capillary refill time to assess circulatory status, the colour and temperature of limbs.

Attention should be paid to the systolic blood pressure, as lowered systolic reading and tachycardia may indicate haemorrhage and/or shock. Tachycardia may indicate that the person is in pain, has fluid overload or is anxious. Hypertension can be the result of the anaesthetic or inadequate pain control.

Some patients are at risk of hypothermia. Shivering can be due to anaesthesia or pyrexia indicative of an infection; a fall in temperature could suggest bacterial infection or sepsis.

Postoperative patients usually respond to verbal stimulation, can answer questions and should be aware of their surroundings prior to being transferred to the ward.

The nurse must record postoperative fluid balance. The following should be recorded on the fluid balance chart: the administration of intravenous fluids, oral intake and urinary output. The presence of nausea and vomiting and the effect of any antiemetics administered should also be recorded. Nasogastric tube drainage, colour and amount of wound drainage are important observations to note and record. Large amounts of fresh blood could be an indication of haemorrhage.

Table 51.3 outlines the issues that the nurse must take into consideration prior to discharging the patient from the recovery room to the ward.

52 Thoracotomy

Figure 52.1 Types of lung surgery

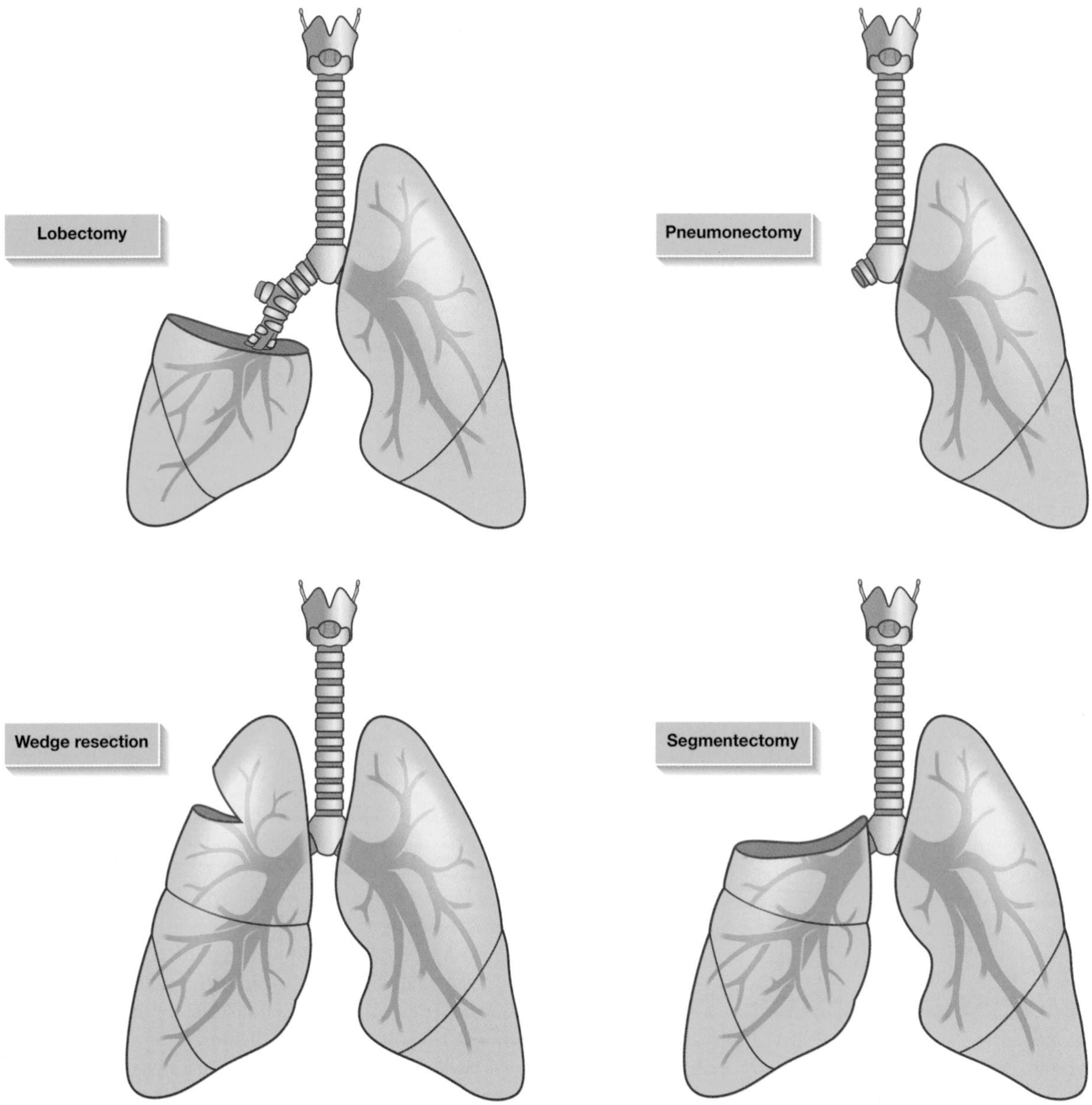

Lobectomy

Pneumonectomy

Wedge resection

Segmentectomy

Table 52.1 Some types of thoracotomy

Procedure	Description
Limited anterior or lateral thoracotomy	An incision is made between the ribs on the front or side of the chest. This allows access to the structures and organs in the front of the thoracic cavity
Posterolateral thoracotomy	An incision across the side and around the back of the chest. This is a larger incision permitting access to more of the chest, including an entire lung
Sternal splitting thoracotomy	An incision down the front of the chest and through the sternum. This allows access to the entire thorax, including both lungs and the heart

Medical-Surgical Nursing at a Glance, First Edition. Ian Peate. © John Wiley & Sons, Ltd. Published 2016 by John Wiley & Sons, Ltd.
Companion website: www.ataglanceseries.com/nursing/medsurg

The surgical opening of the chest cavity is known as a thoracotomy. This is a major surgery process that permits the surgeon to access the throat, lungs, heart, aorta and diaphragm. Usually, a thoracotomy incision is located on the side of the chest; the exact location depends on the disease, disorder or the underlying condition that is being treated. Some types of thoracotomy can be found in Table 52.1.

Surgery of the lung

There are a number of reasons why a person may undergo lung surgery. Some patients require lung surgery because they have emphysema, they may have lung cancer or some other cancer that has spread to the lungs (metastasised). Surgery may also be required to obtain a sample of lung tissue in order to make a diagnosis.

There are several types of interventions that can be suggested if the person is diagnosed with lung cancer. The most appropriate type of treatment is discussed with the patient and the options can include surgery, radiotherapy, chemotherapy, targeted therapies or a combination of treatments.

Surgery can be performed on the lung and pleura. During surgery, some or all of a lung may need to be removed (Figure 52.1); this often occurs if there is emphysema or a tumour.

Lung biopsy

During lung biopsy a small piece of lung is removed with the aim of assisting with a diagnosis. Usually this is performed using minimally invasive surgery (keyhole surgery) where a small incision is made through which the procedure is performed.

Wedge resection

In this type of surgical intervention an aspect of lung tissue (a wedge) is removed if there is a tumour sited close to the outside of the lung.

Metastasectomy

A metastasectomy is the removal of a small part of the lung that contains cancer that has metastasised. In this procedure, the tumour and small area of surrounding tissue is removed. The number of metastases in the lung will vary from person to person and more than one metastasis could be removed during one operation.

Segmentectomy

This involves removal of part of one of the lobes of the lung. Often this is performed for those patients with bronchiectasis. A thoracotomy is required to perform the procedure.

Lobectomy

In this procedure one or more of the lung's five lobes are removed. Those lobes remaining will gradually expand in order to fill the space left by the removed lobe(s).

Sleeve resection

The upper lobe of the lung is removed as well as part of the main airway. The remaining aspect of the lung is then reattached to the main airway.

Pneumonectomy

In this procedure the whole lung is removed.

Video-assisted thoracoscopy (VATS)

Sometimes this is called keyhole surgery and it involves passing a telescopic camera through small cuts in the chest to examine the lungs or pleura under video guidance. One to three small incisions are made by the surgeon on the side of the chest to insert the camera along with surgical tools that are needed to carry out the surgery. All or part of the lung can be removed, fluid or blood that has accumulated may be drained, and other procedures may also be undertaken. This procedure can lead to less pain and also a faster recovery as opposed to other types of open lung surgery.

Sternotomy

A cut is made through the sternum in order to gain access to the chest cavity.

Risk factors

As with all types of surgery, there are a number of potential risks and these include an allergic response to the anaesthetic and other medications as well as the risk of having to undergo a general anaesthetic.

Risks for any surgery include haemorrhage, potential cardiovascular risks including stroke, cardiac arrest, deep vein thrombosis and infection. Lung surgery can result in failure of the lung to expand, damage to the lungs or blood vessels, pain, pneumothorax and accumulation of fluid in the thoracic cavity.

Preoperative care

Preoperative preparation can help to reduce potential postoperative complications. An in-depth physical examination is undertaken along with a comprehensive health history. A range of medical investigations will be required.

Postoperative care

Length of hospital stay will vary depending on the procedure undertaken. For open thoracotomy, hospital stay is usually 5–7 days and 1–3 days after VATS. It is not uncommon for the patient to be cared for in the intensive care unit after surgery.

Mobility should be resumed as soon as possible after surgery (initially sitting on the side of the bed and walking as and when the person's condition dictates).

A chest drain(s) may be *in situ* to drain fluids. The nurse works with the patient to prevent deep vein thrombosis; subcutaneous anticoagulant is usually prescribed.

Pain management is essential and analgesia is initially given intravenously via a patient-controlled analgesic device, enabling the patient to control how much analgesia they use.

Activities to reduce the risk of chest infection are undertaken such as deep breathing exercises. The chest drain(s) are removed when the lung has fully inflated.

53 Chest Drain

Table 53.1 Indications for chest drain insertion

- Pneumothorax (i.e. tension pneumothorax, persistent or recurring pneumothorax, spontaneous pneumothorax)
- Malignant pleural effusion
- Empyema and complications of pleural effusion
- Traumatic haemopneumothorax
- Postoperative (i.e. thoracotomy, oesophagectomy, cardiac surgery)

Figure 53.1 The pleural space

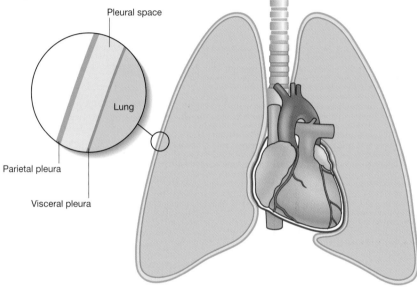

Pleural space

Lung

Parietal pleura

Visceral pleura

Figure 53.2 A chest tube

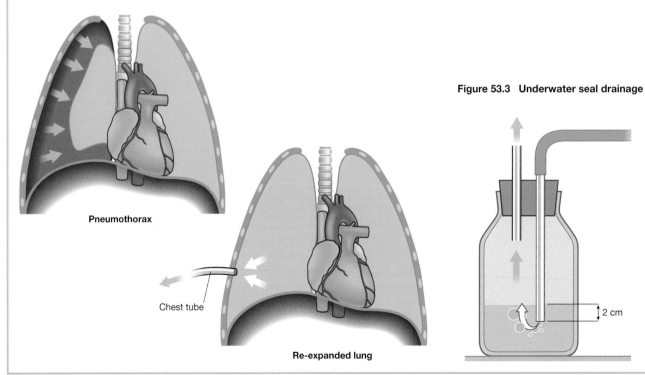

Pneumothorax

Chest tube

Re-expanded lung

Figure 53.3 Underwater seal drainage

2 cm

Medical-Surgical Nursing at a Glance, First Edition. Ian Peate. © John Wiley & Sons, Ltd. Published 2016 by John Wiley & Sons, Ltd.
Companion website: www.ataglanceseries.com/nursing/medsurg

C hest drains (also called chest tubes or underwater seal drains) are used in a variety of clinical settings.

The pleural space

The pleural space (a potential space) is located between the visceral and parietal pleura, held together by a small negative pressure or vacuum, maintaining lung inflation (Figure 53.1). Air or fluid may accumulate in the pleural space. The fluid or air can accumulate rapidly or slowly over a number of days, which can lead to increased difficulty in breathing. Two chest tubes may be required if there is fluid and air in the pleura.

Pleural effusion pertains to fluid collection in the pleura, haemothorax is a collection of blood in the space and if a haemopneumothorax occurs then blood and air are present in this space.

Ventilation

The mechanisms associated with ventilation are concerned with negative intrathoracic pressure drawing air into the lungs, as occurs during spontaneous respiration. This negative pressure is maintained in the pleural space. If there are collections of air, fluid or blood in the pleural space, this will not only compress lung tissue, it will also result in the pleural pressures becoming positive; the consequence of this will be inappropriate ventilation.

Chest tube (Figure 53.2)

A chest tube (or chest drain) drains the contents of the pleural space, which is usually air or blood; there may be other fluids. Indications for chest drain insertion can be found in Table 53.1. The nurse needs to understand how to care for patients with a chest drain *in situ* and how to manage the chest drain in order to maintain respiratory function and haemodynamic stability.

Underwater seal drainage

An underwater seal drain (UWSD) is a particular type of drain which is attached to a chest tube, a long hollow tube inserted between the intercostal spaces and into the pleural space. A combination of intravenous analgesia and local anaesthesia is used for the procedure. Intravenous morphine is often used as the standard analgesia for trauma patients; this should be administered in small doses that are titrated to patient response. It should be remembered that opioids such as morphine may cause respiratory depression. In some instances ketamine can be used as an alternative analgesic.

When the chest tube is inserted and is attached to the UWSD system, the air or fluid will cause 'bubbling' through the water seal that is situated inside the drain. The water seal acts as a one-way valve, preventing the air or fluid flowing back into the pleural space. There are a number of devices available for this.

It is usual for the drainage bottle to be filled with sterile water and the tube must be kept below the water level (2 cm); failure to do this will allow air to enter the pleural cavity during inspiration or if the patient coughs (Figure 53.3). In UWSD the drainage bottle should always be kept below the level of the patient; failure to do this will cause the contents of the bottle to siphon back into the chest cavity. Persistent bubbling of air through the water indicates an air leak from the lung.

The nurse must ensure that chest tubes are never clamped for any reason, so as to avoid the development of a tension pnuemothorax. In some instances, the air outlet of the underwater seal may be connected to moderate suction, which assists in lung re-expansion.

Care and management

The presence of a chest drain can instil fear and anxiety in the patient and family as well as staff (this includes nurses, housekeeping staff and therapists). Understanding the care the person needs as well as the management of the drainage system and offering explanations can help to alieavate these anxieties.

After insertion, the nurse should observe and document the person's respiratory status, the fluid level and amount of any drainage fluid level swing, the presence of underwater bubbling, the dressing site and the patency of the tubing.

Ongoing assessment of the person's overall condition is required, including vital signs such as pulse, blood pressure, temperature, respiration (rate, depth and volume) and SpO_2. Frequency of observations is dictated by the person's condition.

If there is no fluid oscillation, this could signify obstruction of the drainage system caused by clots or kinks, the loss of subatmospheric pressure or a complete re-expansion of the lung.

The person with a chest drain can mobilise as desired (unless this is contraindicated). The nurse must check that all connections are secure and the underwater seal bottle is erect and below the patient's chest. The nurse will be required to assist the person with activities of living they are unable to perform themselves.

Regular pain relief is required for comfort and also to allow the person to complete physiotherapy or mobilise. The nurse should assess pain frequently and document findings and the response to analgesia. Observe for signs of infection and inflammation and document findings; check the dressing is clean and intact and adhere to local policy and procedure. Ensure that sutures remain intact and are secure (this is particularly important in long-term drains where over time sutures could erode).

Physiotherapy referral is required. Regular changes in position are required for those on bedrest to prevent pressure sore formation and to promote drainage, unless there are contraindications.

Removal of the chest drain

The procedure must be explained to the patient. Chest tubes usually remain *in situ* as long as the air or fluid remains in the pleural space. Regular chest X-rays are required to monitor resolution of the problem.

Two people who are competent in the task should undertake removal; one removes the tube and the other occludes the drain site. The tube should be removed either at the end of expiration or at peak inspiration.

The area is cleaned and an occlusive dressing is prepared and held ready. Any stay sutures are removed. The patient should hold their breath, the tube is removed rapidly and the occlusive dressing applied. In some instances a suture is used to close the wound; this may be introduced at the time of drain insertion.

Attend to the patient's comfort and provide analgesia if needed. A chest X-ray should be performed after drain removal. Monitor vital signs closely on removal frequency to be determined based on the person's condition. Document the removal of the drain in the person's notes.

Aftercare

Remove sutures 5 days post drain removal. Dressings remain *in situ* for 24 hours after removal unless dirty. Complications as a result of drain removal include pneumothorax, bleeding and infection of the drain site.

54 Stem Cell Transplantation

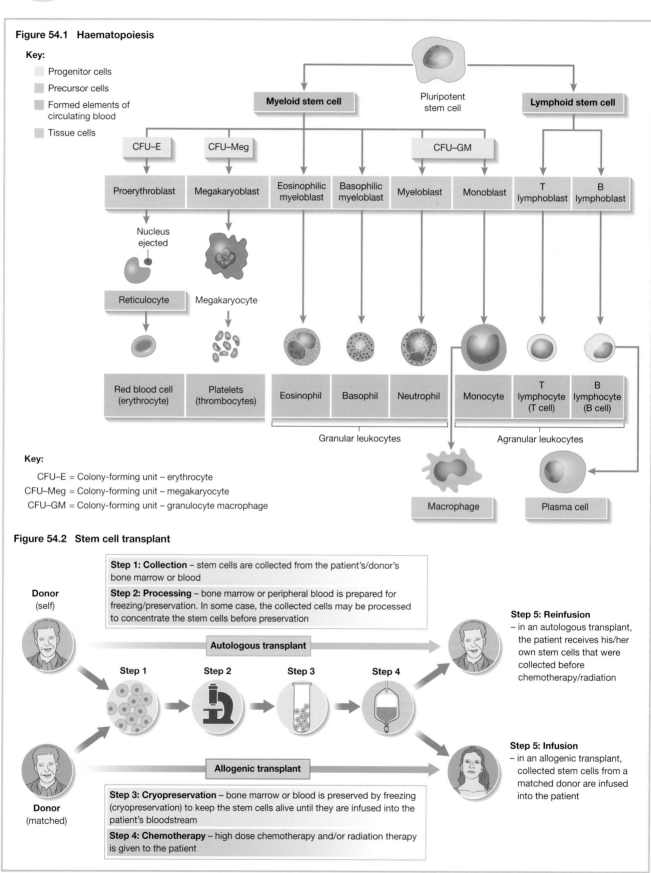

Figure 54.1 Haematopoiesis

Key:
- Progenitor cells
- Precursor cells
- Formed elements of circulating blood
- Tissue cells

Myeloid stem cell

Pluripotent stem cell

Lymphoid stem cell

CFU–E CFU–Meg CFU–GM

Proerythroblast | Megakaryoblast | Eosinophilic myeloblast | Basophilic myeloblast | Myeloblast | Monoblast | T lymphoblast | B lymphoblast

Nucleus ejected

Reticulocyte Megakaryocyte

Red blood cell (erythrocyte) | Platelets (thrombocytes) | Eosinophil | Basophil | Neutrophil | Monocyte | T lymphocyte (T cell) | B lymphocyte (B cell)

Granular leukocytes Agranular leukocytes

Macrophage Plasma cell

Key:
CFU–E = Colony-forming unit – erythrocyte
CFU–Meg = Colony-forming unit – megakaryocyte
CFU–GM = Colony-forming unit – granulocyte macrophage

Figure 54.2 Stem cell transplant

Donor (self)

Autologous transplant

Step 1 Step 2 Step 3 Step 4

Donor (matched)

Allogenic transplant

Step 1: Collection – stem cells are collected from the patient's/donor's bone marrow or blood

Step 2: Processing – bone marrow or peripheral blood is prepared for freezing/preservation. In some case, the collected cells may be processed to concentrate the stem cells before preservation

Step 5: Reinfusion – in an autologous transplant, the patient receives his/her own stem cells that were collected before chemotherapy/radiation

Step 5: Infusion – in an allogenic transplant, collected stem cells from a matched donor are infused into the patient

Step 3: Cryopreservation – bone marrow or blood is preserved by freezing (cryopreservation) to keep the stem cells alive until they are infused into the patient's bloodstream

Step 4: Chemotherapy – high dose chemotherapy and/or radiation therapy is given to the patient

Medical-Surgical Nursing at a Glance, First Edition. Ian Peate. © John Wiley & Sons, Ltd. Published 2016 by John Wiley & Sons, Ltd.
Companion website: www.ataglanceseries.com/nursing/medsurg

A stem cell transplant is sometimes called a blood or marrow transplant. It involves the injection or infusion of healthy stem cells with the aim of replacing damaged or diseased stem cells. A stem cell transplant can also be required when the bone marrow stops producing a sufficient amount of healthy stem cells. The procedure is used to increase the chance of a cure or remission for a variety of cancers and blood dyscrasias. It often involves chemotherapy which is followed by an infusion of stem cells.

Stem cells

In short, stem cells are the body's raw materials. They are the cells from which all other cells with specialised functions are generated. Under the right conditions, stem cells divide to form more cells called daughter cells. The daughter cells either become new stem cells (self-renewal) or they become specialised cells (differentiation) having a more specific function, such as blood cells, kidney cells, heart muscle or bone. Stem cells are the only cells in the body that have the natural ability to generate new cell types. See Figure 54.1 for an overview of haematopoiesis.

Autologous and allogeneic transplantation

Figure 54.2 shows two approaches to stem cell transplantation. In autologous transplantation, the person donates their own blood prior to undergoing treatment (i.e. chemotherapy). In allogeneic transplantation, a donor is matched to the recipient. Stem cells are collected from the donor's bone marrow or blood. Cryopreservation is used to store the collected bone marrow.

Bone marrow transplantation

The bone marrow transplant commences with the harvesting of haematopoietic stem cells from the bone marrow of the person who has cancer when in remission (autologous) or from a donor (allogeneic). The donor may be known, for example, a relative, or unknown; the person has to have closely matched antigens. The procedure is undertaken in the operating theatre by aspiration from the posterior iliac crests. Approximately 1 litre of aspirate is removed, stored and given to the recipient.

Arrangements are made to prepare the recipient for the bone marrow transplant. The aim is to destroy the host's leukaemic cells in the bone marrow; this is achieved by total body irradiation and high doses of chemotherapy via a central line. The cells provided by the donor are then filtered and transfused through the central line, replacing the leukaemic cells.

Allogenic bone marrow transplant carries an additional risk of graft-versus-host disease, in which the transplanted marrow cells see the recipient as foreign and begin to attack the recipient tissue. Antibiotics, immunosuppressant medication and steroids can be given to treat this condition.

As a result of the high doses of chemotherapy and total body irradiation, the patient is susceptible to infections, some of which can be life-threatening. This is more pronounced with allogeneic bone marrow transplant. The patient must be isolated in order to protect them from the risk.

Stem cell transplant

Stem cell transplants may be allogeneic or autologous. In autologous transplants, the person is usually given growth factors to encourage the production of stem cells. When the levels of stem cells are considered to be high enough, the cells are removed, filtered and then stored to be returned to the patient after they have received the high-dose chemotherapy and total body irradiation treatment (see Bone marrow transplant). Allogenic stem cells are taken from a closely matched donor – quite often this is a sibling. There are side effects related to bone marrow or stem cell transplantation.

Care and management

There are several serious risks associated with a stem cell transplant. The main risk is infection. This arises after the extreme chemotherapy and before the bone marrow resumes its usual function. The person will be prone to infection due to low immunity and at this time there is a serious and life-threatening risk of infections. Antibiotics are prescribed and protective isolation is needed until the bone marrow recovers. Isolation may last for 6 weeks; during this time visitors are strictly limited. Keeping the person in touch with their friends and family is essential as the effects of social isolation can have a detrimental impact on the person's health and well-being.

As infection can be a threat to life, the nurse must report any signs of infection or rejection quickly. Potential infection sites should be swabbed and subjected to microscopy. The central line should be treated as a potential source of infection and local policy and procedure must be adhered to; this will include strict aseptic no-touch technique.

As a result of thrombocytopenia, the person is at risk of bleeding after the chemotherapy. Nose bleeds, gums bleeding and bruising may be observed. The patient may notice blood in the stools. If this does occur it must be reported and a platelet transfusion may be needed.

The oral mucous membrane can become extremely fragile and painful after this procedure. Offer ice cubes which can help with oral hygiene; encourage the use of a soft tufted toothbrush, and provide systemic and local analgesia. Mouthwashes may be required. Any oral infections should be reported and treatment instigated.

There may be nausea and vomiting, usually secondary to chemotherapy. Antiemetics should be prescribed prior to commencing the treatment and for the duration of treatment. Along with nausea and vomiting and a sore oral cavity, there may be loss of appetite. The nurse should offer small frequent meals; high-calorie drinks and snacks may be given. For those unable to take anything by mouth. parenteral nutrition may be prescribed, as calories are essential for healing. A fluid balance chart and a food intake chart to monitor the calorie intake should be instigated along with daily weight measurement.

Another essential aspect of post-transplant treatment is rest. Tiredness and fatigue can last for months after transplant, and this should be explained to the patient.

Rehabilitation after stem cell or bone marrow transplant is essential as the transplant process has a damaging impact on the person, which can lead to a longer recovery period. The nurse should encourage exercise (unless contraindicated) and suggest that the person (and, if appropriate, their family) join a support group.

55 Splenectomy

Figure 55.1   The location of the abdominal organs

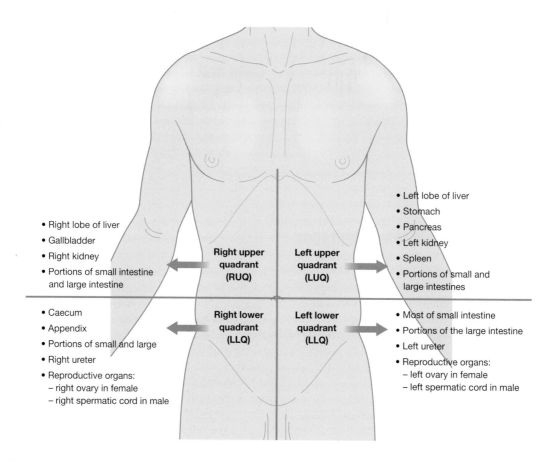

- Right lobe of liver
- Gallbladder
- Right kidney
- Portions of small intestine and large intestine

Right upper quadrant (RUQ)

Left upper quadrant (LUQ)

- Left lobe of liver
- Stomach
- Pancreas
- Left kidney
- Spleen
- Portions of small and large intestines

- Caecum
- Appendix
- Portions of small and large
- Right ureter
- Reproductive organs:
  – right ovary in female
  – right spermatic cord in male

Right lower quadrant (LLQ)

Left lower quadrant (LLQ)

- Most of small intestine
- Portions of the large intestine
- Left ureter
- Reproductive organs:
  – left ovary in female
  – left spermatic cord in male

Table 55.1   Functions of the spleen

- Surveillance for infection
- Circulation of lymphocytes
- Cleaning and filtering of the blood
- Storage of platelets and destruction of old, malformed platelets and red blood cells
- Extraction and storage of iron for the manufacture of haemoglobin

Medical-Surgical Nursing at a Glance, First Edition. Ian Peate. © John Wiley & Sons, Ltd. Published 2016 by John Wiley & Sons, Ltd.
Companion website: www.ataglanceseries.com/nursing/medsurg

The spleen

The spleen is located just under the diaphragm in the left upper quadrant of the abdomen, curving around the anterior aspect of the stomach (Figure 55.1). The spleen is part of the reticuloendothelial system and plays a key role in immunity. The key functions of the spleen, the largest lymphoid organ in the body, are outlined in Table 55.1.

Understanding the basic functions of the spleen will help guide care interventions.

Splenectomy

Splenectomy is the removal of the spleen. The procedure can be performed for a number of reasons, in particular if the spleen has been damaged (such as in a road traffic collision, where there is splenic rupture; the spleen is one of the most frequently injured intraperitoneal organs), if the spleen is diseased, if it contains a growth or tumour or if has become overactive. Some people are born without a spleen (congenital asplenia) or their spleen may be performing poorly (hyposplenism). These people will experience the same problems as someone who has undergone a splenectomy.

Splenectomy may happen in three different ways.

- Elective: where this occurs, prophylactic measures can be instigated to avoid postoperative (and beyond) complications.
- Emergency (traumatic) due to an accident or during surgery.
- Autosplenectomy: the physiological loss of spleen function (hyposplenism); this can be related to sickle cell disease in which the spleen atrophies.

When a splenectomy is performed, the person's immune system becomes significantly compromised. For someone living without the immune function of the spleen, a number of vaccines and antibiotics can be given to help prevent sepsis and other complications.

Incision

The majority of elective splenectomies are undertaken laparoscopically, unless there is severe splenomegaly. The incision will depend on the size of the spleen and the reason for splenectomy as well as surgeon preference. In emergency or trauma situations, it is usual for an upper midline incision to be made as this allows for exposure of the abdominal cavity, can be performed quickly and also provides access for the evaluation and management of other potentially injured organs or structures in the abdominal cavity.

For those patients undergoing splenectomy for a haematological disorder, a left subcostal incision is used to offer clear exposure.

Care and management

It is not usual for a drain to be used unless an injury of the tail of the pancreas is possible or has been confirmed. The abdominal incision is closed with sutures and skin closure may be approximated using staples.

Early postoperative complications include pulmonary complications, for example, atelectasis, pneumonia, subphrenic abscess, paralytic ileus and wound complications (including haematoma and wound infection). Late postoperative complications that may occur include splenosis (begins with splenic rupture, either from trauma or surgical removal; spillage of the damaged splenic pulp into the adjacent pelvic and abdominal cavities occurs) and overwhelming postsplenectomy infection.

The person may have a urinary catheter *in situ* as well as a nasogastric tube and the nurse needs to adhere to local policy and specific postoperative instructions if given. Preoperative intravenous antibiotics will have been given. The person may require a blood transfusion and/or an intravenous infusion after the procedure. This will depend upon the amount of blood lost before, during and after the procedure and is only done as needed. Oxygen therapy may be *in situ* as the person returns from the recovery room.

The nurse will need to administer analgesia as prescribed, monitoring and documenting the effect. The carbon dioxide used in laparoscopic surgery may cause shoulder or chest pain for 1–2 days after surgery.

It is essential to monitor carefully for signs and symptoms that may indicate haemorrhage and shock. Those with preoperative bleeding tendencies will remain at risk postoperatively.

Monitor postoperative temperature elevation. The nurse should note that pyrexia may not be the best indicator of postoperative complications such as pneumonia or urinary tract infection, as pyrexia without associated infection is common following splenectomy. Administer prophylactic antibiotics as prescribed.

Observe dressings for signs of haemorrhage or discharge.

The nurse should report any concerns or abnormalities and ensure that they document their findings.

Unless contraindicated, the patient may start on clear fluids 4–6 hours postoperatively and a regular diet may be commenced the day after surgery.

The patient should be encouraged to mobilise early (unless contraindicated). Referral to a physiotherapist should be made as the location of the incision makes postoperative atelectasis or pneumonia a risk.

Assist the patient with activities of living that they cannot perform for themselves. Provide explanations in such a way that the person understands and thus can cooperate with their plan of care.

Pneumococcal, meningococcal and *Haemophilus influenzae* (Hib) vaccinations are suggested for patients post splenectomy. If the splenectomy is elective then these immunisations should be given at least 14 days prior to the procedure, or after 14 postoperative days for an emergency or unexpected splenectomy. National guidance exists concerning immunisations (the Green Book).

All postsplenectomy patients should be offered education regarding the need to promptly treat any possible infection to pre-empt a more serious sepsis. Patients should also be advised to have a supply of antibiotics available when travelling in anticipation of an infection occurring.

The nurse must explain to the patient the need to report even minor signs or symptoms of infection immediately to the practice nurse or general practitioner. It could be suggested to the patient that they wear a medical alert bracelet. Follow-up appointments will be made where the patient will be asked to attend the outpatient department.

56 Coronary Artery Bypass Graft

Figure 56.1 Coronary artery bypass graft

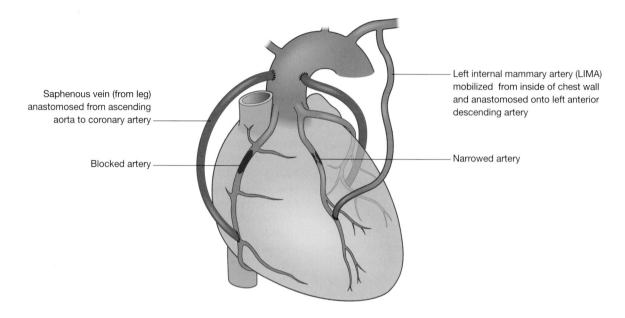

Saphenous vein (from leg) anastomosed from ascending aorta to coronary artery

Blocked artery

Left internal mammary artery (LIMA) mobilized from inside of chest wall and anastomosed onto left anterior descending artery

Narrowed artery

Table 56.1 Potential complications

- Myocardial damage (including myocardial infarction)
- Acute kidney failure
- Ventricular arrhythmias
- Stroke
- Damage to other organs occur
- Haemorrhage
- Cognitive decline

Medical-Surgical Nursing at a Glance, First Edition. Ian Peate. © John Wiley & Sons, Ltd. Published 2016 by John Wiley & Sons, Ltd.
Companion website: www.ataglanceseries.com/nursing/medsurg

Coronary artery bypass graft (CABG) is a major procedure undertaken for coronary artery disease. A number of preoperative investigations will have been undertaken to make a diagnosis of ischaemic heart disease (IHD), confirmed by coronary angiography outlining the obstruction.

Coronary artery bypass grafting may be performed as a primary procedure, if percutaneous coronary intervention has failed, or as a repeat procedure. The key objective is to improve blood flow and oxygen supply to the heart. Blood is diverted around constricted or blocked aspects of the major arteries of the heart.

The procedure involves taking a blood vessel from another part of the body and attaching it to the coronary artery above and below the narrowed area or blockage; this is the graft. The number of grafts depends on how severe the heart disease is and how many coronary blood vessels have become narrowed (Figure 56.1).

Most CABGs are performed on men and most of these are aged over 60 years.

Preoperative care

The nurse should provide routine preoperative care and teaching. Prior to surgery, check and have available the results of any laboratory and diagnostic tests, including (but not limited to) full blood count, coagulation profile, urinalysis, chest X-ray and coronary angiogram. It is important that these baseline data are available for comparison of postoperative results and values. Type and cross-match four or more units of blood as required. Blood should be made available for use perioperatively and postoperatively as needed.

Preparation should be tailored to the needs of the patient. It will also need to take into account the surgeon's preference and local policy and procedure, for example, preoperative body preparation, fasting and administration of premedication.

Teaching related to the procedure and postoperative care is required for the patient and family. Specifically, the following should be addressed: the intensive care unit (cardiac recovery unit) sensory stimuli, who the various members of staff are, noise and alarms and the unit's visiting policy. Information should be given about tubes, drains and general appearance. Monitoring equipment and their functions should be explained, including cardiac and haemodynamic monitoring systems. Respiratory support such as a ventilator, endotracheal tube, suctioning and communication whilst intubated will need to be addressed. Describe the proposed incisions and types of dressings. Explain clearly how pain will be managed.

Preoperative teaching must be done so as not to cause undue distress; if carried out effectively, it can reduce anxiety and prepares the patient and family for the postoperative environment and likely sensations.

Postoperative care

After 24–48 hours post surgery, if stable, the patient will be transferred from the intensive care unit to the ward (cardiac surgical unit); telemetry monitoring will be in place continuously. The nurse should aim to ensure that the patient is haemodynamically stable. This will ensure that the vital organs are sufficiently perfused. Vital signs will be checked, monitored and documented in accordance with local policy and procedure; assess for signs and symptoms of adequate cardiac output. Subtle signs such as tachycardia and cool extremities should be investigated. Other signs of diminished cardiac output include diminished peripheral pulses, changes in cognition, decreased urine output and hypotension.

Dysrhythmias such as tachydysrhythmias (atrial fibrillation) are common after CABG and often occur on the second or third postoperative day.

Those who are hypokalaemic and hypomagnesaemic can become prone to atrial fibrillation.

Pulmonary dysfunction and hypoxaemia can occur after CABG, often due to fluid volume overload, poor inspiratory effort and atelectasis (the latter due to the effect of anaesthetic gases). Common signs of respiratory impairment are shortness of breath and decreased oxygen saturation.

Pleural effusions can result from bleeding secondary to internal mammary artery harvesting. Small effusions may resolve spontaneously. To reduce the risk of postoperative pulmonary complications, assess breath sounds frequently, monitor SpO_2, administer prescribed oxygen and encourage incentive spirometry every hour while awake. Advise the patient to splint the incision when coughing and moving. Keep pain under control and provide individual pain relief to encourage mobility (this will be intravenous in the first instance). When in bed, turn from side to side; physiotherapy and nebulised bronchodilators may be required.

Take steps to prevent venous thromboembolism, administer daily medication and use antithromboembolic hosiery.

Urinary output should be monitored and recorded, daily weight measurement can help guide the use of diuretics.

The patient can be commenced on clear liquids and diet advanced as tolerated. Administer antiemetics if the patient is nauseated. Treat constipation with stool softeners or bulk laxatives as prescribed.

Superficial infections and deep sternal wound infection (mediastinitis) can occur and can have a serious effect on patient morbidity and length of stay. Wound care should be performed according to hospital policy and patient need. Monitor the patient for signs and symptoms of infection, including pyrexia, increased chest wall pain or tenderness, an unstable sternum and purulent discharge from the wound. Administer antibiotics as prescribed.

Care provided must be based on local policy, procedure and protocol but must also reflect individual needs. Care administered should be documented.

Potential complications are shown in Table 56.1.

Discharge

Appropriate discharge planning involves the patient, care givers, nurses, doctors and therapists; a team approach is the best way to address factors that contribute to heart disease. An individual discharge plan is needed and will include detailed information about when to contact the hospital or GP. Advise the patient to seek immediate medical attention if there is chest pain, shortness of breath not relieved by rest, a fast or irregular heartbeat, chills, fever, severe headache, numbness or tingling in the arms or legs, fainting spells, or haemoptysis.

57 Cardiac Valve Surgery

Figure 57.1   Valve replacement

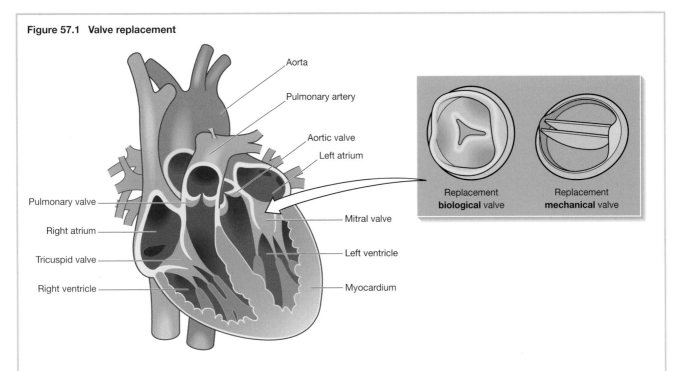

Figure 57.2   Insertion of stent to improve cardiac blood flow

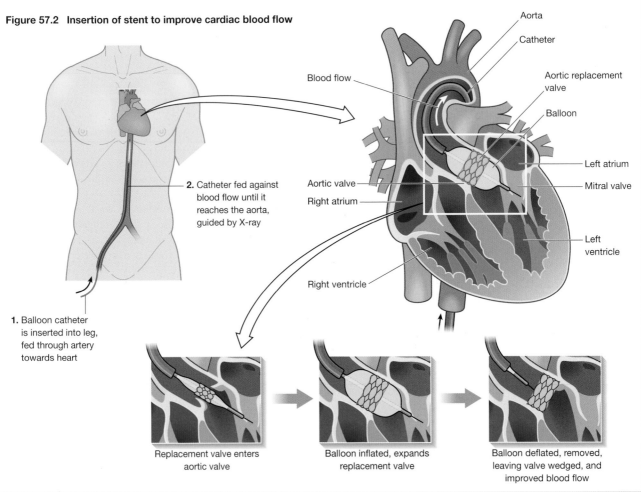

Cardiac valve surgery is usually performed to repair or replace a failing valve. Cardiac valves allow for one-way, low-resistance blood flow. The opening and closing of a valve occur according to pressure gradients between each side of the valve.

Valvular heart disease

Valvular heart disease (VHD) is defined according to the valve or valves affected and the type of functional alteration. Abnormality of the valve is identified as either stenosis (a narrowing or constriction creating a pressure gradient) or regurgitation (incomplete closure of the valve leaflets causes a backflow of blood). The valves must open widely, permitting rapid blood movement and minimal cardiac work; equally, they have to remain tightly closed to prevent a backward flow of blood. Failure of the value to open fully obstructs the flow of blood. When the valve does not close properly, this allows blood to leak backwards.

Causes of valvular heart disease

Valvular heart disease can be congenital or acquired. Congenital factors include a number of congenital malformations. For example, a congenital condition found in adults is Marfan's syndrome, a connective tissue disorder. Acquired causes of valve disease include ischaemic coronary artery disease, degenerative changes related to ageing, rheumatic changes, infective endocarditis as a result of a bacterial infection, cancer or thrombus.

Treatment options

Not everyone with VHD will need surgery; however, surgery on the valve may be indicated. Valvular surgery can improve symptoms and the person's quality of life. Valve repair and valve replacement are the two surgical options available for VHD. Valve repair is commonly undertaken if the mitral valves have become floppy and are leaking but are not extremely damaged and valve replacement is needed for a diseased valve.

The most common types of valve replacement are mechanical (artificial) valves or tissue (animal) valves (Figure 57.1).

There are a number of factors that must be considered before valve surgery is undertaken and these determine whether a repair or a replacement will be needed. The surgeon has to consider what is the cause of the problem, which valve is affected, how seriously the valve is affected, how many valves are affected, the person's symptoms and their overall health status.

The most common valve to be replaced is the aortic valve as it cannot be repaired. The mitral valve is the valve most commonly repaired. Rarely the tricuspid valve or the pulmonary valve is repaired or replaced.

Surgical approaches

The most common approach is open heart surgery, where an incision is made in the sternum (a median sternotomy), enabling the surgeon to access the heart and the aorta. The patient is attached to a cardiopulmonary bypass machine and as the procedure progresses, the work of the heart is carried by the bypass providing oxygen to the tissues and removing carbon dioxide.

Minimally invasive robotic-assisted valve surgery is carried out through much smaller incisions or through a catheter; this is called percutaneous surgery. Several different techniques can be used, including transcatheter aortic valve replacement (TAVR) (also called transcatheter aortic valve implantation (TAVI)).

If the mitral valve can be repaired, ring annuloplasty may be performed, in which the surgeon repairs the ring-like aspect around the valve by sewing a ring of plastic, cloth or tissue around the valve. Valve repair involves trimming, shaping or rebuilding one or more of the valve leaflets (these are the flaps that open and close the valve).

If there is extensive damage to the valve, a new valve will be needed (valve replacement surgery). The diseased valve is removed and a new one replaces it. The main types of new valves are:

- mechanical: a man-made material, for example, stainless steel, titanium or ceramic. These types of valve last the longest
- biological: the valve is made from human or animal tissue; these last for approximately 12–15 years.

The person's own pulmonary valve can be used in some cases to replace the damaged aortic valve. The pulmonary valve is then replaced with an artificial valve.

An aortic valve may not last very long, and it may need to be replaced again by either a mechanical or a biological valve.

Postoperative care

Post valve replacement or repair, the patient will be nursed in the intensive care unit and undergoes close monitoring for 24–48 hours.

Pain control is essential and the person requires regular analgesia. Effects of analgesia are recorded and reported; if it is ineffective, a more detailed assessment of need is required and a stronger analgesic may be required. There may be a chest drain, pacing wires and sensor pads *in situ*.

The nurse needs to provide holistic physical and psychological care. The recovery time varies from person to person but the patient should be able to leave hospital 7–10 days after surgery. Other factors that need to be considered include age, overall health and fitness and previous medical history.

Wound care is undertaken according to local policy and procedure. Prophylactic antibiotics are usually given. The sternum may take around 6–8 weeks to heal; there will be a scar that fades over time. The patient should be advised to wash the wound using mild soap and water when bathing or having a shower. A shower can be taken after pacing wires have been removed (4–5 days). Dissolvable sutures (if used) should disintegrate within approximately 3 weeks. Follow-up is needed if other sutures have been used.

The person (and family) should be offered support and provided with information when being discharged.

Anticoagulants

Those who have had a mechanical valve implanted require lifelong anticoagulation to prevent valve thrombosis. Heparin will be started shortly after surgery and then changed (gradually) to an oral anticoagulant, usually warfarin.

The nurse should advise the patient that they will need to carry an anticoagulant alert booklet with them at all times. This is in case of emergencies and a healthcare professional or doctor needing to know that the person is taking warfarin and at what dose.

58 Varicose Veins

Figure 58.1 Varicose veins

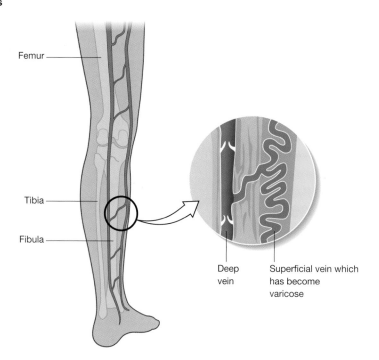

Femur

Tibia

Fibula

Deep vein

Superficial vein which has become varicose

Figure 58.2 Veins of the legs prone to varicosity

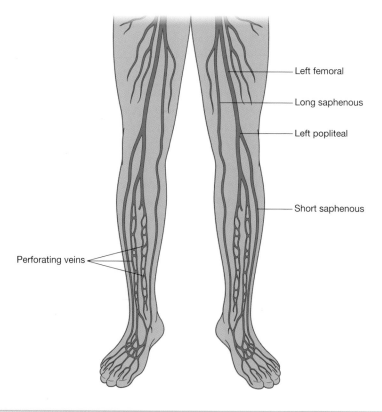

Left femoral

Long saphenous

Left popliteal

Short saphenous

Perforating veins

Medical-Surgical Nursing at a Glance, First Edition. Ian Peate. © John Wiley & Sons, Ltd. Published 2016 by John Wiley & Sons, Ltd.
Companion website: www.ataglanceseries.com/nursing/medsurg

Under normal circumstances, blood is collected from superficial venous capillaries and is then directed upward and inward through a series of one-way valves into the superficial veins. In turn, these then drain into veins of the muscle fascia (a flat band of tissue) into deeper veins that are located under the fascia. If the valves fail to function effectively, leakage occurs, resulting in backflow into the vein. Superficial veins are different from deep veins, which are thick-walled and enclosed by fascia; the superficial veins are unable to cope with high pressure and they will eventually become dilated and tortuous. When one of the valves fails, this puts pressure on those veins that are in close proximity (their neighbours), causing retrograde flow affecting the entire local superficial venous network (Figure 58.1).

Varicose veins can cause significant clinical problems and are not just a cosmetic issue; they signify underlying chronic venous insufficiency with subsequent venous hypertension. The venous hypertension can lead to a range of clinical signs, from symptoms to superficial findings such as varicose veins, reticular veins, telangiectasias, swelling, skin discoloration and ulceration.

It is usually the superficial veins in the legs that are involved; these veins are prone to experience hydrostatic pressure as a result of gravity (Figure 58.2). Hydrostatic pressure is one pathological process; there are others that can also be implicated, for example an innate weakness of the wall of the vein.

Pregnancy can be a contributing factor as well as obstruction to venous outflow such as a deep vein thrombosis, trauma or compression from a surrounding structure, for example, a tumour or cirrhosis of the liver.

Varicose veins are extremely common; they also become more prevalent with increasing age.

Risk factors

There are a number of factors that increase a person's risk of developing varicose veins. The risk of varicose veins increases with age. Women are more likely to develop this condition. Hormonal changes during pregnancy, premenstruation or menopause can be a factor as female hormones may cause relaxation of the walls of the veins. Hormone replacement therapy or the contraceptive pill can also increase risk. There is a greater chance of developing the condition if other family members had varicose veins. Obesity and overweight can result in added pressure on veins. Standing or sitting for long periods of time may cause blood flow problems as well as stagnation or pooling of the blood.

Signs and symptoms

Symptoms may be purely aesthetic and the patient wants treatment due to the unsightly varicosities. Often the person will present with pruritus, discomfort and heaviness of the legs; there may be night cramps, oedema, burning sensations, numbness, an aversion to exercise or restless legs. In larger varicose veins, pain is usually described as a dull ache and is worse after long periods of standing.

Investigations and diagnosis

A detailed history should be undertaken where questions concerning a history of venous insufficiency are asked.

A general assessment of cardiovascular status and abdominal examination to exclude secondary causes, for example, tumours, should be undertaken. Varicosities are examined with the patient standing; gentle pressure is applied to a swelling to determine if this is a varicosity; the vein will empty and then refill. The skin should be inspected for signs of chronic venous insufficiency.

Two tests can be used to assess valvular competency (Trendelenburg's test) and deep venous patency (Perthes' test). Other non-invasive investigations include imaging tests such as hand-held Doppler, duplex ultrasound and colour flow imaging. Physiological tests can also assess venous function.

Care and treatment

The nurse, working with the patient, should suggest lifestyle changes, such as weight loss and exercise; this may help in preventing complications, as opposed to reversing the disease process. The person should be advised to avoid prolonged standing and when possible keep the legs elevated.

Varicose veins can be managed conservatively with stockings and compression. Other management options can be considered if the person is concerned about their cosmetic appearance, worsening symptoms regardless of conservative management, or if the patient requests surgical management.

Usually procedures to treat varicose veins can be elective and emergency treatment is often reserved for varicosities that are bleeding or if there is suspicion of deep vein thrombosis.

National policy exists that will help guide treatment options from a surgical perspective. Conventional surgery such as stripping and ligation is still performed for confirmed varicose veins. Other minimally invasive procedures include radiofrequency ablation, endovenous laser therapy and foam sclerotherapy. If foam sclerotherapy is unsuitable, then consideration should be given to conventional surgery. In avulsion technique, small incisions are made over each varicosity and that part of the vein is then excised. Stripping is where a wire, plastic or metal rod is passed through the lumen of the saphenous vein and pulled until the vein is stripped out of the leg.

Ambulatory phlebectomy can be performed, using local anaesthetic. In this procedure, many small incisions are made in the skin overlying the vein, which is then hooked out. Injection sclerotherapy was previously used as first-line treatment for new varicosities, but is used less frequently now and is only indicated for below-knee varices that are persistent or recurrent after surgery; foam sclerotherapy has commonly replaced this technique.

After treatment, a compression stocking is applied and patients are advised to maintain or increase their normal activity levels; local policy and procedure should guide the instruction given to the patient. Activity is a strong protective factor against venous stasis. Analgesia should be taken as prescribed. The person should be given details of follow-up treatment and contact details of the hospital.

59 Craniotomy

Figure 59.1 Craniotomy

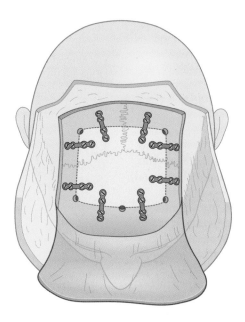

Table 59.1 Some indications for craniotomy

- Clipping of cerebral aneurysm
- Resection of arteriovenous malformation
- Resection of brain tumour
- Biopsy of tissue
- Removal of abscess
- Evacuation of haematoma
- Insertion of implantable hardware (such as deep brain stimulators)

Figure 59.2 The protective coverings of the brain

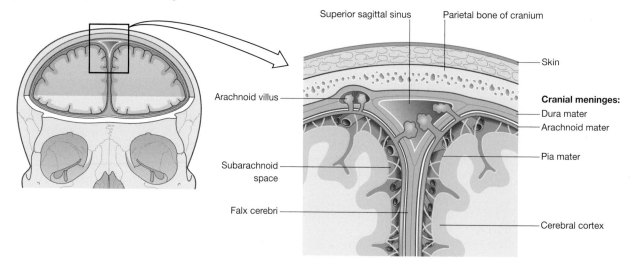

Medical-Surgical Nursing at a Glance, First Edition. Ian Peate. © John Wiley & Sons, Ltd. Published 2016 by John Wiley & Sons, Ltd.
Companion website: www.ataglanceseries.com/nursing/medsurg

Generally, craniotomy refers to a surgical procedure where a section of the skull is removed in order for the surgeon to access the intracranial compartment. The segment of skull that is temporarily removed is known as a bone flap (or a window flap). After the procedure this is put back into its original position, usually secured into place with plates and screws (Figure 59.1). Figure 59.2 shows the meninges covering the brain.

A stereotactic craniotomy refers to those craniotomies that use a three-dimensional co-ordinated approach (usually with the aid of imaging and computer-based navigational software).

Craniotomy is usually undertaken in specialist care settings where there is a range of neurosurgical and neurological services available.

Indications

There are a number of reasons why a craniotomy may need to be performed. Performing a craniotomy provides the primary means by which a neurosurgeon can enter the intracranial space. Diseases that affect the brain and its parts can include conditions of the brain parenchyma, vasculature, meninges and bone; in all cases this requires an opening in the skull as the first step via craniotomy. See Table 59.1 for a list of some indications for a craniotomy.

Preoperative preparation

There are legal, physical and psychological aspects that must be considered, as is the case with all proposed surgery. All surgical procedures have potential complications and careful preparation of the patient (and if appropriate the family) will be required.

An admission history and holistic assessment provide a database and baseline for planning care against which postoperative examinations are compared. Full neurological assessment with cognitive status examination and cranial nerve, motor, sensory and cerebellar examinations should be performed. The nurse needs to address psychosocial aspects with the patient and family, such as fears and anxieties, worries about disability, loss of independence, changes in personality characteristics and fear of alterations in physical appearance.

Obtaining informed consent is central and local policy and procedure must be followed. The responsibility to inform the patient of the purpose of surgery, possibility of alternative treatments, risks, benefits, complications and expected outcomes lies with the surgeon. The nurse's presence during the informed consent discussion can help in clarifying and reinforcing the information provided to the patient and family.

Institution-specific preoperative requirements should be addressed. The patient may be prescribed corticosteroids to reduce the risk of cerebral oedema and anticonvulsant medications to decrease risk of intraoperative and postoperative seizures.

Prophylactic antibiotics are given to reduce the risk of postoperative infection. Deep vein thrombosis prophylaxis along with a sequential compression device or thromboembolic stockings are needed as well as preoperative imaging if needed (i.e. MRI scan).

Potential postoperative complications

Postoperative complications can often lead to permanent neurological damage if these go unrecognised. Prompt recognition of postoperative neurological decline by the nurse and timely diagnosis and intervention by the multidisciplinary team can improve patient outcome as well as quality of life.

The specific potential postoperative complications are usually associated with the type of surgery performed. Postoperative craniotomy complications can be divided into early and late stages. The complications lead to an alteration in neurological status.

Most early complications occur within the first 6 hours after surgery. Early complications include haemorrhage and haematoma formation resulting in a depressed level of consciousness or a focal neurological deficit presenting within a few hours after surgery. Evacuation of the haematoma is usually required.

If wound closure is incomplete, cerebrospinal fluid (CSF) leak can occur, and the introduction of a CSF shunt may be needed. Cerebral infarct (stroke) may be caused by damage to a major artery or vein. Air can enter the cranium (pneumocephalus), introduced through the craniotomy site, causing confusion, lethargy, headache, seizures and nausea and vomiting. Late complications will include infection, and late seizure may also occur.

Postoperative nursing care

The patient will be nursed in an intensive care unit postoperatively. Local policy and procedure must be adhered to in the immediate postoperative phase which will include, for example, airway management, management of fluid intake and pain control. Postoperative neurological evaluation focuses on two features – consciousness and focal neurological findings. Objective scoring instruments such as the Glasgow Coma Scale can help to determine changes in consciousness and focal neurology; any change or concern should be reported immediately. Observations should be compared to previous findings with the aim of detecting changes. Raised intracranial pressure is a real concern and this can occur rapidly or may be insidious.

Specifically, postoperatively, the nurse needs to consider wound care and the management of any drains. Postoperative imaging such as MRI or CT scan may be indicated. Monitor cardiac rate and rhythm along with blood pressure and maintain ordered parameters. Respiratory rate, rhythm and depth should be noted along with SpO_2 and assessment of arterial blood gases and any concerns or changes reported. It is essential to prevent atelectasis or chest infection; prescribed oxygen therapy is required.

The person will need assistance with all the activities of living. If tolerated, begin with clear liquid diet and progress to regular diet as tolerated. Early mobility (unless contraindicated) is key to preventing negative effects of bedrest, such as chest infection, pneumonia and deep vein thrombosis. Assess pain using visual analogue scales and administer prescribed pain medication as needed, recording and noting the patient's response. Postoperative nausea and vomiting should be addressed.

Follow-up appointments are required and there may be a need for neurorehabilitation sessions. The nurse plays an important role in ensuring that the discharge process is smooth and seamless, acting as the keystone in co-ordinating services such as speech, physiotherapy and occupational therapy and social services, if needed.

60 Neurosurgical Clipping

Figure 60.1   Clipping of an aneurysm

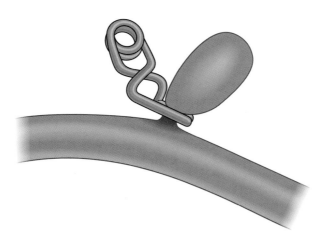

Figure 60.2   Aneurysms of the brain

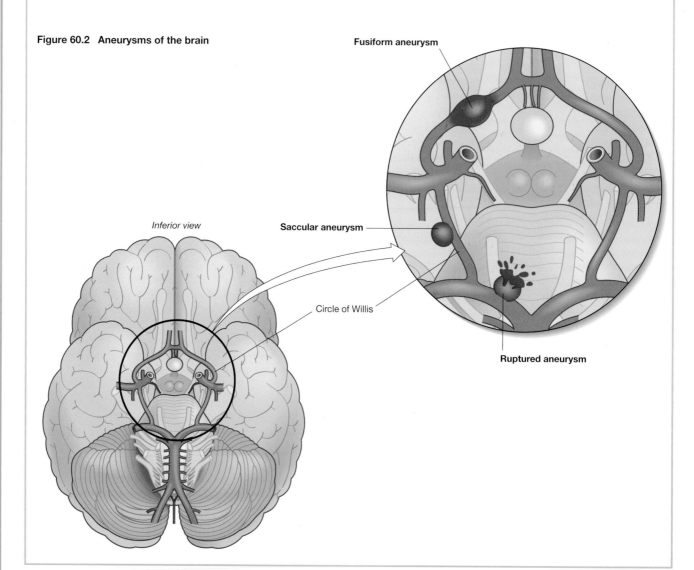

Fusiform aneurysm

Saccular aneurysm

Ruptured aneurysm

Inferior view

Circle of Willis

Medical-Surgical Nursing at a Glance, First Edition. Ian Peate. © John Wiley & Sons, Ltd. Published 2016 by John Wiley & Sons, Ltd.
Companion website: www.ataglanceseries.com/nursing/medsurg

There are many reasons why neurosurgical clipping is undertaken. Neurosurgical clipping is a surgical procedure performed most often to treat a balloon-like bulge of an artery wall known as an aneurysm. As an aneurysm grows, it becomes thinner and weaker. There is a real possibility that it will leak or rupture, and as it does, it releases blood into the spaces around the brain. Often this causes a subarachnoid haemorrhage.

In the procedure, the neurosurgeon places a tiny clip across the neck of the aneurysm to halt or prevent bleeding (Figure 60.1).

Aneurysm

An aneurysm is a bulge or weakening of an artery. Blood to the brain is supplied by four major blood vessels (two carotid and two vertebral arteries) that join together at the circle of Willis located at the base of the brain. Smaller branch arteries leave the circle to supply brain cells with oxygen and nutrients. Artery junction points can become weak, resulting in ballooning of the blood vessel wall that can form an aneurysm.

Signs and symptoms

Not all aneurysms leak or rupture but those that do cause symptoms from severe headache to stroke-like features (such as hemiparesis, facial weakness, diplopia and changes in pupil size) or death.

Causes

Causes include hypertension and atherosclerosis, trauma, heredity component and abnormal blood flow at the junction where arteries come together. Other rare causes include mycotic aneurysms caused by infections of the artery wall; tumours and trauma can also cause aneurysms to form.

Diagnosis

Diagnosis is made by taking an in-depth history of the present condition, asking the patient about headache, type of headache, any neck stiffness and any acute onset of the headache. A computed tomography (CT) scan of the head is required and consideration will be given to the performance of a lumbar puncture (LP).

Types of aneurysm

Aneurysms vary in size and shape (Figure 60.2). Saccular aneurysms possess a neck at their origin on the main artery and a dome; these can expand and grow like a balloon. Saccular aneurysms are the easiest to apply a clip across. There are some aneurysms that have a wide neck or are fusiform in shape with no definable neck; this type is more difficult to place a clip across. Clips are made in a variety of shapes, sizes and lengths.

Treatment

Treatment for a symptomatic aneurysm is to repair the blood vessels. As with any type of surgical intervention, there are a number of risks which must be given serious consideration by the patient (and the nurse may need to act as advocate) and surgeon.

There are two treatment options: clipping and coiling. The aim of surgical clipping is to isolate an aneurysm from the normal circulation without blocking any of the small perforating arteries that are located close by. Under general anaesthesia, a craniotomy is performed and the brain is retracted in order to locate the aneurysm. A small clip is placed across the base, or neck, of the aneurysm, blocking the normal blood flow from entering (thereby preventing growth of the aneurysm and potential rupture). The clips are made of titanium and stay on the artery permanently.

Coiling requires a neurosurgeon or interventional radiologist to thread a tube through the arteries (as with angiogram), identify the aneurysm and fill it with coils of platinum wire or latex, preventing further blood from entering the aneurysm.

The choice of aneurysm treatment must be weighed against the risk of rupture and the overall health of the patient. Because clipping involves the use of anesthesia and surgically entering the skull, patients with other health conditions or who are in poor health may be treated with observation or coiling.

Postoperative care and recovery

Postoperatively, the person will be nursed in the neurosurgical intensive care unit for observation and monitoring. Analgesia is provided as required and antiemetics are also given. There may be nausea and headache after surgery.

Those with an unruptured aneurysm are discharged from the hospital in 3–4 days. Ruptured aneurysm patients stay in hospital longer, depending on postoperative progress and the presence of complications such as vasospasm; signs of vasospasm include arm or leg weakness, confusion, sleepiness or restlessness.

General complications related to neurosurgery include infection, allergic reactions to anaesthesia, stroke, seizure and cerebral oedema. Specific complications include vasospasm, stroke, seizure, haemorrhage and an imperfectly placed clip which may not completely block off the aneurysm or unintentionally block a normal artery.

Aneurysms which have been completely clipped have a very low risk of regrowth. However, with partially clipped aneurysms the patient needs to have periodic angiograms to ensure that the aneurysm is not growing.

Those who have undergone aneurysm clipping may suffer short-term and/or long-term deficits due to the result of a rupture or treatment. Over time some of these deficits can disappear with healing and therapy. It can take months or years for the person to regain function.

The person can wash their hair after all the sutures have been removed. The nurse should encourage early activity (unless this is contraindicated). A multidisciplinary approach is advocated and the nurse works with the physiotherapist and occupational therapist which is the cornerstone of recovery. Both hospital and home rehabilitation after individual assessment will be required in the postoperative period. Those with unruptured aneurysms usually return to full activity over a period of 2–6 weeks. Fatigue is said to be the key complaint.

Titanium and platinum coils are MRI compatible. Certain types of intracranial aneurysm clips are contradicted in MRI procedures. The person needs to be given information concerning the coil or clip type prior to MRI.

As most aneurysm clips are made of titanium, they are not detected by security gates. The patient must inform the Driver and Vehicle Licensing Agency if they have had a cerebral aneurysm.

61 Appendicectomy

Figure 61.1 Appendicitis

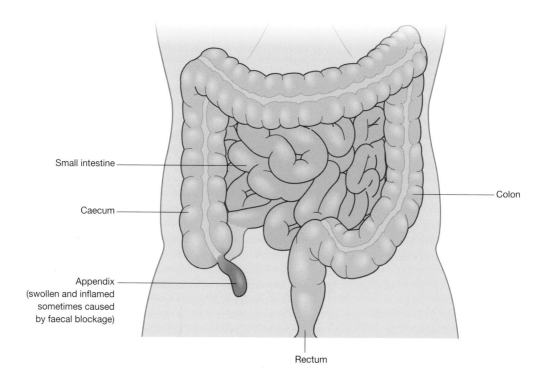

Small intestine

Caecum

Appendix
(swollen and inflamed
sometimes caused
by faecal blockage)

Colon

Rectum

Figure 61.2 The risk of developing appendicitis with age

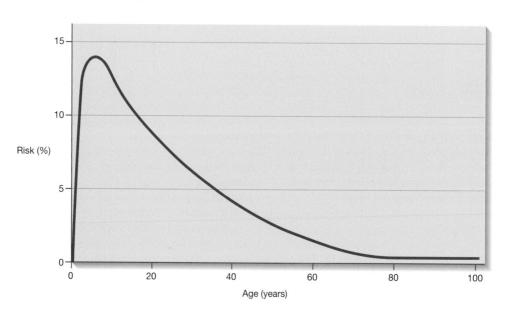

Risk (%)

Age (years)

Medical-Surgical Nursing at a Glance, First Edition. Ian Peate. © John Wiley & Sons, Ltd. Published 2016 by John Wiley & Sons, Ltd.
Companion website: www.ataglanceseries.com/nursing/medsurg

The appendix

The appendix is a small, narrow, tube-like dead-end pouch attached to the caecum (the caecum is the first part of the large intestine), usually about 5–10 cm long. The appendix has no fixed position and no known function in humans. The appendix is made up of some immune tissue and it may play a part in providing immunity. The appendix can be removed without any ill effects.

Appendicitis

Appendicitis refers to inflammation of the appendix (Figure 61.1). Appendicitis is usually caused by a bacterial infection, although the reason the appendix becomes infected is unknown. The appendix can become obstructed by a lump of faeces, calcium salts and faecal debris (called faecoliths) or rarely a tumour, leading to inflammation and infection. Swelling and inflammation lead to infection, blood clot or rupture of the appendix.

Appendicitis is a surgical emergency requiring prompt surgery to remove the inflamed appendix. If the condition is left untreated, the inflamed appendix may otherwise perforate, leaking toxic, infectious materials into the abdominal cavity. This can lead to peritonitis (a serious inflammation of the peritoneum). Peritonitis can be fatal unless it is treated quickly with antibiotics.

The most common cause of an acute abdomen in the UK is appendicitis. The condition can occur at any age but is most common in those between the ages of 10 and 20 years (Figure 61.2), and is more common in men than women.

Signs and symptoms

There is no single sign, symptom or diagnostic test that can accurately confirm the diagnosis of appendicitis. In young children, pregnant women and the elderly, the classic symptoms often do not appear and the diagnosis is particularly easy to miss in these groups.

The classic history is associated with anorexia and periumbilical pain followed by nausea and vomiting with right lower quadrant pain but this may not be present in all cases. The person may have diarrhoea or they may be constipated.

The most common symptom of appendicitis is abdominal pain, which usually begins as periumbilical or epigastric pain that can migrate to the right lower quadrant of the abdomen.

Often the patient lies down, they are still, flexing their hips and drawing their knees up to reduce movement and trying not to worsen their pain. Movement, deep breathing and coughing can exacerbate the pain.

Initially the person's temperature and pulse are normal; a low-grade pyrexia then develops and an increase in pulse rate can be an indication of peritonitis. There can be localised tenderness, guarding and rebound tenderness developing in the right iliac fossa.

Investigations and diagnosis

A diagnosis of appendicitis is usually made on observation, physical examination and the taking of a detailed medical history. However, there are a number of other differential diagnoses that can mimic appendicitis and these need to be ruled out, such as ectopic pregnancy, gastrointestinal obstruction and perforated peptic ulcer.

Urinalysis should be undertaken to exclude urinary tract infection. A pregnancy test should be undertaken to eliminate ectopic pregnancy.

There are no laboratory tests specific for appendicitis, but they may be helpful in confirming a diagnosis in those with an atypical presentation. A full blood count may demonstrate an elevated white cell count (a normal white cell count does not exclude appendicitis). C-reactive protein (an inflammatory marker) may be raised; a normal level does not exclude a diagnosis of appendicitis.

Imaging studies, such as ultrasound, can help where the diagnosis is doubtful. CT scanning is more accurate when diagnosing acute appendicitis.

Care and treatment

The nurse is required to provide physical and psychological care and consideration must be given to the fact that most cases are emergencies. Despite the urgent nature of the condition, the physical, psychological and legal aspects of care must be addressed.

Appendicectomy is the treatment of choice and this is increasingly performed as a laparoscopic procedure (keyhole). Appendicitis can resolve spontaneously, but early operative intervention remains the treatment of choice; currently surgical treatment is the acknowledged standard.

If there are cases of diagnostic doubt then a period of 'active observation' may be useful.

The patient will need to receive intravenous fluids and opiate analgesia; the patient should receive nothing by mouth. Antibiotics given in the preoperative period can provide a reduction in surgical site infections. In some instances, postoperative antibiotics may be given. The person may require an antiemetic; the nurse should offer mouthcare, and provide the person with a receiver and tissues.

Postoperative care

The postoperative care needs of the patient will depend on a number of factors such as the type of surgical incision (open or laparoscopic) and if the appendix was ruptured or not.

The morning after surgery (where the person has an unruptured appendix), clear liquids are offered. The diet progresses to solid food if clear fluids are tolerated. When the patient is eating and drinking, the intravenous infusion is removed. The person is encouraged to mobilise gently (unless contraindicated). Prescribed analgesia is given as required and the effect documented. The nurse continues to monitor the patient for signs of infection (pyrexia, tachycardia, discharge on dressing or from wound). Those with an uncomplicated peri- and postoperative course are usually discharged from the hospital 1–2 days following surgery.

Those who are recovering from surgery where the appendix was perforated will have a longer hospital stay. During surgery, a drain will have been inserted and this remains in place until the drainage ceases. Intravenous antibiotics will continue and on discharge, oral antibiotics are prescribed and should be taken as directed. The patient may be discharged with the drain still *in situ* and nurses in the primary/community care setting care for this.

Complications can include wound infection, dehiscence, bowel obstruction and abdominal/pelvic abscess. Paralytic ileus may occur; this is more common when the appendix has perforated.

62 Right-sided Hemicolectomy

Figure 62.1   The large bowel

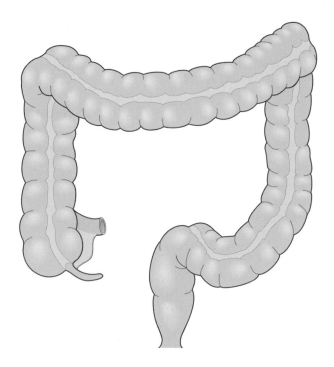

Figure 62.2   Right sided hemi colectomy

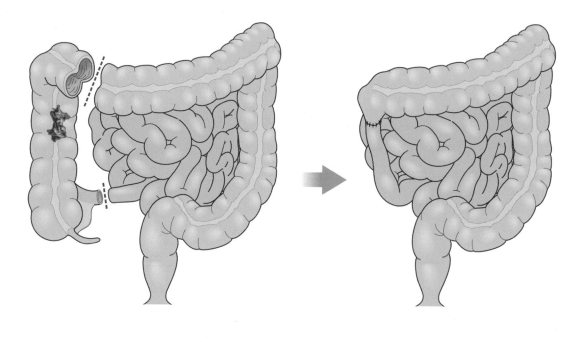

The large bowel

The gastrointestinal (GI) tract extends from the mouth to the anus. The lower GI tract includes the small intestine, large intestine (including the appendix), caecum, colon, rectum and anus. The large intestine is approximately 1.5 meters; it absorbs water as well as any remaining nutrients from partially digested food passed from the small intestine. The large intestine changes waste products from liquid to solid matter – faeces. Faeces pass from the colon to the rectum. The rectum is 10–15 centimeters in length and is positioned between the final part of the colon, called the sigmoid colon, and the anus (Figure 62.1).

Colonic surgery

There are different types of colonic surgery. The majority of surgery on the colon is performed as a result of bowel cancer. The type of surgical intervention depends on where the cancer is in the colon, the type and size and if there is any metastatic spread.

Local resection is performed if the cancer is very small and is at an early stage. The cancer may be removed from the surface of the bowel with a border of healthy tissue.

If the cancer is larger, the part of the bowel containing the cancer is removed and the two ends are joined back together again; this is called an end-to-end anastomosis (Figure 62.2). Local abdominal lymph nodes will also be removed. Rectal cancer often involves the removal of the mesentery. A temporary colostomy or ileostomy may be required.

Laparoscopic resection (keyhole) has undergone much refinement over the years. In this approach, early-stage bowel tumours are removed through a number of small incisions in the skin and muscle. Laparoscopic surgery can reduce hospital stay and discomfort following surgery and may minimise scarring.

Preoperative care

For open right hemicolectomy, thorough preparation of the bowel is required. Local policy and procedure must be followed. Standard bowel preparation may be conducted over a 24-hour period either prior to or after admission. Usually the patient drinks only clear liquids for 24 hours, and bowel preparation requires the person to drink 4 L of polyethylene glycol solution (a laxative) taken over 2–3 hours in the afternoon of the day before the procedure. A sodium phosphate enema may be administered on the night before the operation.

Prophylactic antibiotic therapy may be given. Electrolyte levels are checked and again on the night before surgery.

To prevent venous thromboembolism, preoperative anticoagulant therapy is commenced (for example, heparin, tinzaparin or dalteparin); this is also maintained for a number of weeks postoperatively. The nurse, working with other members of the multidisciplinary team, teaches the patient how to perform leg exercises to lower the risk of blood clot formation; antithromboembolic stockings will be provided. Preassessment tests will include a number of blood tests, a chest X-ray to check lungs are healthy and an ECG.

The nurse needs to act as the patient's advocate, providing explanations for any questions asked and offering the person and their family physical and psychological support. Referral to a colorectal clinical nurse specialist may be required.

Postoperative care

On return to the ward, the person will usually have an intravenous infusion *in situ*, a urinary catheter, a wound drain and a nasogastric tube. Vital signs are monitored (such as blood pressure, temperature, pulse, respiration rate and depth, oxygen saturation, urinary output) according to local policy and the patient's condition. Prescribed oxygen therapy may be required. The nurse must report any concerns or deterioration in the person's condition to the nurse in charge. Pain will be controlled with prescribed analgesia (nurse administered, epidural or patient controlled) and the nurse must assess and document efficacy of administered medication.

Nasogastric aspiration is maintained as per instruction usually until the paralytic ileus has resolved. Clear liquids are commenced when the patient is no longer feeling nauseous or vomiting and normal bowel sounds have returned and when the person passes flatus. If liquids are tolerated well, normal intake can commence, depending on the patient's condition. Intravenous fluids are usually discontinued when the patient is tolerating normal oral intake. The urinary catheter may be removed 2–3 days postoperatively.

The patient will require assistance with the activities of living and will be encouraged to take part in their care when their condition improves. Mobility is encouraged unless contraindicated. At all stages of care provision, the nurse should explain all actions and activities in a language the person understands. Time should be set aside for the person (and family) to ask questions or to seek clarification of any issues. It must be remembered that people recover at different rates, but the average stay in hospital is 4–8 days.

Potential postoperative complications

All surgery carries risk with the potential of postoperative complications. Hemicolectomy (open or laparoscopic) is a major operation.

For anastomotic leak, antibiotics are given and the bowel is rested (the patient remains nil by mouth and the nasogastric tube is aspirated); however, further surgery may be required.

Paralytic ileus (where the bowel is slow to recommence activity) can cause vomiting; the patient remains nil by mouth and the nasogastric tube is aspirated and intravenous fluids are indicated.

Chest infection can occur, so encouraging deep breathing exercises may help prevent this; referral to a physiotherapist may be required. There is a risk of wound infection so antibiotics are given. Deep vein thrombosis (and subsequent pulmonary embolism) can occur as a result of major surgery and immobility so pre- and postoperative anticoagulant therapy are prescribed and early mobilisation is encouraged. If haemorrhage occurs, this may require a blood transfusion and the nurse must be alert to any changes in the person's condition that may indicate haemorrhage. Further surgery may be required.

Risks increase with age and are also higher in those who have pre-existing conditions such as heart, chest or other medical conditions, for example diabetes, or if the person is obese or overweight.

63 Bariatric Surgery

Figure 63.1 Types of gastric bypass

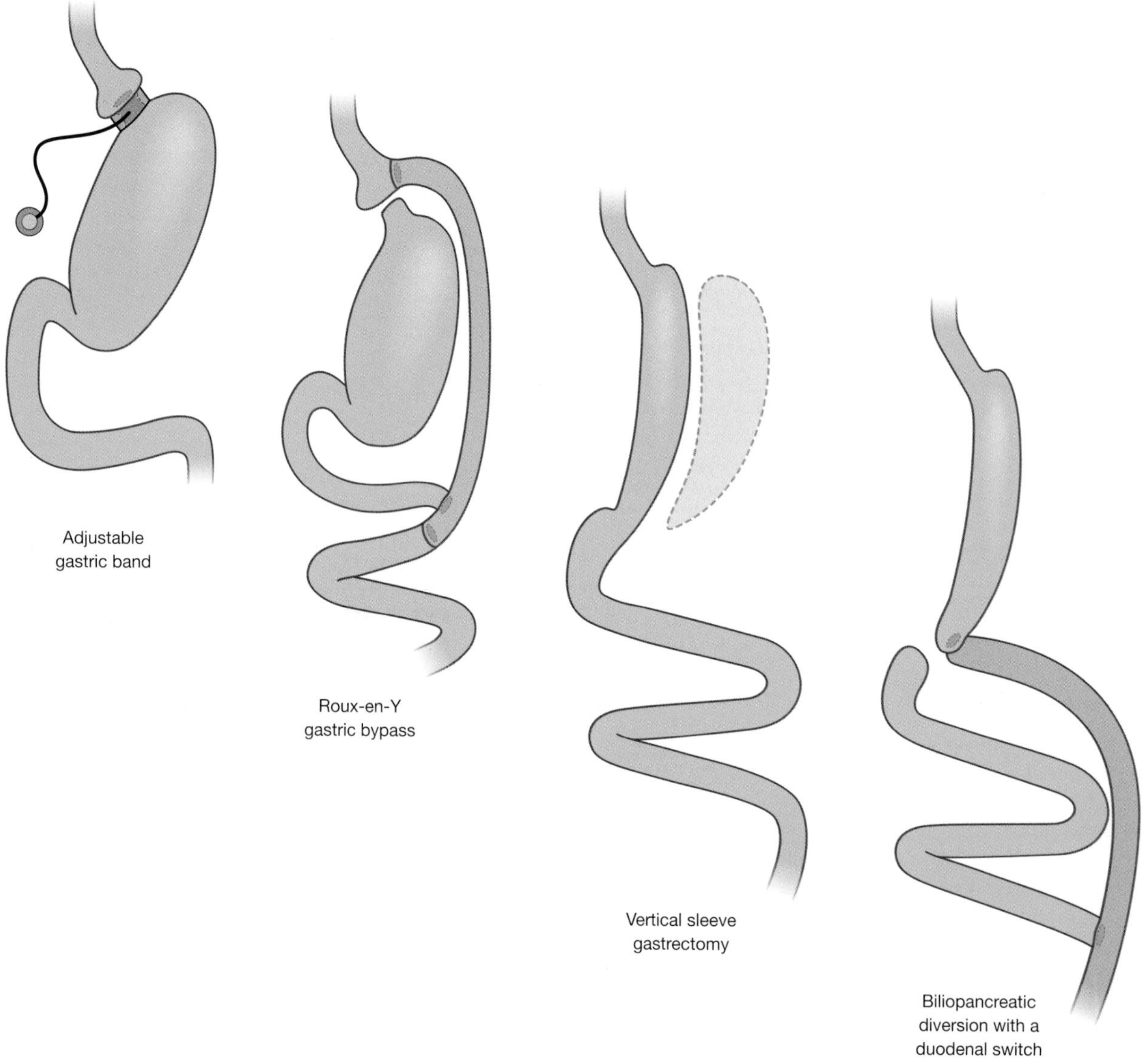

Adjustable
gastric band

Roux-en-Y
gastric bypass

Vertical sleeve
gastrectomy

Biliopancreatic
diversion with a
duodenal switch

Table 63.1 Other forms of gastric surgery

Approach	Description
Duodenal switch	Biliopancreatic diversion is occasionally performed with a duodenal switch. A short distal length of small intestine is formed, and this severely limits absorption of calories
Gastric stimulation	Uses an implanted pacemaker-type device that generates electrical gastric stimulation
Intragastric balloon	This is not a surgical procedure it is an endoscopic procedure, an inflated silicone balloon is placed in the stomach producing a sense of satiety. This is a new procedure and as such data is limited concerning efficacy and side effects

Bariatric surgery (also known as weight loss surgery) is used as a last resort to treat people who are severely obese. The procedure works by reducing intake or the absorption of calories. This type of surgery is used to treat people with potentially life-threatening obesity when other treatments, such as lifestyle changes, have not worked. Indications include:

- having a body mass index (BMI) of 40 or above
- having a BMI of 35 or above and having another serious health condition that could be improved if weight is lost, for example, type 2 diabetes or hypertension
- other non-surgical methods have failed to maintain weight loss for at least 6 months
- the person is generally fit to undergo anaesthetic
- the person commits to long-term follow-up.

Weight loss surgery has proved to be effective in significantly and quickly reducing excess body fat for those who meet the above criteria. Bariatric surgery must always be undertaken in a specialist centre with long-term follow-up of patients. There are national guidelines available regarding bariatric surgery. Contraindications would include those who are unfit for surgery and people with an uncontrolled alcohol or drug dependency.

Types of surgery

There are a number of types of bariatric surgery.

- Adjustable gastric band
- Gastric bypass (Roux-en-Y)
- Vertical sleeve gastrectomy
- Biliopancreatic diversion

See Figure 63.1.

Adjustable gastric banding

The surgeon places a constricting ring around the stomach, below the gastro-oesphageal junction. The band contains an inflatable balloon that permits the size of the ring to be adjusted. The specialist nurse or surgeon can control the size of the ring by inflating or deflating it with saline (this is done subcutaneously).

Gastric bypass (Roux-en-Y)

A small gastric pouch is created and joined to the jejunum, which bypasses the duodenum and proximal jejunum. This restricts food intake as well as decreasing the absorption of food.

Sleeve gastrectomy

In this procedure (which is irreversible), the majority of the stomach is removed (gastrectomy) and a sleeve-shaped cylinder of stomach remains, thus reducing capacity.

Biliopancreatic diversion

This is complex bariatric surgery and is a more extensive form of the gastric bypass. In this procedure, the gastric pouch is joined to the ileum and an even more extreme form of malabsorption occurs. A decrease in the amount of food, vitamins and minerals absorbed produces the possibility of long-term problems, such as anaemia and osteoporosis.

Other types of gastric surgery can be performed; details can be found in Table 63.1.

The type of surgery will depend on a number of factors and a detailed holistic physical and sometimes psychiatric assessment is required, with the surgeon working with the patient to determine the most appropriate approach. The procedure may be performed as an 'open case', which requires an abdominal incision, or as a laparoscopic procedure via 1 cm puncture holes for the insertion of surgical instruments and a camera. Laparoscopic surgery has a number of advantages (smaller incision, less tissue damage, earlier discharge) but it must be noted that all types of surgery bring risk.

Potential complications

Whilst there are a number of advantages associated with bariatric surgery, there are also complications; this is why preoperative discussion is essential. There must be clarity concerning expectations as some patients may have unrealistic ideas concerning the amount of weight that they are likely to lose, how much time it may take to lose weight and the need for follow-up as well as the potential complications.

As is the case for any abdominal surgery, perioperative complications exist and include venous thromboembolism. Prophylaxis reduces the incidence of deep vein thrombosis and pulmonary embolism.

Potential problems associated with the band are band slippage, leakage, infection or migration. Bypass surgery also has potential complications including leakage or stenosis of the stoma, gastrointestinal ulcers or bleeding, small bowel obstruction as well as hernia.

Nausea and vomiting and dumping syndrome may occur. Malnutrition as a result of micronutrient deficiency is a potential problem and is particularly associated with malabsorptive procedures.

If the original operation fails, revisional surgery may be needed. This should only be undertaken in specialised centres, by a surgeon with extensive experience.

Recommendations

In order to reduce mortality and morbidity associated with bariatric surgery, a national enquiry recommends the following.

- Any surgeon performing the procedure must undergo a minimum number of procedures prior to being permitted to perform the operation unsupervised.
- The provision of services should be restricted to a number of accredited centres, with a set minimum number of procedures carried out each year.
- Those undergoing the procedure must have access to the full range of specialised professionals required to meet their needs in accordance with national guidelines.
- Psychological support should be introduced at an earlier stage in the process.
- Consent should be a two-stage process and should not be taken on the day of surgery.
- The GP should be provided with a clear discharge plan as soon as possible; this will include detailed dietary advice.
- If required, postoperative psychological advice should be made available.

64 Arthroscopy

Figure 64.1 Arthroscopy

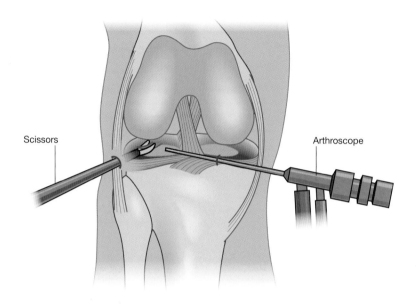

Scissors

Arthroscope

Figure 64.2 The meniscus and cruciate ligaments

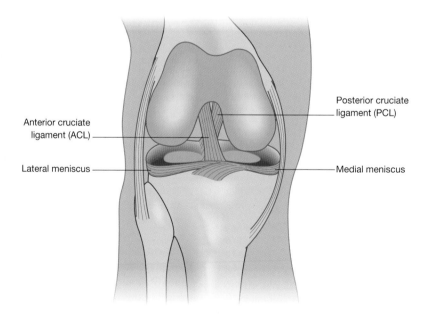

Posterior cruciate
ligament (PCL)

Anterior cruciate
ligament (ACL)

Lateral meniscus

Medial meniscus

Medical-Surgical Nursing at a Glance, First Edition. Ian Peate. © John Wiley & Sons, Ltd. Published 2016 by John Wiley & Sons, Ltd.
Companion website: www.ataglanceseries.com/nursing/medsurg

Arthroscopy falls within the domain of minimally invasive orthopaedic surgery. The procedure permits direct visualisation of the interior of a joint via an endoscope (Figure 64.1). The procedure is most commonly performed on the knee but it can also be carried out on other joints such as the shoulder, hip, ankle and wrist.

The meniscus and cruciate ligaments

The medial meniscus is located on the inside of the knee and the lateral meniscus is on the outside. They act to deepen the articular surfaces of the fairly flat tibial plateau that accommodate the relatively round femoral condyles. The superior surfaces are concave and connect with the femoral condyles; the inferior surfaces are flat and conform to the tibial plateaus.

The menisci are capable of absorbing a substantial amount of compressive load from the medial and lateral femoral condyles. They have a degree of mobility, permitting the tibia to roll and glide back on the femur during flexion.

Several muscles and ligaments control the motion of the knee as well as protecting it from damage at the same time. Two ligaments on either side of the knee, the medial and lateral collateral ligaments, stabilise the knee from side to side. In the centre of the knee joint is the anterior cruciate ligament, one of a pair of ligaments forming a cross. There is an anterior cruciate ligament and a posterior cruciate ligament, which stabilise the knee from front to back during normal and athletic activities. The ligaments of the knee ensure that the weight transmitted through the knee joint is centred within the joint, reducing the amount of wear and tear on the cartilage inside the knee.

Meniscal injury of the knee

Medial meniscus tears are often related to a stable knee joint, as opposed to lateral meniscal tears that may be concurrent with damage to the anterior cruciate ligament. Menisci tears usually happen as a result of twisting of the weight-bearing knee and also as a result of trauma. A severe type of knee injury involving the collateral or cruciate ligaments is usually caused by a twisting movement with a flexed knee and planted foot.

One of the procedures most frequently used for the diagnosis and treatment of knee injuries is knee arthroscopy.

Making a diagnosis

Most meniscal injuries can be diagnosed by obtaining a detailed history from the patient. Significant points to uncover will include the mechanism of injury (such as twisting, squatting, changes in position) and the type of pain experienced. Note should be taken of any mechanical complaints reported by the patient such as clicking, locking, pinching or a sensation of giving way. Note also the presence of oedema, possibly as a result of effusion. There may be impairment in range of movement.

In order to make a definitive diagnosis or to confirm the type of knee injury, a series of imaging studies may be considered and these can include a plain radiograph and magnetic resonance imaging (MRI). Arthroscopy is the best tool for making a meniscal tear diagnosis. It is both therapeutic and diagnostic, providing the person with immediate treatment of most disorders.

Conservative management

In all but the most severe cases, conservative treatment should be attempted. During the acute phase, treatment may include the following: outpatient physiotherapy appointments, rest with activity modification, the application of ice packs and the administration of non-steroidal anti-inflammatory drugs. If this approach does not lead to resolution, then surgical treatment is considered.

Knee arthroscopy

The key aim of meniscus surgery is to save the meniscus. Those tears with a high probability of healing with surgical intervention are repaired but some tears are not repairable and resection must be restricted to only the dysfunctional portions, preserving as much normal meniscus as possible.

The surgical options will include partial meniscus repair, partial meniscectomy and meniscus repair. Depending on individual circumstances, the procedure can be carried out using an open or laparoscopic approach. The latter is the standard option; it is a minimally invasive day case procedure and has many advantages over open meniscal surgery.

The most commonly associated condition of the ligaments is complete tear of the anterior cruciate ligament. The principles of repair include smoothing and abrading the torn edges and the bordering synovium to encourage bleeding and healing.

Arthroscopy can be performed under local, regional or general anaesthesia through a number of small incisions. The surgeon inserts the arthroscope into the knee joint; this sends the images to a screen, enabling the surgeon to visualise the structures of the knee in detail.

A sterile solution is instilled via one of the ports of the arthoscope, filling the joint and removing any cloudy fluid. When the surgeon is able to visualise the knee clearly, a diagnosis can be made. If surgical treatment is required, instruments are inserted via another small incision (for example, scissors, motorised shavers or lasers). The procedure usually lasts 30 minutes to over an hour depending on the findings and the treatment. The incisions are closed with a suture or Steri-Strips and covered with a soft bandage.

Recovery and discharge

Whilst recovery from knee arthroscopy is faster than recovery from open knee surgery, it is important to provide the patient with information to promote recovery on discharge.

The leg must be elevated as much as possible for the first few days after surgery to prevent swelling. An ice pack can be used to relieve swelling and pain. The wound should be kept clean and dry; the surgeon will determine when the person can shower or have a bath and when the dressing should be changed.

Crutches are usually required and the nurse teaches the person how to use these safely. The person should not fully bear weight, strain or overuse the joint in the first few days.

A number of factors have to be considered regarding driving. The decision is based upon individual needs but typically, the person should refrain from driving for approximately 2 weeks post procedure.

Outpatient physiotherapy appointments are needed to strengthen the joint. The person should be advised to rest, with activity modification; the application of ice packs and the administration of non-steroidal anti-inflammatory drugs may help with pain and discomfort.

A follow-up appointment to see the orthopaedic surgeon is required.

65 Lower Limb Amputation

Figure 65.1 Levels of lower limb amputation

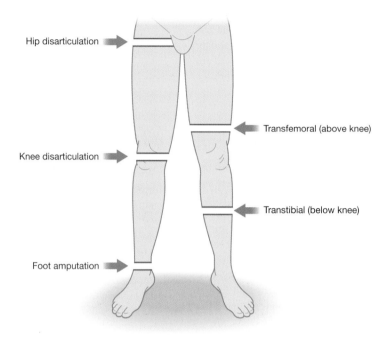

- Hip disarticulation
- Transfemoral (above knee)
- Knee disarticulation
- Transtibial (below knee)
- Foot amputation

Table 65.1 Common level amputations

- **Symes or ankle disarticulation** – amputation of the foot
- **Transtibial** – amputation at mid calf
- **Knee disarticulation** – amputation through the knee joint
- **Transfemoral** – amputation at mid thigh
- **Hip disarticulation** – amputation through the hip joint
- **Transpelvic (hindquarter)** – amputation of the whole leg and the pelvis on the same side

Table 65.2 Dressing types

Type	Description
Soft dressings	These dressings do not control postoperative oedema
Soft dressing with pressure wrap	Requires an even distribution of pressure to avoid possible limb strangulation
Semi-rigid dressings	These include plaster splints and paste bandages held in place with a stockinette. Same advantages of rigid dressings, but no immediate postoperative prosthesis can be used
Rigid dressings	Many rigid dressings are commercially available, and intraoperative prosthetic assistance may be required, these can have the potential advantage of residual extremity maturation, decreased oedema, less pain, wound protection and early mobilisation in combination with an immediate postoperative prosthesis. However, there is poor access to the wound and excessive pressure, leading to wound necrosis

Medical-Surgical Nursing at a Glance, First Edition. Ian Peate. © John Wiley & Sons, Ltd. Published 2016 by John Wiley & Sons, Ltd.
Companion website: www.ataglanceseries.com/nursing/medsurg

Types of amputation

The majority of limb amputations are performed on the lower limbs. The most common reason for lower limb amputation is peripheral vascular disease associated with diabetes mellitus and ensuing gangrene. Severe trauma, malignancy and congenital conditions are also implicated. Injuries as a result of shrapnel and land mines in military and civilian personnel can also result in amputation.

Upper extremity amputation is often the result of thermal or electrical burns or severe crush injuries. Malignant, vasospastic disease and infection can also require an upper limb amputation.

The surgeon decides the level of amputation. Common amputation levels are shown in Figure 65.1; see also Table 65.1.

Amputation

Patients and their family must be aware of their options and be provided with information concerning realistic expectations of the potential outcome of surgery. This is essential if informed decisions (and as such informed consent) are to be achieved concerning amputation.

One major challenge facing a person undergoing amputation is overcoming the psychological stigma associated with the loss of a limb. Following the removal of a limb and the application of a suitable prosthesis, many patients can remain active members of society, maintaining an independent lifestyle.

Surgery has to be performed in such a way as to ensure that the patient can wear a prosthesis comfortably. The patient, working with the multidisciplinary team (nurse, prosthesist, therapist, doctor and social worker), must learn to walk with a prosthesis, attach and remove the prosthesis, care for the prosthesis, monitor the skin and be alert to any pressure points.

The decision to carry out a lower limb amputation comes after all other options have been exhausted. This is a final decision that once begun cannot be reversed. The only contraindication to amputation is poor health that impairs the patient's ability to tolerate anaesthesia and surgery. The removal of the diseased limb is needed to eradicate systemic toxins and as such save the person's life.

Preoperative care

A key concern is wound healing as many amputations are performed as a result of compromised circulation. A full blood count is required (and standard preoperative laboratory studies) and other tests may be necessary, depending on the patient's condition. Specifically, C-reactive protein (CRP) (an inflammatory marker) is an indicator of infection. Haemoglobin assessment is required, as well-oxygenated blood is necessary for wound healing. Lymphocyte count can determine immune deficiency which increases the possibility of infection. Low serum albumin level implies malnutrition and reduced ability to heal the wound. Blood transfusion and supplementary nutritional support may be indicated.

A range of imaging studies is required including radiography, CT scan, bone scan and Doppler ultrasonography.

As well as the physical preparation, those undergoing amputation should be evaluated for cognitive abilities (psychological assessment may be needed). Phantom limb sensations that occur in the amputated limb are not uncommon and are associated with the peripheral nervous system and spinal cord. The patient needs to be made aware of this possibility and if this does occur they should make this known.

A multidisciplinary approach will involve consultation with a physiotherapist (muscle strengthening exercises may be undertaken to help with postoperative ambulation), social worker and perhaps a psychiatrist. Introducing the patient to someone who has undergone an amputation may also prepare them for future expectations and provide answers to questions the patient may not have considered. Preoperative and postoperative care must be tailored to meet the individual needs of the patient.

Postoperative care

The person may be cared for in the intensive care unit postoperatively where their condition is monitored closely and any potential or actual problems can be dealt with quickly. Major concerns in the postoperative period are haemorrhage and oedema.

The type of postoperative dressings and treatments regimen will vary. If there is a pressure dressing in place, this is usually removed 48–72 hours after the procedure has been performed. The stump is elevated to prevent oedema and haemorrhage (in lower limb amputations this should not exceed 24 hours as there is a risk of hip contraction). The dressing covering the stump must be checked to ascertain if there is excessive bleeding; if this is the case or there are signs of fresh bleeding, this must be reported immediately. Other signs and symptoms that may indicate haemorrhage include tachycardia, hypotension, restlessness, increased pain and pallor. Local policy may require a surgical tourniquet be left at the patient's bedside in case of haemorrhage.

Prophylactic antibiotic therapy may be given pre-, peri- and postoperatively. There will be a wound drain *in situ* and this is managed as per local policy and procedure. Pain relief may be in the form of a patient-controlled analgesia system, intravenous infusion and transcutaneous electrical nerve stimulation.

The various types of postoperative dressings have advantages and disadvantages. There are four types of postoperative dressings available (Table 65.2). When dressings are removed the nurse should take the opportunity to assess the skin, identifying any actual or potential skin breakdown problems; findings should be documented in the care plan and action taken if needed.

Assistance with the activities of living will be required. Correct positioning is required to prevent abduction contractures and a range of movement exercises should be carried out and the patient encouraged to do these independently when able. Teaching for self-care should begin as soon as possible. Physiotherapy for transfers and assistance with mobility are initiated.

The degree of mobility in the postoperative period is at the discretion of the surgeon and physiotherapist, depending on the patient's rehabilitation potential. Cautionary instructions regarding falling are provided to the patient to avoid the potential of injuring and opening the postoperative wound.

There may be a need for referral concerning psychosocial and emotional issues. The success of surgery is multifaceted in terms of function and emotional satisfaction. The aim is to achieve a useful residual limb in a person who is active with a positive attitude, who accepts the need for amputation and who continues to be a productive member of the community.

66 Laminectomy

Figure 66.1 Conditions that may require laminectomy

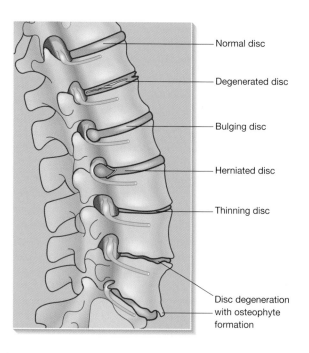

- Normal disc
- Degenerated disc
- Bulging disc
- Herniated disc
- Thinning disc
- Disc degeneration with osteophyte formation

Table 66.1 Types of back surgery

Type	Description
Laminectomy	The bony coverings of the spine are removed and any thickened ligaments, joints and bone spurs (overgrowths of bone) are shaved back. This widens the spinal canal relieving pressure that has built up around the spinal nerves
Discectomy	One or more of the discs are removed through a small insicion in the back. Part of the bony coverings of the spine (lamina), along with a section of ligament is removed
Spinal disc replacement	The procedure aims to restore disc height and movement between the vertebrae. The affected discs are removed and replaced with artificial ones
Foraminotomy	The surgeon performs a keyhole procedure to widen the foramina (the bony holes through which spinal nerves branch off from the spinal cord) and reduce pressure on the spinal nerves
Vertebroplasty	Through a small incision on the back and using X-rays as guidance, a cement-like mixture is injected into the vertebrae to stabilise the spine
Spinal fusion	Two or more of the vertebrae are joined together using a bone graft and a type of metal scaffolding made of screws, rods or plates

Medical-Surgical Nursing at a Glance, First Edition. Ian Peate. © John Wiley & Sons, Ltd. Published 2016 by John Wiley & Sons, Ltd.
Companion website: www.ataglanceseries.com/nursing/medsurg

Back surgery

A laminectomy is a surgical procedure undertaken with the aim of accessing the spinal cord through the spine. This is often carried out to prevent any further degeneration and in so doing can help to relieve back and leg pain that is caused by a number of conditions, for example, a prolapsed or herniated disc and spinal stenosis (Figure 66.1).

The procedure is commonly performed on the cervical, thoracic or lumbar sections of the spine, depending on the condition. Cervical, thoracic and lumbar laminectomy is often performed on people with spinal stenosis. Also known as open decompression, this surgical procedure removes a small portion of the vertebra called the lamina. The lamina is found on the back or dorsal aspect of the vertebra, the area that covers the spinal canal. See Table 66.1 that outlines the various types of back surgery.

Lumbar laminectomy

This procedure is performed for a number of reasons; the most common is for back pain caused by a herniated disc.

The most common site of back pain is in the lower back; the back pain may be due to a herniated disc with associated nerve pain transmitted down a lower extremity (sciatica). When a disc herniates, the jelly-like nucleus pushes through the annulus (harder outer ring), putting pressure on the adjacent nerve root, which can cause varying degrees of pain.

Cauda equina syndrome is the most serious problem and occurs where there is compression at the point where roots of all the spinal nerves are located. All nerve function below the area of compression is lost and this includes loss of bowel and bladder control. Cauda equina syndrome is a surgical emergency necessitating immediate decompression.

Laminectomy is only undertaken if conservative medical treatment for a herniated disc has failed; surgery can produce gratifying relief. Surgery is considered for people with frequently recurring sciatica, and if the pain impedes the person's ability to work or carry out the activities of living.

Progressive loss of nerve function, for example, the person may lose a certain reflex and later begin to lose strength gradually, is another indication for surgery. Far more commonly, people go to a doctor with an acute lack of nerve function.

The decision to undergo surgery must be a joint decision between the patient and the doctor.

Risks and complications

All operative procedures carry risk and there are some risks associated with back surgery. The possible complications include an unexpected reaction to the anaesthetic, excessive bleeding or development of a deep vein thrombosis.

A specific complication of back surgery is spinal cord or nerve damage, leading to numbness, pain, paralysis and loss of muscle, bladder or bowel control. Other complications are specific to the type of operation performed; for example, postoperative surgery for a slipped, herniated or bulging disc may result in another slipped disc requiring further treatment. If an implant has been fitted, the screws or implants in the back may come loose and further surgery may be needed.

Preoperative care

The person must be given all the information they need in order to make an informed decision and the nurse may be required to provide physical and psychological support to the person during the decision-making process, acting as an advocate. During this time, an opportunity should be provided for the patient to understand what is being proposed.

A detailed medical history is obtained, as is the case for all types of surgery. A baseline neurological examination is undertaken and the outcome documented.

A series of imaging tests such as x-rays and MRI scan will be done. Other tests such as ECGs and routine blood tests are carried out. Local policy and procedures regarding fasting protocols will be adhered to. Antithromboembolic medication may be given and the person may be asked to wear compression stockings.

The procedure can be undertaken using a general anaesthetic or spinal anaesthetic.

Postoperative care

On return to the ward, the patient will normally lie on their side or back. There may be a urinary catheter *in situ* and a drain in place.

Vital signs as per hospital policy are undertaken. Pain control is required and the nurse responds to the person's needs concerning pain, assessing, evaluating and recording care outcomes. Assess for site of pain, characteristics of pain and degree of pain using a pain scale. Pain must be re-evaluated after analgesia is given.

A key concern postoperatively is to ensure that the spinal column is kept in alignment in order to encourage healing and to prevent any further injury occurring. Pillows are used to support the patient. The surgeon will direct if the patient can be moved from side to side; log rolling is required to avoid twisting of the spine, and at all times the nurse must inform the patient of what is happening.

When allowed out of bed (and this depends on individual circumstances), a back brace or corset may be required. The nurse, working with the patient and the physiotherapist, support the patient with regard to mobility. The patient should not sit or stand for any period of time and ongoing physiotherapy sessions are required. The patient is assisted with the activities of living.

The nurse must assess sensation, checking the extremities for numbness and tingling, and should determine that the patient is able to move shoulders, arms, legs, hands and feet. Muscle strength is assessed by asking the person to push their hand against yours whilst you apply gentle downward pressure to the extremity.

Check the wound, noting drainage (if there is a drain in place), amount and characteristics; observe for any signs of cerebral spinal fluid.

All care provided and results of assessment must be documented, and any concerns must be reported without delay.

Discharge advice is provided on an individual basis. An outpatient physiotherapy appointment is required. The sutures or staples will need to be removed approximately 2 weeks after surgery.

67 Pituitary Surgery

Figure 67.1 The pituitary gland and the organs it acts on

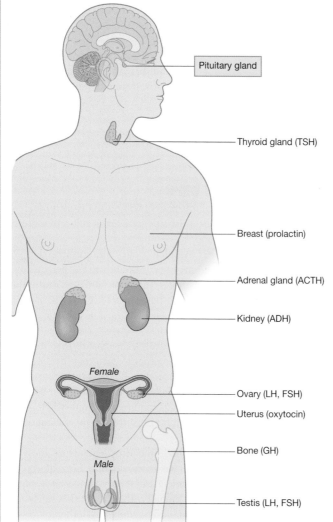

- Pituitary gland
- Thyroid gland (TSH)
- Breast (prolactin)
- Adrenal gland (ACTH)
- Kidney (ADH)
- *Female*
- Ovary (LH, FSH)
- Uterus (oxytocin)
- Bone (GH)
- *Male*
- Testis (LH, FSH)

Table 67.1 The hormones of the anterior and posterior pituitary gland

The anterior pituitary produces six hormones:

1. Growth hormone (GH), controlling growth

2. Prolactin that stimulates the production of breast milk postpartum

3. Adrenocorticotrophic hormone (ACTH) stimulates the production of hormones from the adrenal glands

4. Thyroid-stimulating hormone (TSH), which stimulates the production of hormones from the thyroid gland

5. Follicle-stimulating hormone (FSH) and luteinizing hormone (LH), which stimulate the ovaries and the testes

The posterior aspect of the pituitary gland produces:

1. Anti-diuretic hormone (ADH), this reduces the amount of urine produced by the kidneys

2. Oxytocin, which stimulates the contraction of the uterus during childbirth and the release of breast milk for breastfeeding

Figure 67.2 Transphenoidal surgery

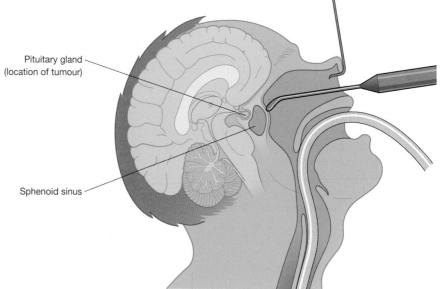

- Pituitary gland (location of tumour)
- Sphenoid sinus

Pituitary gland

The pituitary gland is situated at the base of the brain; it is a small but important gland about the size of an acorn and is sometimes referred to as the 'master gland' as it releases hormones that control the basic functions of growth, metabolism and reproduction. The pituitary gland produces hormones that control and regulate the other glands in the body (Figure 67.1). The gland has two parts: anterior and posterior (Table 67.1).

Pituitary surgery

The most common treatment for pituitary tumors is transsphenoidal surgery; this approach is the most common way to remove pituitary tumours and is also less invasive. Transsphenoidal means that the surgery is undertaken through the sphenoid sinus, a hollow space in the skull posterior to the nasal passages and below the brain. The back wall of the sinus covers the pituitary gland (Figure 67.2). For larger or more complicated pituitary tumours, a craniotomy may be required. Most pituitary tumours are benign.

Transsphenoidal hypophysectomy

A number of disorders and tumours, such as Cushing's syndrome, acromegaly and advanced metastatic carcinoma of the breast and prostate gland, have been treated by transsphenoidal hypophysectomy (TSH) (also known as endoscopic transsphenoidal resection).

Endoscopy can be used to assist and guide the surgeon with this procedure via the sphenoid sinus and into the pituitary fossa. The endoscope and accompanying instrumentation provide minimally invasive access to the pituitary gland. Avoiding a craniotomy reduces its associated slight risks of damage to the brain and potential epilepsy.

Preoperative preparation

A number of investigations and tests are required prior to performing TSH in order to find out about the type, position and size of the tumour.

Eye tests are required to detect pressure on the optic nerve. A range of vision tests are needed to assess visual fields. Blood tests are needed to determine the levels of the various pituitary hormones.

Treatment is planned with the multidisciplinary team (including an endocrinologist, neurosurgeon, neurologist, oncologist, special nurses, therapists) and the patient is involved in all decisions made.

Understanding that the patient may find the idea of brain surgery very frightening can help them express their fears and anxieties with the intention of providing information and advice that may alleviate worries and concerns. Care provision will centre on the physical as well as the psychological needs of the patient (and if appropriate the family also).

The benefits and disadvantages of treatment must be explained and this has to be done on an individual basis, taking the person's holistic needs into account. The person usually stays in hospital 3–9 days after surgery with time off work between 4 and 6 weeks but this should be assessed in relation to the person's individual needs.

Postoperative care

There are two elements associated with postoperative nursing care; the first occurs when the person is cared for in the intensive care unit and their condition is closely monitored and assessment of pituitary function is carried out. It is essential to check visual acuity, visual fields and extraocular movements in the first 24 hours post surgery.

The second aspect occurs when the patient has been transferred from the intensive care unit to the neurosurgical ward. Vital signs and neurological observations are carried out as per hospital policy and any deviation is noted and reported.

Headache is a chief complaint after surgery and the nurse may be required to administer opiates, for example, intravenous morphine. Pain control is required and the nurse responds to the person's needs with regard to pain. Assess pain using a pain scale (assess site, type and level of pain), provide pain relief, evaluate efficacy of care interventions and record outcomes. If pain control is ineffective then reassessment and a new plan of care are required.

If there is nausea and/or vomiting, the prescribed antiemetic should be administered and its usefulness recorded. Eating and drinking commence as soon as the person is able to tolerate fluids and diet.

The nurse will be required to assist the person with those activities of living that they cannot perform independently. The role of the nurse is to maintain a safe environment, provide comfort and identify any deterioration in the patient's condition, making this known to the person in charge immediately.

Depending on the approach, sutures are inserted in the upper gum or in the nostril and are usually soluble. Where an incision has been made under the lip, oral care should be performed as per hospital policy. The wound usually heals within 3 weeks and complete absorption of the stitches may take 3 months. There may be some numbness around the front teeth and for some people this might be permanent. The nasal pack is removed on the second or third day; this procedure may be uncomfortable for the patient and they need to be told this. The patient should not blow the nose, use an incentive spirometer, cough hard or sneeze forcefully through the nose due to the risk of dislodging the surgical repair or forcing air into inflamed sinuses.

The patient should be encouraged to get out of bed to walk with supervision on the first postoperative day if there are no contraindications or complications.

Discharge and follow-up

The outcome of TSH is usually very successful. Hypopituitarism (hormone deficiency caused by the inadequate secretion of one or more of the hormones usually secreted by the pituitary gland) may occur and some people have to continue taking hormone replacements, often for the rest of their lives. There is a need for regular check-ups with an endocrinologist, which can continue for several years. The patient will also be followed up by the neurosurgeon. Check-ups can involve further scans, blood tests will be required in order to monitor hormone levels, and eye tests are required.

The patient should be advised not to lift weight over 10 kg over the first 4 weeks post surgery and to refrain from underwater diving as these may place pressure on the sinuses. Air travel should also be avoided during this period.

68 Thyroidectomy

Figure 68.1 Types of thyroid surgery

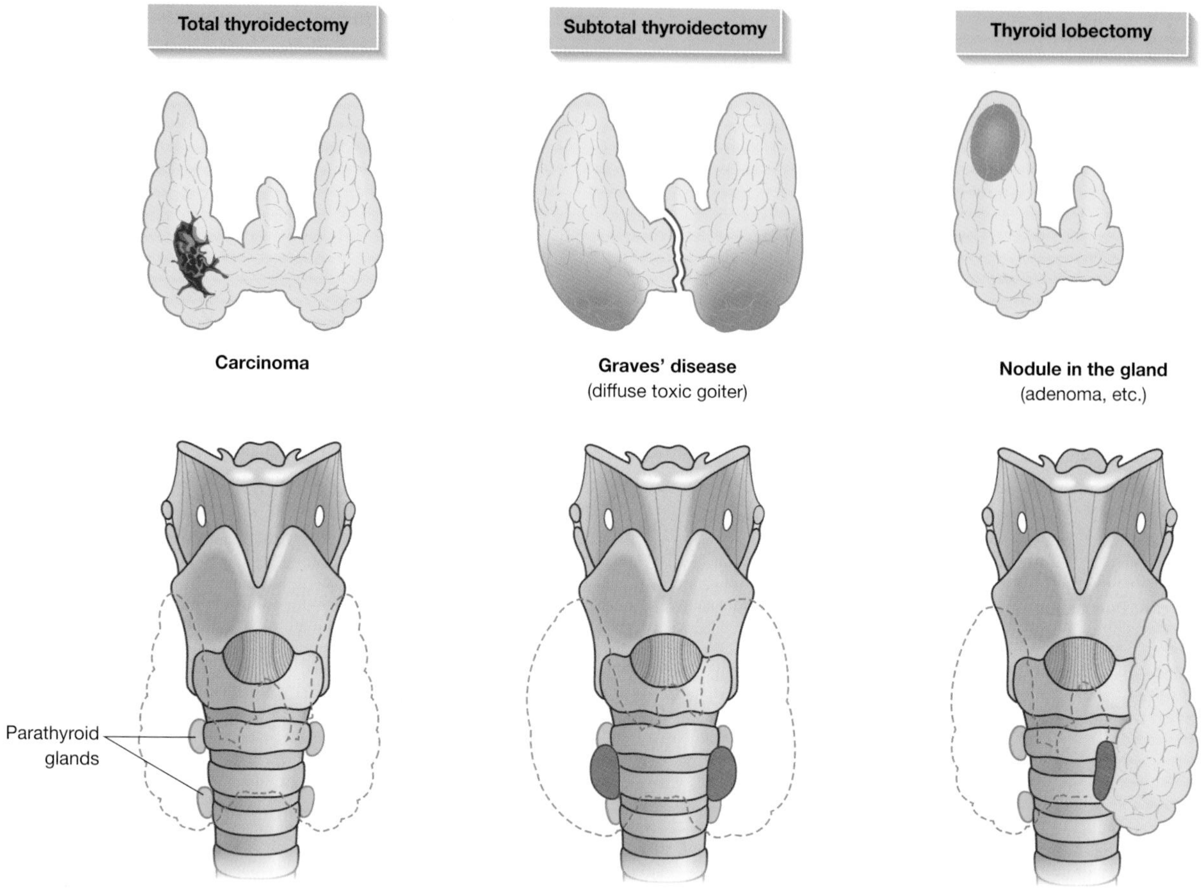

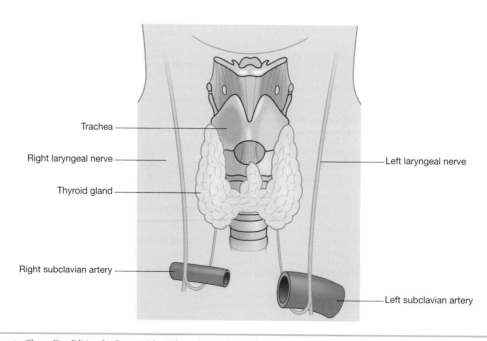

| Total thyroidectomy | Subtotal thyroidectomy | Thyroid lobectomy |

Carcinoma

Graves' disease
(diffuse toxic goiter)

Nodule in the gland
(adenoma, etc.)

Parathyroid
glands

Figure 68.2 Laryngeal nerves and the thyroid gland

Trachea

Right laryngeal nerve

Left laryngeal nerve

Thyroid gland

Right subclavian artery

Left subclavian artery

Disorders of the thyroid gland

Complaints of the thyroid gland are categorised as either hypersecretion of thyroid hormones (excessive thyroid gland activity – hyperthyroidism) or hyposecretion of thyroid hormones (reduction in thyroid gland activity – hypothyroidism). Thyroid disorders can be categorised further by the underlying mechanism causing the change in thyroid hormone secretion.

- Primary – as a result of a disorder of the thyroid gland.
- Secondary – due to alterations in thyroid function caused by an increase of decrease in the production of either thyrotropin-releasing hormone (TRH) from the hypothalamus or thyroid-stimulating hormone (TSH) from the pituitary gland.

Hyperthyroidism

Excessive production and release of thyroid hormone is known as hyperthyroidism; it is commonly caused by an autoimmune disorder known as Graves' disease. Other causes of hyperthyroidism include thyroid cancer, thyroid nodules (usually non-cancerous), viral thyroiditis, postpartum thyroiditis and those patients who are taking iodine-containing drugs, for example, amiodarone.

Types of thyroid operations

- Thyroid lobectomy to remove a nodule or goitres (swellings in the neck resulting from enlargement of the thyroid gland) that occur in one lobe.
- Partial thyroid lobectomy removes a solitary nodule in one specific part of the gland.
- Thyroid lobectomy with isthmectomy for benign Hürthle cell tumours and for non-aggressive thyroid cancers.
- Total thyroidectomy for thyroid cancers.

See Figure 68.1.

Patients who do not respond to medications used to help control the effects of an overactive thyroid gland, those who are unable to take radioactive iodine, those with a thyroid malignancy or who have an unsightly enlarged thyroid are suitable for thyroid surgery.

Open surgery is usually performed but newer techniques/procedures are being used such as robotic minimally invasive surgery.

Preoperative care

There are a number of specific preoperative actions that need to be undertaken. Those patients who are thyrotoxic should be treated with the beta-blocker propranolol and/or carbimazole (a drug used to reduce thyroid function) to ensure they are euthyroid (a normally functioning thyroid) at operation.

Prior to thyroid surgery, due to a possibility of operative damage to the recurrent laryngeal nerve, the vocal cords should also be checked (See figure 68.2).

Potential postoperative complications

Surgery is a last resort as it brings with it potential complications, including collections of serous fluid; poor scar formation; haemorrhage that may result in tracheal compression; laryngeal nerve damage; hypoparathyroidism resulting in hypocalcaemia; thyrotoxic storm (hyperpyrexia, dehydration, tachycardia, with or without arrhythmias); hypotension; heart failure; nausea; jaundice; vomiting; diarrhoea; abdominal pain. There may be confusion, agitation, delirium, psychosis, seizures or coma. Infection occurs in 1–2% of all cases. Perioperative antibiotics are not recommended for thyroid surgery. Hypothyroidism (insufficient secretion of thyroid hormones) can result.

A number of patients will need long-term thyroid replacement therapy as a result of surgery.

Postoperative care

After recovery from anaesthetic, the patient is nursed in an upright position; the head should be supported with pillows.

Administer prescribed analgesia and monitor effectiveness. Common complaints are a sore throat and discomfort with swallowing; this usually lasts a few days.

Perform vital signs as per hospital policy, monitoring for complications, assess dressing (and drain if *in situ*) and the area under the neck and shoulders for drainage. Monitor blood pressure and pulse for an indication of hypovolaemic shock. The danger of haemorrhage is greatest in the first 12–24 hours postoperatively.

Assess respiratory rate, rhythm, depth and effort. Provide prescribed humidified oxygen, assist the patient with coughing and deep breathing. Suction equipment, oxygen and a tracheostomy set must be available for immediate use.

Assess for the ability to speak aloud, documenting quality and tone of voice. There may be hoarseness due to oedema or the perioperative endotracheal tube; this will subside but permanent hoarseness or loss of vocal volume is a possible danger.

The nurse should assess the person for signs of calcium deficiency, including tingling of toes, fingers and lips, muscular twitches, positive Chvostek's and Trousseau's signs and a decrease in serum calcium. Calcium gluconate or calcium chloride should be made available for immediate intravenous use if required. Note that tetany can occur 1–7 days post thyroidectomy.

The patient should be encouraged to mobilise, walking around on the evening of surgery. The wound is covered with skin glue and there are no sutures to be removed so the patient may shower the next day.

Discharge and follow-up

Most patients are discharged after 24 hours, unless there are any complications, and can return to work about a week after surgery if their job does not involve manual work. If the patient has a physically demanding job, return to work is usually after 2 weeks.

Normal activity is resumed as soon as comfort levels allow. The patient may drive when they can safely and comfortably operate a car, usually within 2 days. The only restrictions on activity are no exercise or athletics until the postoperative follow-up visit approximately 2 weeks post surgery.

Patients undergoing a total thyroidectomy will be hypothyroid following the operation. Medical management of hypothyroidism and continued monitoring are essential. Those with thyroid cancer should also be monitored and followed up for disease recurrence.

Prior to discharge, patients should be given information on signs of hypocalcaemia (i.e. numbness or tingling of the digits or perioral area). Should the person develop signs of hypocalcaemia or neck swelling or difficulty breathing, they should go immediately to the nearest accident and emergency department.

69 Orchidectomy

Figure 69.1   Orchidectomy

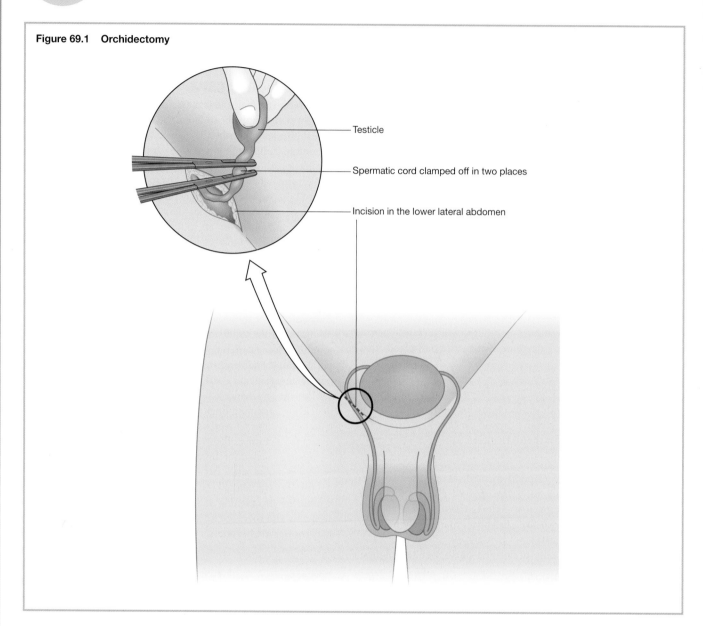

Testicle

Spermatic cord clamped off in two places

Incision in the lower lateral abdomen

Often orchidectomy (also called orchiectomy) is performed as part of the treatment for cancer; other reasons include the need to reduce the amount of testosterone (the primary male sex hormone).

Orchidectomy is the usual treatment if there is a tumour within the testicle; it may also be performed to treat prostate cancer or cancer of the breast, as these cancers are testosterone dependent and have the propensity to metastasise.

Bilateral orchidectomy is commonly performed as one stage in male-to-female gender reassignment surgery. This is to lower the levels of male hormones and to prepare the genital area for later operations to construct a vagina and external female genitalia.

Types of orchidectomy

There are three types of orchidectomy: simple, subcapsular and inguinal (or radical). Simple or subcapsular orchidectomy can be performed under local anaesthesia; the procedure takes approximately 30 minutes. Inguinal orchidectomy is usually performed under general anaesthesia and may take up to an hour to complete.

Simple orchiectomy

Performed as part of palliative treatment for advanced cancer of the prostate as well as part of gender reassignment surgery. An incision is made in the midpoint of the scrotal sac and through the underlying tissue. The testicles and parts of the spermatic cord are removed through the incision. The incision is closed with two layers of sutures and this is covered with a surgical dressing. If the man desires a prosthetic testicle, it can be inserted prior to closure of the incision to give the appearance of a normal scrotum from the outside.

Subcapsular orchidectomy

This procedure is also performed for treatment of prostate cancer and is similar to a simple orchidectomy but glandular tissue is removed from the lining of the testicles as opposed to the whole testicle being removed. This is usually undertaken with the aim of keeping the appearance of a normal scrotum.

Inguinal orchidectomy

Sometimes this is called a radical orchidectomy; undertaken for testicular cancer, it can be unilateral or bilateral. An incision is made in the inguinal canal as opposed to the scrotum. The entire spermatic cord as well as the testicle is removed (Figure 69.1). The rationale for this complete removal is that testicular cancers can spread from the spermatic cord into adjacent lymph nodes.

Various layers of tissues and skin are closed with several types of sutures. The wound is covered with a sterile dressing.

Preoperative care

The patient may be asked to attend a preoperative assessment clinic. The procedure will be discussed with the man and opportunity given to ask any questions or seek clarification of any issues he may have. Informed consent is required after providing the man with information concerning the procedure and potential risks and side effects.

A physical examination and comprehensive health history will be needed, including current medications and any known allergies. A range of blood tests and other investigations are undertaken prior to surgery, depending on the man's individual needs, such as ECG and X-ray. The man will be asked to discontinue aspirin-based medications for a week prior to surgery and all non-steroidal anti-inflammatory drugs (NSAIDs) 2 days before the procedure takes place.

Depending on the type of anaesthetic, the man may need to stop eating and drinking. Local policy and procedure should be adhered to concerning fasting as well as skin preparation. The man will be asked to shower or bathe on the morning of surgery.

Those men who are undergoing orchidectomy should consider banking sperm if they have plans to have children after surgery. It is possible to father a child if only one testicle is removed but it is recommended to bank sperm as a precaution in case the other testicle should, at a later date, develop a tumour.

In those men who have requested an orchidectomy as part of male-to-female gender reassignment, specific care is required concerning their medication (they may have been taking hormones for several months to several years prior to surgery). Standards of care for gender reassignment require a psychiatric diagnosis as well as a physical examination. The nurse must plan care that responds to the unique needs of the individual.

Postoperative care

After leaving the recovery room, care may be provided on the ward or in the day surgery unit, depending on the patient's condition and type of surgery.

The man's vital signs are recorded as per local policy and any deviation from the norm should be acted upon and reported. The nurse observes the dressing for any signs of excessive bleeding. Analgesia is provided as required and the outcomes are recorded and reported; an antiemetic may be given if there is nausea and/or vomiting.

Sips of water should be offered as soon as the man is able to drink unless there is nausea and/or vomiting. When he is fully awake he can eat and drink as normal.

A scrotal support (jock strap) or support pants should be provided to keep the dressing secure. Dissolvable sutures are used with a scrotal incision; with an inguinal incision staples are used.

Discharge and follow-up

The man should be advised to wear the scrotal support or tight-fitting underwear until he is pain free. The light dressing may be removed and changed 24 hours after the surgery and he may then shower. Some bruising and swelling is normal; this will subside over a few weeks. Excessive swelling is not normal and help should be sought.

The man should be advised to look at the wound daily and if it becomes hard, red or there is excessive swelling, to visit the practice nurse or GP. If bleeding occurs within 24 hours of discharge, advise the man that he should contact the hospital; after this time he should contact his GP. An appointment will be given to have the skin staples removed, if these have been used.

The man can return to work and undertake all other activities when he feels able. If a further appointment is required this should be sent to the patient.

70 Vasectomy

Figure 70.1 Vasectomy

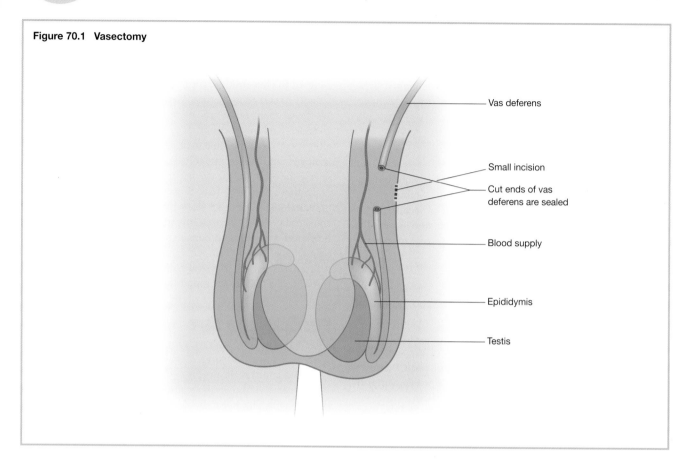

- Vas deferens
- Small incision
- Cut ends of vas deferens are sealed
- Blood supply
- Epididymis
- Testis

A vasectomy is a surgical procedure undertaken for male sterilisation; it is a permanent birth control method. In a vasectomy the two vasa deferentia are severed and closed off. Post vasectomy, the man will still produce sperm but they do not move out of the testicles. In the majority of cases, vasectomy is successful. A vasectomy can be reversed by reattaching the ends of the vasa deferentia in a procedure known as a reverse vasectomy; this is a more complicated procedure than a vasectomy and is not always successful.

Types of vasectomy

There are two types of vasectomy.

- Conventional (incisional).
- No-scalpel vasectomy (non-incisional).

Conventional vasectomy

During a conventional vasectomy, the skin of the scrotum is anaesthetised with local anaesthetic. Two small incisions approximately 1 cm long are made on either side of the scrotal sac. The surgeon is then able to access the vasa deferentia and sever them and a small section is removed. The ends are then closed, either by tying them using a ligature or applying diathermy, causing them to seal.

The incisions are sutured using dissolvable sutures that dissolve within a week.

No-scalpel vasectomy

The non-incisional approach (no-scalpel vasectomy) is carried out under local anaesthetic. During a no-scalpel vasectomy the vasa deferentia are palpated through the scrotum and held in place using a small clamp.

A special instrument (vas fixating ring forceps) is used to make a small puncture hole in the skin of the scrotum. Small forceps are used to open up the hole, providing the surgeon with access to the vasa deferentia and avoiding the need to cut the skin with a scalpel. The vasa deferentia are closed in the same way as in an incisional vasectomy, by tying or sealing.

During this procedure, there will be little bleeding and need for sutures. It is less painful and less likely to result in complications compared to the conventional vasectomy.

Risks

There are few risks associated with vasectomy. There are potential complications and these are often related to bleeding (haematoma formation) or infection. Prolonged pain may occur as a result of inflammation along the vasa deferentia causing sperm granuloma (sperm leakage) or congestion of sperm at the epididymis resulting in epididymitis. With rest and the administration of anti-inflammatory medications, these conditions will usually resolve.

Preoperative care

As vasectomy is an irreversible form of contraception, it is essential that the man provides informed consent. The man should be encouraged to give much consideration to having the procedure performed and it should only be considered if the man and his partner are sure they do not want children, or any further children or if there are any major problems in the man's relationship with his partner. It is not a legal requirement to gain the man's partner's permission prior to performing a vasectomy. Prior to opting for a vasectomy, a couple should give serious consideration to other alternative methods of contraception.

Vasectomy is usually performed using local anaesthetic but if the man is having general anaesthetic or sedation he may be asked to attend a preoperative assessment before the operation. This may include a blood test, a blood pressure check or a chest X-ray. There are restrictions to eating and drinking in the preoperative period; usually the man must not eat anything from 6 hours before the operation and may only drink sips of water until 2 hours before.

Postoperative care

Any discomfort is usually mild and analgesia will be given to combat this. After an hour or so the local anaesthetic will begin to wear off. The following are general guidelines aimed at promoting a speedy recovery.

Wrap an ice pack or a package of frozen peas in a towel and apply to the scrotum for the first 24 hours after the procedure.

The man should be advised to avoid walking or standing as much as possible for a couple of days. He should wear snug cotton briefs or a scrotal support for the first week or two after the procedure and avoid heavy lifting or exercise for at least 2–3 days. The man usually returns to work within 1–2 days unless the job involves physical exertion. Generally he should avoid activities that can cause discomfort.

Should the man experience any severe pain or is concerned about his condition, he should be encouraged to contact the hospital or clinic where the procedure was performed or visit his GP. He should contact the doctor if any of the following symptoms develop.

- Temperature and chills
- Large or developing black and blue areas
- An increase in pain
- Leakage (drainage) from the wound
- A growing mass (swelling)
- Excessive swelling of the scrotum
- Other concerns

Postvasectomy semen analysis

Failure rates with vasectomy are low. Sterility is not instantaneous and the nurse needs to explain this carefully to the man. Postvasectomy semen analysis is required to assure azoospermia before the man and his partner stop using other forms of birth control.

The time taken to lose sperm motility is 3 weeks post procedure and the time to azoospermia is 10 weeks. The absence of any sperm 12 weeks after the procedure is a reliable prediction of long-term sterility. It is usual for two negative semen samples to be provided 4–6 weeks apart to determine sterility but local policy must be adhered to.

It is important for the man and his partner to use some form of birth control until the man is informed specifically that he is sterile.

71 Dilation and curettage

Figure 71.1 The hysteroscope

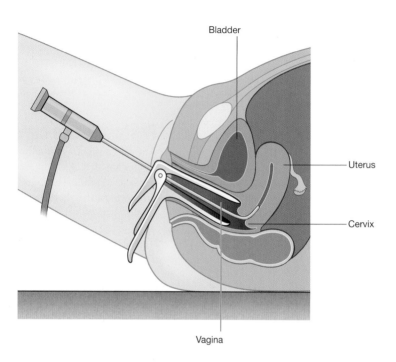

Bladder

Uterus

Cervix

Vagina

Figure 71.2 Dilation and curettage

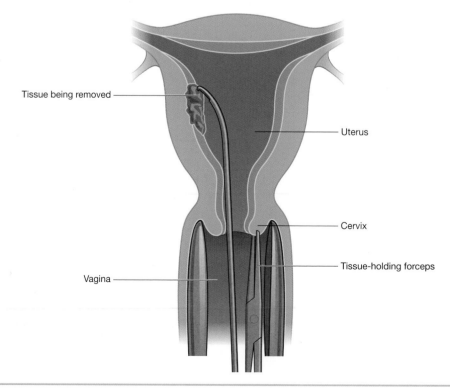

Tissue being removed

Uterus

Cervix

Tissue-holding forceps

Vagina

Medical-Surgical Nursing at a Glance, First Edition. Ian Peate. © John Wiley & Sons, Ltd. Published 2016 by John Wiley & Sons, Ltd.
Companion website: www.ataglanceseries.com/nursing/medsurg

Dilation and curettage (D&C) is a surgical procedure undertaken to remove tissue from the endometrium and takes approximately 10–15 minutes to perform. New techniques are now available to assist with assessment of the uterine cavity and the endometrium.

Dilation and curettage

The procedure is carried out for a number of reasons. Often it is carried out for diagnostic purposes or in association with a variety of pelvic conditions, for example, abnormal uterine bleeding or if there is any suspicion of endometrial carcinoma. Causes of abnormal bleeding include the presence of abnormal tissues, for example, fibroid tumours (myomas), polyps or cancer of the endometrium or uterus. A D&C may be used after a miscarriage to remove the fetus and other tissues if they have not all been passed naturally. If these tissues are not completely removed this can result in infection or heavy bleeding. This kind of D&C can also be called a surgical evacuation of the uterus or a D&E.

Occasionally after childbirth, small pieces of the placenta can remain adhered to the endometrium and are not passed and this can cause bleeding or infection. A D&C removes these fragments, encouraging endometrial healing.

There are two parts of the procedure.

1 Dilation –the cervix is dilated.
2 Curettage –aspects of the endometrium are removed using a sharp instrument.

This is often used in combination with a hysteroscope (Figure 71.1) when carrying out the operation; this enables the gynaecologist to assess for any abnormalities that may be present such as fibroids or polyps (Figure 71.2).

Usually the procedure is undertaken on an outpatient basis (in the day surgery unit or an ambulatory care setting), using a general anaesthetic; it is unusual for the woman to be kept in hospital overnight.

The procedure is performed through the vagina; the cervix is dilated using rods and a small, sharp scraping instrument known as a curette; this is passed into the uterus to gently scrape off the endometrium. If this is a diagnostic procedure then the tissue that has been removed (biopsy) is transported to a laboratory to be analysed and tested.

Potential risks associated with D&C

Dilation and curettage is usually very safe and complications are rare. However, as is the case with any surgical procedure, there are risks which include the following.

• Perforation of the uterus. This occurs when a surgical instrument perforates the uterus. This is more likely to happen in those women who were recently pregnant and also in women who have gone through menopause. The majority of perforations will heal spontaneously. If a blood vessel or another organ (such as the bowel) is damaged, then a second procedure may be required to repair it.
• Damage to the cervix. If the cervix is torn during the procedure, pressure is applied or the woman is given medication to stem the bleeding, or sutures are used to close the wound.
• Scar tissue (adhesions) on the uterine wall. Rarely, after D&C scar tissue can develop in the uterus which occurs most often

when the D&C is carried out after a miscarriage or delivery. This can cause abnormal, absent or painful menstrual cycles, future miscarriages and infertility.
• Infection after a D&C is possible, but this is rare.
• There may be other risks depending on the woman's specific medical condition.

The woman should inform the nurse if she:

• is allergic to or sensitive to medications, iodine or latex
• is pregnant or suspects that she may be pregnant
• has a vaginal, cervical or pelvic infection.

Preoperative care

Prior to the procedure, a detailed medical history is taken and a complete physical examination is performed in order to ensure that the woman is in good health. A series of blood tests are required as well as other diagnostic tests.

The procedure is explained to the woman and she is offered the opportunity to ask any questions concerning the procedure. A consent form will need to be signed.

If the procedure requires general anaesthesia, the woman will need to fast prior to the operation and this should be done in alignment with local policy and protocol. If performed under local anaesthesia, instructions concerning fasting are needed.

Postoperative care

The woman's postoperative nursing care and the recovery process will vary depending on the type of procedure performed and type of anaesthesia that was administered. If a general anaesthetic has been given, the woman is taken to the recovery room for observation. Once the blood pressure, pulse and breathing are stable and the woman is alert, she is transferred to the ward prior to discharge.

After a D&C the woman should rest for about 2 hours before going home. Analgesia may be required for cramping or soreness but aspirin should be avoided as this may increase the chance of bleeding. She can have normal diet and fluid as tolerated.

A sanitary pad should be provided for bleeding; it is normal to have some spotting or light vaginal bleeding for a few days after the procedure. The woman may experience cramping for the first few days after a D&C. She should be advised not to douche, use tampons or have intercourse for 2–3 days after a D&C or as recommended by the doctor. Other restrictions on activity, including no strenuous activity or heavy lifting, may be needed.

Inform the woman that because a D&C removes the lining of the uterus, the lining must regenerate and her next menstrual period may begin earlier or later than usual. Inform her that she should contact the doctor if she experiences any of the following post D&C.

• Bleeding that is heavy enough that she has to change pads every hour.
• Light bleeding lasting longer than 2 weeks.
• Temperature.
• Cramps that last more than 48 hours.
• Pain that gets worse as opposed to getting better.
• Foul-smelling discharge from the vagina.

A follow-up appointment will be required.

72 Cone Biopsy

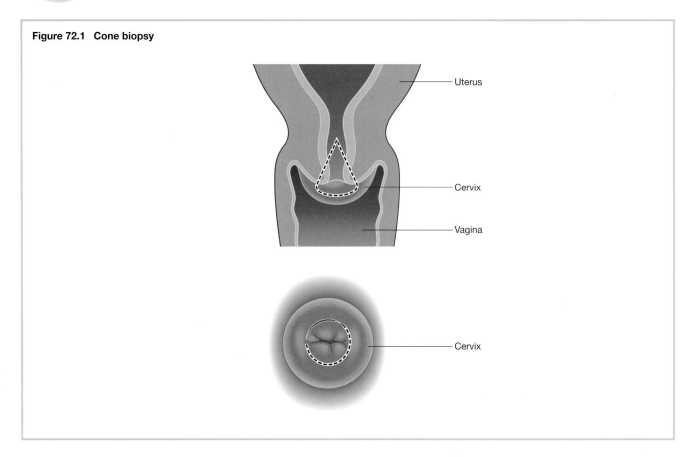

Figure 72.1 Cone biopsy

A cone biopsy is undertaken in order to remove abnormal cells from the cervix (Figure 72.1). The woman's previous cervical smears will have already shown an abnormality necessitating further investigation. This procedure allows for the removal of the abnormal cells to be microscopically examined. As part of the procedure, the nurse specialist or doctor can also see where the abnormal cells are and how extensive the area of abnormality is. The procedure can be used to diagnose cervical cancer or as a treatment to remove precancerous cells.

Cone biopsy

The cone biopsy may remove all of the abnormal tissue and if this is the case, this means that no further treatment is required apart from follow-up cervical smears.

The edges of the cervical tissue removed can contain abnormal cells, meaning that abnormal tissue may be left in the cervix. The cone biopsy may be repeated to remove the remaining abnormal cells. If follow-up tests demonstrate normal cells, then no further treatment is required. If abnormal cells remain, the gynaecologist and the woman may discuss other treatments, such as hysterectomy.

The cone biopsy may reveal that the cancer has grown deep into the cervical tissue and if this is the case, further treatment may be suggested, for example, surgery, radiotherapy or chemotherapy.

The procedure is usually performed under general anaesthesia; it is unusual for the woman to have to spend the night in hospital. Care provision must be designed to meet the individual woman's needs.

A cone-shaped piece of tissue is removed from the cervix using:

- a scalpel
- a carbon dioxide laser
- a loop electrosurgical excision procedure (LEEP).

A cone biopsy is an extensive form of a cervical biopsy. By undertaking a cone biopsy, abnormal tissue that is high in the cervical canal can be removed. A cone biopsy can:

- remove a thin or a thick cone of tissue from the cervix, depending on how much tissue is required for examination
- be used to diagnose and occasionally to treat abnormal cervical tissue. The abnormal tissue is removed and sent to a laboratory to be examined.

A lubricated speculum is inserted into the woman's vagina, allowing the inside of the vagina and the cervix to be examined. A cone biopsy using LEEP may be performed using a local anaesthetic.

Potential risks associated with cone biopsy

As with all surgery, there are potential risks, for example:

- serious haemorrhage requiring further treatment
- cervical stenosis (narrowing of the cervix)
- inability of the cervix to stay closed during pregnancy, which brings with it an increased risk of miscarriage or preterm delivery.

Preoperative care

The woman should be encouraged to stop smoking as this increases the risk of wound infection, as well as increasing the possibility of abnormal cells returning as smoke impacts negatively on the immune system.

The woman will need to fast if a general anaesthetic is to be administered. Local policy and procedure must be followed concerning fasting; this is typically 6 hours prior to surgery.

In order to gain informed consent, the woman needs to be provided with information that she understands regarding the procedure, what will happen before, during and after. The nurse acts as advocate and an opportunity must be given for the woman to ask questions regarding the procedure. A consent form will need to be signed.

Preoperative assessment will have been undertaken prior to admission for the procedure, including blood tests (and other tests and investigations if needed) and baseline assessment of vital signs. A past medical history is obtained and physical examination will have been performed.

Postoperative care

Immediately after surgery the woman is cared for in the recovery room where she is monitored and observed. When stable, she is transferred to the day surgery unit or the ward, where the nurse continues to monitor and observe the woman, assessing vital signs and reporting and documenting any abnormality. Specific postoperative instructions may have been given by the gynaecologist.

Prescribed pain relief may be required. The woman may have a vaginal pack *in situ* to help stop any bleeding; there may also be a urethral catheter and these will be removed prior to discharge.

Discharge advice

The woman will need to arrange for someone to drive her home.

Usually it takes about 4 weeks to make a full recovery from cone biopsy, but this varies between individuals.

Paracetamol or ibuprofen can be used as pain relief once discharged. There may be some light vaginal bleeding and discharge for up to 4 weeks after the procedure and this is normal. A sanitary towel as opposed to a tampon should be worn during this period.

Strenuous exercise and sexual intercourse should be avoided for around 4 weeks after the procedure. Douching should not be undertaken.

The woman should be advised to call the hospital or see the practice nurse/GP if she has:

- a temperature
- moderate to heavy bleeding (more than she usually has during a menstrual period)
- increasing pelvic pain
- bad-smelling or yellowish vaginal discharge.

Follow-up and further treatment may be needed and the nurse informs the woman of this when she is discharged.

73 Burns

Table 73.1 Types of burn

Type	Source
Radiation	Sunburn, radiotherapy and radiation
Electrical	From high voltage electricity
Thermal	From excessive heat, steam, extreme cold, liquids and surfaces
Chemical	Corrosive substances such as acid and alkali

Figure 73.1 The Rule of Nines

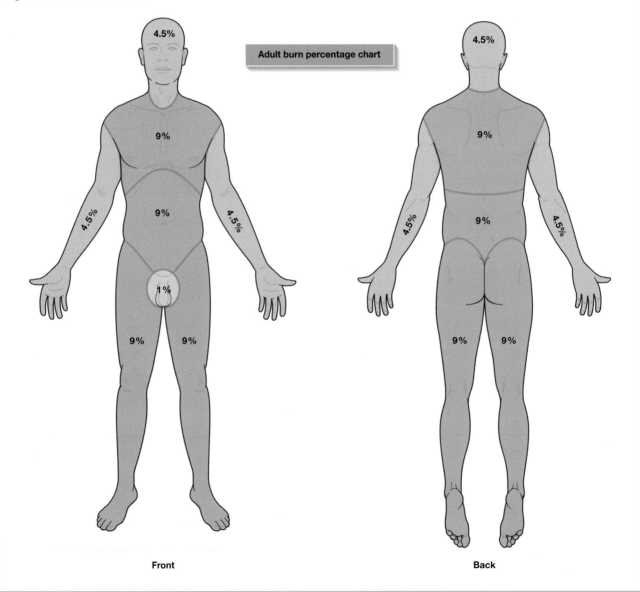

Adult burn percentage chart

Front

Back

Medical-Surgical Nursing at a Glance, First Edition. Ian Peate. © John Wiley & Sons, Ltd. Published 2016 by John Wiley & Sons, Ltd.
Companion website: www.ataglanceseries.com/nursing/medsurg

Burns have the potential to impact on all body systems, in particular the cardiovascular and renal systems. Caring for people with burns can set a unique challenge to the nurse as they pose a threat to the person's physical and emotional well-being.

A burn is an injury to the skin caused by heat, electricity, chemicals, radiation or friction and is a cause of significant morbidity. The majority of burns are accidental and many involve children, the older person, adults who are obese and those who have cardiovascular and neurological disorders. Even a minor burn can result in pain, scarring and infection.

Whilst most interventions are based on meeting the patient's physiological needs during the immediate and emergency phase of care, the nurse must also remember that the nature of the injury can present as a crisis for the individual and their family. Emotional support should be offered to the person (and if appropriate their family); the nurse must provide explanations for all procedures being undertaken, and provide comfort. Referral to other health and social care professionals may be needed.

The successful treatment of burns and the ongoing care of those people with severe burns require careful management, including the appropriate selection of dressings to support wound healing, and to achieve positive patient outcomes.

Types of burn

The origin of tissue destruction caused by a burn or a scald must be identified, as each type of burn requires a different management strategy. Hot liquids or steam cause scalds; fire, chemicals or electricity causes burns. See Table 73.1 for types of burns and source.

How the burn was sustained (the mechanism) may provide clues about its potential severity. Burns resulting from radiation are rare, apart from sunburn (ultraviolet light). Generally, the higher the temperature of the heat source and the longer the exposure, then the greater the damage to the skin as well as the underlying structures. However, damage may also occur at extremely low temperatures.

Scald injuries are dependent on temperature, volume and duration of the contact. The degree of skin damage is related to the thickness of the skin; hot oil, for example, causes deeper burns than water. Burns resulting from exposure to flames tend to cause deep damage and electrical burns usually result in full-thickness injuries. This type of burn can produce an entry and exit point. More than one reaction may take place at the same time with a chemical burn.

After first aid measures have been carried out, assessment of the patient with a burn may include the 'A, B, C, D, E, F' approach: A Airway maintenance, B Breathing, C Circulation and control of haemorrhage, D Disability – neurological status, E Exposure and environmental safety, F Fluid replacement and resuscitation. Adopting such a systematic approach may help the nurse to identify other injuries or complications posing a more immediate threat to the person than the burn itself.

Classification of burns

Burns are classified according to the depth of tissue damage (the total body surface area). Full-thickness burns involve all layers of the skin, extending into the adipose, muscle, connective tissue and bone layers. Deep partial-thickness burns involve the epidermis and dermis, hair follicles, sebaceous glands and sweat glands. Partial-thickness burns affect the epidermis, dermis and the papillae of the dermis. Superficial burns only affect the epidermis.

Other important information concerning the burn includes the history of the burn, time of injury, causative agent, any early treatment given, age and body weight. Initially on arrival, the person with a burn may be awake, but in a major burn injury conscious states can alter quickly and so these questions should be asked straight away.

Injury to the surface area is measured by body parts affected. The Rule of Nines divides the body into five surface areas (Figure 73.1); only partial- or full-thickness burns are included in the estimation. Any person with a burn who meets any of the following criteria should be transferred to a specialist burns unit for further management.

- Burns to the face, hands or feet.
- Burns to a person aged 5 years and under, and 60 years and over.
- Burns circumferential to a joint.
- Chemical and electrical burns.
- Inhalation injuries.
- More than 10% body surface in an adult.
- Any burn that has not healed in 14 days.

Nursing care

First aid for minor burns includes reducing the heat by placing the affected area under running cold water, wrapping the burn in cling-film, covering with a towel and applying ice to continue the heat reduction. Loose skin should be removed, leaving blisters intact to minimise the risk of infection. A non-adhesive dressing should be applied directly to the affected area and covered with an occlusive absorbent dressing. Review takes place after 24 hours. Pain relief should be provided. If there is infection then antibiotics will be required.

Preventing further fluid loss by wrapping the burns in cling-film is required for a major burn. Cold water or ice should not be applied to major burns as this can cause hypothermia. These patients should be referred immediately to a specialist burns unit after being medically resuscitated and stabilised.

With chemical burns, irrigation of the chemical is required for long periods using large amounts of water. A urine dipstick is used against the wet skin over the burn to help identify when irrigation has been sufficient (aiming to achieve a pH of 5.5). Irrigation will also be needed if eyes have been affected.

The person may need protective nursing and may need to be isolated due to the body's defence mechanism (the skin) being breached. A multidisciplinary team approach is required as the patient with burns goes through three phases of care: emergency, intermediate and rehabilitative.

74 Skin Grafts

Figure 74.1   Common sites of skin graft collection

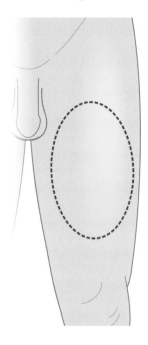
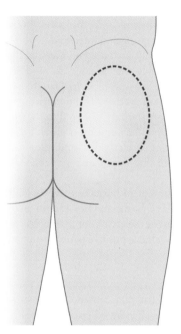

Figure 74.2   A full thickness graft with vein and artery

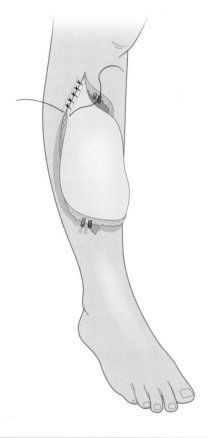

Medical-Surgical Nursing at a Glance, First Edition. Ian Peate. © John Wiley & Sons, Ltd. Published 2016 by John Wiley & Sons, Ltd.
Companion website: www.ataglanceseries.com/nursing/medsurg

Skin flaps

There are a number of reasons why a person may require a skin graft; for example, following burns surgery, those discharged from a specialist burns unit may require reconstruction of a burn wound. Just as there are a number of reasons why surgery is performed, there are also various types of flaps performed (as a part of plastic or reconstructive surgery).

A skin flap is a unit of tissue that is relocated from the donor site to the recipient site, at the same time maintaining its own blood supply (Figure 74.1).

Flaps range from simple advancements of skin to combinations of different types of tissue. These composites do not only consist of soft tissue, but can include skin, muscle, bone, fat or fascia.

A flap is transferred with its blood supply still intact, while a graft is a transfer of tissue without its own blood supply. The survival of the graft is therefore entirely dependent on the blood supply from the recipient site.

Flap classification

There are many methods that have been used to classify flaps; often they are complex and varied. There are three commonly used classifications.

- Type of blood supply
- Type of tissue to be transferred
- Location of donor site

Blood supply

Flaps, like any living tissue, must receive a sufficient blood flow to survive. A flap can maintain its blood supply in two main ways. A random flap is one that receives its blood supply from many unnamed vessels as opposed to a recognised artery. Numerous local cutaneous flaps fall into this category. When the blood supply comes from a recognised artery or group of arteries, this is known as an axial flap. The majority of muscle flaps have axial blood supplies. Figure 74.2 shows a full-thickness graft with vein and artery.

Tissue to be transferred

Generally, flaps can include, in part or in whole, nearly any part of the human body but there has to be an adequate blood supply to the flap once the tissue has been transferred. Flaps can be made up of just one type of tissue or several different types.

Those flaps that are composed of one type of tissue include skin, fascia, muscle, bone and viscera (such as colon, small intestine, omentum). Multiple flaps include fasciocutaneous (radial forearm flap), myocutaneous (transverse rectus abdominis muscle flap), osseocutaneous (fibula flap), tendocutaneous (dorsalis pedis flap) and sensory/innervated (dorsalis pedis flap with deep peroneal nerve).

Hence, an alternative way of classifying flaps is to describe the different kinds of tissue being used in the flap.

Location of donor site

Tissue can be transported from an area next to the defect, known as a local flap. These types of flaps are described based on their geometric design, and include rotation, transposition and interpolation.

Tissue that has been transferred from a non-contiguous anatomical site (from a different part of the body) is called a distant flap; these may be either pedicled (transferred while still attached to their original blood supply) or free (physically detached from their natural blood supply and then reattached to vessels at the recipient site).

Anastomosis is usually undertaken using a microscope and is referred to as a microsurgical anastomosis.

Performing flap surgery

The fundamental aim of plastic and reconstructive surgery is to provide restoration of function and aesthetic form.

As with any surgical procedure, flap surgery is not without risk. Complications can be devastating and a number of fundamental principles apply before, during and after surgery with the aim of improving outcome and decreasing operative morbidity.

The defect should be replaced like for like, for example, bone for bone, muscle for muscle, hairless skin for hairless skin. If it is not possible to replace like with like then the next most similar tissue substitute should be used. The aim is to conceal the reconstruction as much as possible.

Postoperative care and discharge

A skin flap may put a person at risk of infection or there may be haemorrhage. Antibiotics may be given for infection. Scars may form on both the donor site and recipient site and the skin may not look or feel the same.

In the first few weeks, the skin can become raised as the healing process occurs; usually this will settle down on its own and will eventually appear as a fine white line. After a skin graft the area will be a dusky pink colour and appear as a dent; this will improve as blood vessels grow into the skin from underneath (angiogenesis), but a dent may remain. The person may choose to wear make-up once the wound has become dry. The cosmetic appearance of the skin will continue to improve for up to 18 months. Massaging a moisturiser, for example E45 or Vaseline, into the flap/graft twice daily for 2–3 months can assist with the healing process.

The wound may be tender 1–2 hours after the excision as the effect of the local anaesthetic wears off. The dressing should be left in place for 48 hours or as advised by the dermatologist. The person should avoid strenuous exertion and stretching of the area until the sutures are removed and for some time afterwards. If bleeding occurs, advise the person to press on the wound firmly with a clean folded towel without removing the existing dressing or looking at it for 20 minutes. If bleeding continues after this time then medical attention should be sought.

The wound should be kept dry for 48 hours, and then can be gently washed and dried. If the wound becomes increasingly red or painful, the practice nurse or GP should be contacted.

Follow-up will be required and it is usual for sutures to be removed 5–10 days after the procedure.

75 Cosmetic and Plastic Surgery

Figure 75.1 Full abdominoplasty

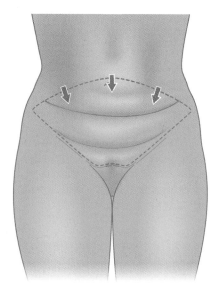 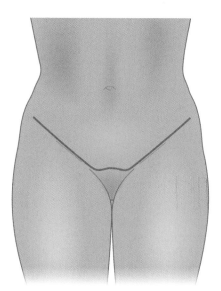

Table 75.1 Some potential complications post abdominoplasty

- Haemorrhage

- Ischaemia and subsequently poor wound healing and skin grafting may be required

- Scaring and abnormal skin alignment

- Shape of the anterior abdominal wall is changed causing other areas of the body to become more prominent, particularly the hips and the flanks

- Deep vein thrombosis and pulmonary embolism

- Paraesthesia over anterior abdominal wall

- Infection

Cosmetic surgery and plastic surgery are closely related specialties, but they are not the same. The terms are often incorrectly used interchangeably. Cosmetic surgery and plastic surgery have different goals. Whilst both cosmetic surgery and plastic surgery deal with improving a person's body, the overarching philosophies that guide the education, research and goals for patient outcomes differ.

Cosmetic surgery

The procedures, techniques and principles of cosmetic surgery concentrate on enhancing a patient's appearance. The key goal in this type of surgery is to improve aesthetic appeal, symmetry and proportion. Cosmetic surgery can be performed on all areas of the head, neck and body. As those areas to be treated usually function properly, cosmetic surgery is seen as elective surgery. The scope of the various cosmetic surgery procedures includes:

- breast enhancement: augmentation, lift, reduction
- facial contouring: rhinoplasty, chin or cheek enhancement
- facial rejuvenation: facelift, eyelid lift, neck lift, brow lift
- body contouring: abdominoplasty (tummy tuck), liposuction, gynaecomastia treatment
- skin rejuvenation: laser resurfacing, Botox®, filler treatments.

Plastic surgery

Plastic surgery is seen as a surgical specialty dedicated to the reconstruction of facial and body defects as a result of birth disorders, trauma, burns and disease. The aim of plastic surgery is to correct dysfunctional areas of the body and is by its nature reconstructive. Plastic and reconstructive surgeons are one in the same thing. These are some examples of plastic surgery procedures.

- Breast reconstruction
- Burn repair surgery
- Congenital defect repair: cleft palate, extremity defect repair
- Lower extremity reconstruction
- Hand surgery
- Scar revision surgery

Abdominoplasty

Abdominoplasty aims to remove excess fat and skin and in many cases can restore weakened or separated muscles to create an abdominal profile that is smoother and firmer. This procedure is not a substitute for weight loss nor can it correct stretch marks (striae), although these may be removed or improved if located on the areas of excess skin that will be excised.

Abdominoplasty is major surgery and is performed under general anaesthetic and can take between 2 and 5 hours. The person will need to be in hospital for 2–3 days. There are several types of abdominoplasty procedures available which are tailored to meet a person's needs and wishes.

Full abdominoplasty

This procedure is best suited for patients who have significant skin laxity (this may be the result of massive weight loss), excess fat and separation of the muscles; a full abdominoplasty is the most common procedure.

During the procedure, an incision is made above the symphysis pubis (hip to hip), below any existing scar line and around the umbilicus. The excess skin and fat are excised from the umbilicus to just above the pubic hair. The muscles below and above the umbilicus are tightened (Figure 75.1). The skin is then sutured to provide a circular scar around the umbilicus and a long scar across the lower aspect of the abdomen. This approach leaves a large scar but it does provide the greatest improvement in abdominal shape. Women contemplating pregnancy should not undergo this procedure.

Mini abdominoplasty

For those with only a small amount of excess skin, a lesser form of abdominoplasty may be more appropriate. This type of surgery will still require a general anaesthetic.

A wedge of skin and fat is excised from the lower aspect of the abdomen, leaving a horizontal scar above the pubic hair. The muscles may also be tightened. There is no scar left around the umbilicus but this may be stretched slightly, taking on a different shape.

Preoperative care

An assessment of the person's general medical condition is undertaken prior to the operation. A comprehensive medical history is taken which includes an assessment of the medications the person is taking. The person should be advised to stop smoking prior to surgery. Prophylactic antithromboembolic medications may be prescribed and the nurse must advise the person concerning local policy regarding fasting.

Postoperative care

The patient is nursed in the recovery room postoperatively until stable and is then transferred to the ward. Ongoing monitoring of vital signs is needed and any abnormalities must be reported to the nurse in charge.

The surgeon will have provided instructions concerning the position in which the patient is to be nursed. Specific positioning aims to take the pressure off the abdominal muscle to help with postoperative pain and discomfort.

Analgesia should be administered as prescribed and the effect recorded. If there are any drains *in situ*, these should be managed as per local policy; the nurse needs to note and report amount and type of drainage. An abdominal dressing will be in place, and the nurse observes this for signs of excessive oozing. If a Velcro fastening is used this can be loosened based on patient wishes and surgeon's instructions.

An intravenous infusion provides fluids until the patient is able to eat and drink. Small amounts of fluids should be commenced when the person feels able and this is gradually increased. The nurse promotes circulation and prevents clot formation in the veins of the legs by encouraging the patient to move the legs and to take regular deep breaths, expanding the lungs. The person is encouraged, with assistance, to mobilise gently over the next few days. Assistance is provided with the activities of living.

On discharge, the person should avoid doing any heavy lifting, straining or bending. The physiotherapist will provide advice on how to get up from a sitting position and how to roll as opposed to sitting straight up out of bed.

The wounds can be cleaned when they are sealed, usually from about a week. A firm corset is provided that should be worn at all times to reduce swelling and ease discomfort. Individual advice is given regarding wound care and taking a shower.

Some potential complications are listed in Table 75.1.

76 Cataract

Table 76.1   Some changes in vision that can occur with cataracts

- Cloudy, fuzzy, or foggy vision

- Glare from lamps or the sun, difficulty driving at night as a result of glare from car headlights

- The need for frequent changes to glasses prescription

- Diplopia in one eye

- Near vision may improve for a short time, this temporary improvement is known as second sight

Figure 76.1   Normal lens (a) **and lens affected by cataract** (b)

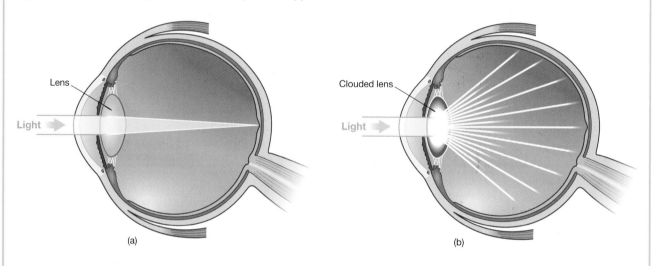

Lens

Light

(a)

Clouded lens

Light

(b)

Figure 76.2   Phacoemulsification

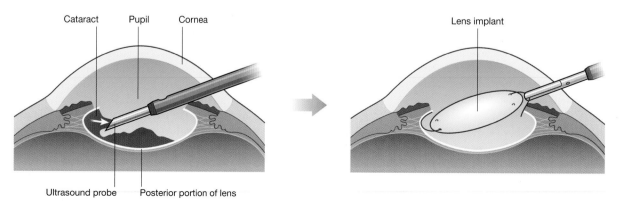

Cataract   Pupil   Cornea

Lens implant

Ultrasound probe   Posterior portion of lens

Medical-Surgical Nursing at a Glance, First Edition. Ian Peate. © John Wiley & Sons, Ltd. Published 2016 by John Wiley & Sons, Ltd.
Companion website: www.ataglanceseries.com/nursing/medsurg

A cataract is a painless, cloudy area in the lens of the eye which blocks the passage of light to the retina (Figure 76.1). The retina is the nerve layer located at the back of the eye; the nerve cells here detect the light that enters the eye, sending signals to the brain about what the eye is seeing. Cataracts block this light and so this can cause vision problems. Table 76.1 outlines the ways in which cataracts can effect vision.

Cataracts can occur as a result of a number of things. The ageing process (although ageing does not always lead to cataracts) and exposure to sunlight can cause cataracts. Cataracts may also happen following eye injury, for example as a result of eye disease, or as a result of some health problems, such as diabetes. Some children may be born with cataracts.

Treatment for cataract

Cataracts can be removed surgically which is the only effective method of treating them. Surgery is undertaken when the lost vision impacts on a person's quality of life. Surgery removes the cataract (the clouded lens of the eye). It is possible to replace the lens with an artificial one known as an intraocular lens implant (IOL); most people have a lens implanted. If an IOL cannot be used then contact lenses or, in some cases, glasses can make up for the implant.

For those who have bilateral cataracts, it is not usual to perform surgery on both eyes at the same time; the first eye needs to recover. An assessment is made to determine how much eyesight has improved prior to surgery being done on the second eye.

Types of surgery

There are two types of cataract surgery, both performed on an outpatient basis. Locally injected anaesthetic is used or the instillation of anaesthetic eye drops. The choice of surgical intervention will depend on what kind of cataract the person has.

Phacoemulsification (small-incision surgery)

This is the most common method of performing cataract surgery. Small incisions are made and ultrasound (sound waves) is used to break down the lens into small pieces (Figure 76.2).

Standard extracapsular cataract extraction (ECCE)

Here the lens and the anterior aspect of the lens capsule are opened and the lens is removed in one piece.

Preoperative care

Preoperative assessment is required; the aim is to ensure the person is fit for surgery and put a care plan in place. A detailed visual history will be undertaken along with a complete ophthalmic history. The impact of cataract on the patient's lifestyle should be evaluated. A full medical history should be taken with particular emphasis on medications that the person is taking that may increase the risk of surgery and any medical conditions that could make positioning or lying supine problematic.

In the preoperative period, it is essential that the nurse take into account the patient's social circumstances, for example, the availability of transport and provision of help at home.

Discussion must take place with the patient concerning risks and benefits of surgery, including any risks specific to them, along with type of anaesthesia and type of IOL. Time should be allowed for the person to ask questions. Informed consent should be obtained.

On the day of surgery, pupillary dilation through the administration of dilating drops (short-acting mydriatics) is needed, as adequate pupillary dilation is essential for cataract surgery. Other preoperative checks include identification of the patient and identification of the eye for surgery.

Postoperative care

After surgery and on return to the day care unit, the patient should be discharged when:

- the patient is comfortable and has no pain
- there are no problems (for example hyphaema) with the eye when examined by an ophthalmologist if called to see the patient.

Postoperative written advice, medications, appointments and emergency contact details are given to the patient. A discharge summary should be provided to the patient who will take this to their GP.

First-day postoperative review usually takes place over the telephone with an experienced nurse who contacts the patient to determine if there are any postoperative complications and to reinforce any advice offered after surgery. A first-day review visit may be required:

- where surgery was complicated
- where there is co-existing eye disease such as glaucoma or uveitis
- for patients with only one eye.

Follow-up is required for those patients not seen on the first postoperative day and a review appointment is necessary to:

- review progress and medication
- consider second eye surgery where applicable
- organise follow-up for co-existing eye disease
- provide guidance on spectacle prescription (which can be prescribed approximately 4 weeks after phacoemulsification).

Eye care after cataract surgery includes using the prescribed eye drops, protecting the eye and being alert to signs of infection. The patient should be advised to contact the doctor promptly if they notice any signs of complications, such as:

- decreasing vision
- increasing pain
- increasing redness
- swelling around the eye
- any discharge from the eye
- any new floaters, flashes of lights or changes in the field of vision.

The person should be advised that it is normal to have blurred vision and some swelling after surgery and that it takes time for the swelling to go down.

77 Mastoidectomy

Table 77.1 Advice for those recovering from ear surgery

- Nose blowing, sneezing and coughing should be avoided if possible. If the patient needs to cough or blow the nose this should be done gently, continue this approach for a week after surgery

- Do not drink through a straw for 2–3 weeks post operatively, avoid drinking from the mouth of a plastic bottle

- Limit physical activity for a week after surgery

- Avoid exercise and sports for 3 weeks or until the surgeon discharges the patient

- Keep the ear dry for 4–6 weeks

- Keep a cotton wool ball in the ear after the dressing is removed, change this daily

- Avoid contact with people who have coughs and colds

- Do not fly until the surgeon permits this

- If exposed to loud noise or working in loud environments wear ear protectors

Medical-Surgical Nursing at a Glance, First Edition. Ian Peate. © John Wiley & Sons, Ltd. Published 2016 by John Wiley & Sons, Ltd.
Companion website: www.ataglanceseries.com/nursing/medsurg

The mastoid

One of the most important structures of the inner ear is the mastoid bone. Whilst it is called a bone, the mastoid does not have the characteristic structures associated with bones. Rather than being solid and rigid like most bones, the mastoid is composed of air sacs and resembles a sponge.

The mastoid, the tympanic, squamous and petrous bones make up the temporal bone. There are several critical structures that are located within or traverse the temporal bone. The temporal bone is situated between the occipital bone posteriorly, the parietal bone superiorly, the sphenoid bone anteromedially and inferiorly the soft tissues of the neck. The mastoid is made up of a cortical osseous covering of changeable thickness and is filled with very thin osseous septations, which form an air cell system.

Indications for mastoidectomy

Chronic otitis media with or without cholesteatoma (an abnormal skin growth) is one of the most common reasons for performing a mastoidectomy. Those people with chronic otitis media often have otorrhoea (discharge from the ear) and progressive hearing loss. A mastoidectomy allows access to remove cholesteatoma or any diseased air cells, and can provide access to the temporal bone. Mastoidectomy is also one of the key steps required in placing a cochlear implant. The procedure is often a first step in removal of lateral skull base tumours.

Preoperative care

It is usual for a mastoidectomy to be performed under general anaesthesia. A preoperative temporal bone CT scan is required as this provides useful information concerning the anatomy of the temporal bone, particularly if this has been notably distorted by disease or previous surgery. Routine blood tests, chest X-ray and ECG may be required.

A detailed medical history is undertaken and this is usually done at a preoperative assessment clinic. The person should be advised that if they use ear drops, they should continue taking these unless otherwise advised by a doctor. Local policy with regard to fasting should be adhered to. Time should be given to the patient at the assessment clinic or on the day of the operation to ask questions if they need to. Informed consent must be gained.

Physical preparation may involve the removal of some of the scalp hair from around the ear. Those with long hair will need to have this secured so that it does not interfere with the operative site (behind the ear).

Postoperative care

On return to the ward, the position in which the patient is nursed is dictated by the surgeon, but the nurse needs to ensure that the airway is protected and patent. There will be a dressing and in some cases a drain may have been inserted.

The nurse is responsible for monitoring, recording and reporting vital signs as well as observing for any signs of damage that may have occurred to the facial nerve, which include the inability of the patient to:

- close the eyes
- wrinkle the forehead
- pucker the lips.

Fluids and food are gradually introduced when the patient is able to tolerate them. They may, however, be nauseous and may vomit, so prescribed antiemetics must be given.

The nurse should also protect the patient from injury. The patient may experience dizziness and loss of balance as a result of disturbance to the apparatus that controls equilibrium. When the person gets up from lying flat, this should be done slowly; they should sit first and then assume the upright position after any dizziness has passed. The nurse must advise the person about this as well as providing support to them.

Mastoid dressings vary depending on surgeon preference. The dressing is usually removed 24 hours post surgery. The patient should be advised to keep the operative ear dry; they can achieve this by covering it with a cup or placing a petroleum jelly-covered cotton wool ball over the external ear canal whilst taking a shower or washing their hair.

Postoperative care usually requires a visit to remove ear packing 1–2 weeks after surgery. Topical antibiotic drops will be prescribed on the following postoperative day after surgery. The drops have a dual purpose: they decrease the risk of a postsurgical infection as well as keeping the packing moist, which will facilitate easy removal of the pack. When the pack is removed will depend on the type of surgery. See Table 77.1 for patient advice suggestions.

Potential complications following surgery

There are a number of potential complications that may occur after surgery; infection and scar formation are two. The patient needs to be aware of the complications in order to give informed consent. Some other potential complications can include the following.

Facial nerve injury

A transient facial weakness can be seen in the immediate postoperative period, which usually settles within 2–4 hours. Postoperative facial nerve paralysis that does not resolve after a few hours requires exploration in the operating theatre.

Hearing loss

A temporary conductive hearing loss is common post mastoidectomy, as a result of blood, serous fluid and packing filling the middle ear space. A significant hearing loss is rare.

Vertigo

Vertigo and/or dizziness are frequent occurrences in those undergoing ear surgery. Permanent vestibular symptoms (vertigo/dizziness) are rare after mastoidectomy.

Change in taste

Patients usually notice an altered sensation of taste, often described as a metallic or sour taste on the affected side. This sensation can be persistent but it often resolves over a period of months.

Vascular injury

Blood vessels can be injured with a drill or microinstruments. During surgery, gentle, continuous pressure is needed over the vessel until the bleeding is controlled.

Dural damage

On rare occasions leakage of cerebral spinal fluid may occur, especially when there is abnormal anatomy and the disease process has involved the dura and this has become damaged.

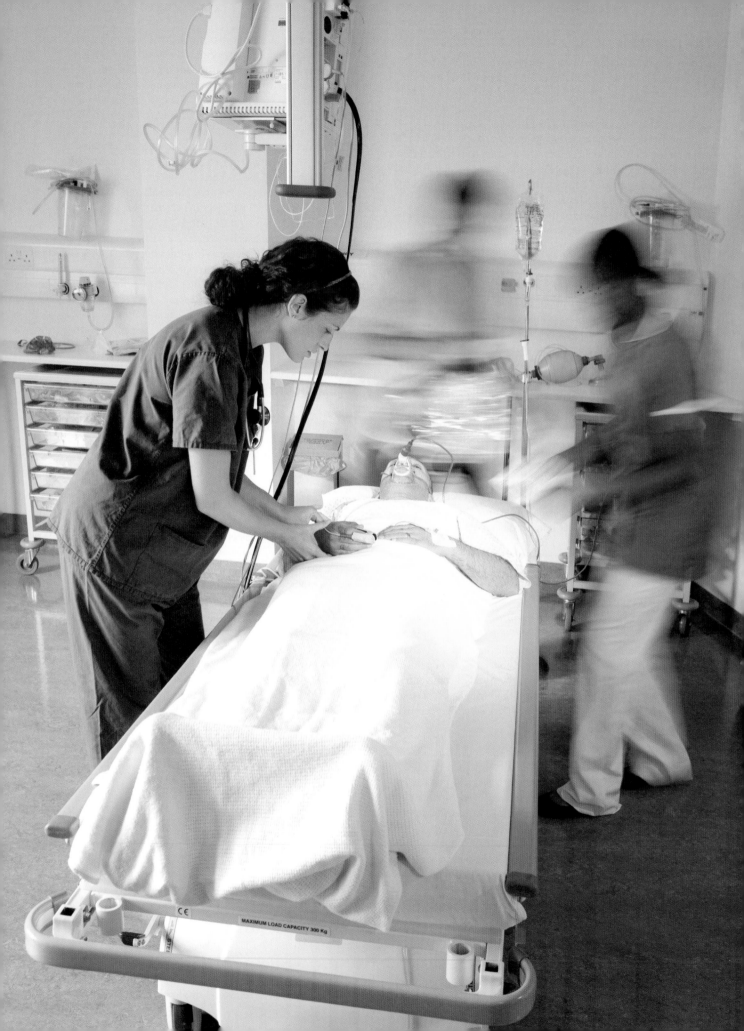

Appendix 1: Normal Values

Haematology

Full blood count
Haemoglobin (males) 13.0–18.0 g/dL
Haemoglobin (females) 11.5–16.5 g/dL
Haematocrit (males) 0.40–0.52
Haematocrit (females) 0.36–0.47
Mean corpuscular volume (MCV) 80–96 fL
Mean corpuscular haemoglobin (MCH) 28–32 pg
Mean corpuscular haemoglobin concentration (MCHC)
  32–35 g/dL
White cell count $4–11 \times 10^9$/L

White cell differential

Neutrophils $1.5–7 \times 10^9$/L
Lymphocytes $1.5–4 \times 10^9$/L
Monocytes $0–0.8 \times 10^9$/L
Eosinophils $0.04–0.4 \times 10^9$/L
Basophils $0–0.1 \times 10^9$/L
Platelet count $150–400 \times 10^9$/L
Reticulocyte count $25–85 \times 10^9$/L or 0.5–2.4%

Erythrocyte sedimentation rate

Westergren under 50 years:
  Males 0–15 mm/1st hour
  Females 0–20 mm/1st hour

Over 50 years:
  Males 0–20 mm/1st hour
  Females 0–30 mm/1st hour

Plasma viscosity

(25°C) 1.50–1.72 mPa/s

Coagulation screen

Prothrombin time 11.5–15.5 s
International normalised ratio <1.4
Activated partial thromboplastin time 30–40 s
Fibrinogen 1.8–5.4 g/L
Bleeding time 3–8 min

Coagulation factors

Factors II, V, VII, VIII, IX, X, XI, XII 50–150 IU/dL
Factor V Leiden:
Von Willebrand factor 45–150 IU/dL
Von Willebrand factor antigen 50–150 IU/dL
Protein C 80–135 IU/dL
Protein S 80–120 IU/dL
Antithrombin III 80–120 IU/dL
Activated protein C resistance 2.12–4.0

Fibrin degradation products <100 mg/L
D-dimer screen <0.5 mg/L

Haematinics

Serum iron 12–30 µmol/L
Serum iron-binding capacity 45–75 µmol/L
Serum ferritin 15–300 µg/L
Serum transferrin 2.0–4.0 g/L
Serum B_{12} 160–760 ng/L
Serum folate 2.0–11.0 µg/L
Red cell folate 160–640 µg/L
Serum haptoglobin 0.13–1.63 g/L

Haemoglobin electrophoresis

Haemoglobin A >95%
Haemoglobin A2 2–3%
Haemoglobin F <2%

Chemistry

Serum sodium 137–144 mmol/L
Serum potassium 3.5–4.9 mmol/L
Serum chloride 95–107 mmol/L
Serum bicarbonate 20–28 mmol/L
Anion gap 12–16 mmol/L
Serum urea 2.5–7.5 mmol/L
Serum creatinine 60–110 µmol/L
Serum corrected calcium 2.2–2.6 mmol/L
Serum phosphate 0.8–1.4 mmol/L
Serum total protein 61–76 g/L
Serum albumin 37–49 g/L
Serum total bilirubin 1–22 µmol/L
Serum conjugated bilirubin 0–3.4 µmol/L
Serum alanine aminotransferase 5–35 U/L
Serum aspartate aminotransferase 1–31 U/L
Serum alkaline phosphatase 45–105 U/L (over 14 years)
Serum gamma glutamyl transferase 4–35 U/L (<50 U/L in males)
Serum lactate dehydrogenase 10–250 U/L
Serum creatine kinase (males) 24–195 U/L
Serum creatine kinase (females) 24–170 U/L
Creatine kinase MB fraction <5%
Serum troponin I 0–0.4 µg/L
Serum troponin T 0–0.1 µg/L
Serum copper 12–26 µmol/L
Serum caeruloplasmin 200–350 mg/L
Serum aluminium 0–10 µg/L
Serum magnesium 0.75–1.05 mmol/L
Serum zinc 6–25 µmol/L
Serum urate (males) 0.23–0.46 mmol/L
Serum urate (females) 0.19–0.36 mmol/L
Plasma lactate 0.6–1.8 mmol/L
Plasma ammonia 12–55 µmol/L

Serum angiotensin converting enzyme 25–82 U/L
Fasting plasma glucose 3.0–6.0 mmol/L
Haemoglobin A1 C 3.8–6.4%
Fructosamine <285 μmo/L
Serum amylase 60–180 U/L
Plasma osmolality 278–305 mosmol/Kg

Urine

Albumin/creatinine ratio (untimed specimen):
  Males <3.5 mg/mmol
  Females <2.5 mg/mmol

Lipids and lipoproteins

The target levels will vary depending on the patient's overall
  cardiovascular risk assessment.
Serum cholesterol <5.2 mmol/L
Serum LDL cholesterol <3.36 mmol/L
Serum HDL cholesterol >1.55 mmol/L
Fasting serum triglyceride 0.45–1.69 mmol/L

Blood gases (breathing air at sea level)

Blood H+ 35–45 nmol/L
pH 7.36–7.44
PaO_2 11.3–12.6 kPa
$PaCO_2$ 4.7–6.0 kPa
Base excess ± 2 mmol/L

Carboxyhaemoglobin

Non-smoker <2%
Smoker 3–15%

Immunology/rheumatology

Complement C3 65–190 mg/dL
Complement C4 15–50 mg/dL
Total haemolytic (CH50) 150–250 U/L
Serum C-reactive protein <10 mg/L

Serum immunoglobins

IgG 6.0–13.0 g/L
IgA 0.8–3.0 g/L
IgM 0.4–2.5 g/L
IgE <120 kU/L
Serum beta-2 microglobulin <3 mg/L

Cerebrospinal fluid

Opening pressure 50–180 mm H_2O
Total protein 0.15–0.45 g/L
Albumin 0.066–0.442 g/L
Chloride 116–122 mmol/L
Glucose 3.3–4.4 mmol/L
Lactate 1–2 mmol/L
Cell count ≤5 mL[1]
Differential:
  Lymphocytes 60–70%
  Monocytes 30–50%
  Neutrophils None
  IgG/ALB ≤0.26
  IgG index ≤0.88

Urine

Glomerular filtration rate 70–140 mL/min
Total protein <0.2 g/24 h
Albumin <30 mg/24 h
Calcium 2.5–7.5 mmol/24 h
Urobilinogen 1.7–5.9 μmol/24 h
Coproporphyrin <300 nmol/24 h
Uroporphyrin 6–24 nmol/24 h
Delta-aminolaevulinate 8–53 μmol/24 h
5-hydroxyindoleacetic acid 10–47 μmol/24 h
Osmolality 350–1000 mosmol/kg

Faeces

Nitrogen 70–140 mmol/24 h
Urobilinogen 50–500 μmol/24 h
Fat (on normal diet) <7 g/24 h

Appendix 2: Glossary of Terms

Abdominoplasty   A surgical procedure used to remove excess fat and skin

Acquired   An acquired disorder is a medical condition which develops after birth

Acute   Of sudden onset

Aetiology   The cause of a disease or condition

Aggregate   Clumping together in the blood

Allergen   Substance that can produce hypersensitivity reactions in the body

Analgesia   Pain killer

Anaphylaxis   A severe, systemic allergic response characterised by vasodilation and bronchoconstriction

Aneurysm   A bulging in the weak wall of an artery

Annuloplasty   A surgical technique to repair leaking mitral valves

Anorexia   Loss of appetite

Anoxia   Total depletion of oxygen

Antiemetic   Antisickness medication

Antigen   Substance (often protein) causing formation of an antibody that reacts specifically with that antigen

Anuria   No urine produced

Aphasia   Without speech

Aplastic anaemia   Disease in which the bone marrow, and the blood stem cells that reside there, are damaged, resulting in reduced blood cells

Arteries   Blood vessels that transport blood away from the heart

Ascites   Accumulation of fluid in the peritoneal cavity

Asepsis   The state of being free from disease or contaminants

Atheromatous plaque   A deposit or degenerative accumulation of lipid-containing plaque on the innermost layer of the artery wall

Atrophy   Decrease in size

Autoimmune disease   A disease resulting from a disordered immune reaction in which antibodies are produced that damage components of one's own body

Autologous   Obtained from the same individual

Basophil   A type of white blood cell

Benign   Non-malignant

Beta-blocker   A class of drug often used to treat cardiac arrhythmias

Brudzinski's sign   Flexion of the neck that causes hip and knee to flex

Calculi   Stones

Capillaries   Small blood vessels where exchanges between blood and tissue cells occur

Carcinogen   Cancer-causing substance

Carcinoma   A malignancy originating in epithelial tissues

Cardiac output   Volume of blood pumped out every minute by the ventricles

Chronic   A disease developing gradually and lasting longer than 3 months

Cilia   Hair-like projections that sweep dust and other foreign particles out

Colonoscopy   An examination that views the inside of the colon (large intestine) and rectum, using a tool called a colonoscope

Congenital   A condition existing at birth and often before birth

Coronary revascularisation   The restoration of perfusion to the coronary arteries as a result of ischaemia

Cyanosis   Blue discoloration, usually of the lips and fingers

Cytomegalovirus   A viral genus of the viral family known as herpesviridae

Cytotoxic drug   Chemotherapy drug

Defaecate   To pass stool (motion)

Demyelination   To destroy or remove the myelin sheath (of a nerve fibre), as through disease

Diaphoresis   Excessive sweating

Dyspepsia   Indigestion

Dyspnoea   Difficulty in breathing

Dysrhythmia   An abnormal cardiac rhythm

Embolus   A detached travelling mass (could be blood or fat)

Endoscope   A device designed to look inside body cavities

Engulfing   Swallowing up

Enzymes   Proteins that speed up chemical reactions in a cell

Eosinophil   A type of white blood cell

Epididymo-orchitis   An inflammation of the epididymis or testes

Epigastric   Relating to the abdominal region lying between the hypochondriac regions and above the umbilical region

Erythema   Redness

Erythropoietin   A hormone that stimulates the production of red blood cells in the bone marrow

Exacerbation   An increase in the severity of a disease or any of its signs or symptoms

Fatigue   Extreme tiredness

Fibrinogen   A protein in the blood plasma that is essential for the coagulation of blood and is converted to fibrin by the action of thrombin in the presence of ionised calcium

Fistula   An abnormal connection between an organ, vessel or intestine and another structure

Genetics   Concerns the process of trait inheritance from parents to offspring

Haematemesis   Vomiting of blood

Haematoma   A swelling containing blood (bruising)

Haemopoiesis   The formation of blood cells in the living body (especially in the bone marrow)

Haemoptysis   Coughing of blood

Hemiparesis   Weakness of the entire left or right side

Hepatomegaly   Enlarged liver

Hydronephrosis   A condition where one or both kidneys become stretched and swollen as a result of a build-up of urine inside the kidney(s)

Hypercalcaemia   High levels of calcium in the blood

Hyperkalaemia   High levels of potassium in the blood

Hyperplasia   Increase in cell number

Hypersensitivity reaction   An altered immunological response to an antigen resulting in a pathological immune response upon re-exposure

Hypertrophy   To increase in size

Hypoalbuminaemia   A medical condition where levels of albumin in blood serum are abnormally low

Hypoglycaemia   Low blood glucose

Hypokalaemia   Low levels of potassium in the blood

Hyponatraemia   Low levels of sodium in the blood

Hypoperfusion   Decreased blood flow through an organ, as in hypovolaemic shock; if prolonged, it may result in permanent cellular dysfunction and death

Hypothermia   A condition where the core body temperature is below 35°C

Hypoxaemia   A lower than normal oxygen content of the blood as measured in an arterial blood sample

Idiopathic   Having no demonstrable cause

Immune response   A defence function of the body that produces antibodies to destroy invading antigens and malignancies

Immunoglobulins   Antibodies

Immunosuppressants   Powerful medicines that dampen down the activity of the body's immune system

Inflammation   A biological response

Inflammatory response   Tissue reaction to injury or to an antigen; can include pain, swelling, itching, redness, heat and loss of function

Inotrope   A drug that alters the force or energy of muscular contractions

Ischaemia   Insufficient perfusion of oxygenated blood to a body organ or part

Kernig's sign   Inability to extend the knee while the hip is flexed at a 90° angle

Laryngitis   Inflammation of the larynx

Laxative   Substance used to loosen stools and increase bowel movements

Lethargy   Lack of energy

Ligament   Fibrous tissue that connects bones to other bones

Lobectomy   Removal of a lobe

Lymphadenopathy   Abnormally sized lymph glands

Macrophage   A cell which ingests and destroys microbes and foreign matter

Malaise   A vague feeling of bodily discomfort, as at the beginning of an illness

Mast cell   A cell found in the connective tissue that releases histamine during inflammation

Melaena   Black faeces that may be associated with a gastric bleed

Metastasis   Spread of tumour cells

Microemboli   Tiny blood clots

Mucoprotein   Any of a group of organic compounds, such as the mucins, that consist of a complex of proteins and glycosaminoglycans and are found in body tissues and fluids

Mutation   Alteration or change

Myalgia   Muscle pain

Necrosis   Death of cells or tissues through injury or disease, especially in a localised area of the body

Negative feedback mechanisms   Mechanisms that usually result in a response that balances a change in system

Neoplasia   Growth of cells and tissue into new areas, resulting in a tumour. Can be benign or malignant

Oesophagus   Gullet

Oliguria   Reduced urine output

Orthostasis   Maintenance of an upright standing posture

Palliation   To make the effects of something less harmful

Palpate   To feel

Pathogenesis   Events leading to the development of a disease and the signs and symptoms occurring as the disease progresses

Pathology   The study of changes in cell/tissue structure related to disease or death

Pathophysiology   The study of the disturbance of normal mechanical, physical and biochemical functions, either caused by a disease or resulting from a disease or abnormal syndrome or condition

Percutaneous   Access via the skin

Peripheral   The outer aspect

Peritonitis   Inflammation of the peritoneal cavity

Petechiae   Pinpoint-sized reddish-purple spots on the skin

Petechial rash   Small spots

Phagocytes   White blood cells

Phagocytose   To envelop and destroy bacteria and other foreign material

Phlebectomy   Surgical treatment to remove superficial varicose veins

Phonophobia   A fear of loud sounds

Photophobia   Aversion to light

Polycystic   Containing many cysts

Polyps   A small growth, usually benign and with a stalk, protruding from a mucous membrane.

Proctitis   Inflammation of the rectum

Prophylactic   In prevention of

Prosthesis   A device designed to replace a missing part of the body

Psychosocial   Involving the psychic and social aspects of a person

Pyrexia   Raised temperature

Pyuria   Pus in the urine

Sclera   The white of the eye

Septicaemia   Blood infection

Shock   A condition of severely inadequate blood flow to the body's peripheral tissues, associated with life-threatening cellular dysfunction; also known as hypoperfusion

Sigmoidoscopy   A procedure used to see inside the sigmoid colon and rectum

Sinusoids   Small blood vessels, similar to capillaries

Speculum   An instrument used for the investigation of body orifices

Stenosis   Narrowing of any canal or opening, for example, the intestine, a blood vessel, a heart valve

Syndrome   A collection of signs and symptoms

Synovitis   Inflammation of the synovia

Systemic   A condition that affects the entire body

Tachycardia   Rapid heart rate[100 beats per minute]

Tachypnoea   Rapid breathing[20 breaths per minute]

Thromboxane   A substance made by platelets that causes blood clotting and constriction of blood vessels

Thrombus   A blood clot forming in a vessel and remaining there

Tinnitus   The perception of a noise in one or both ears, for example, a ringing in the ears

Uraemia   Accumulation of waste products, normally excreted in the urine, in the blood; causes severe headaches, vomiting

Vasculitis   Inflammation of the wall of a blood vessel

Venules   Small veins

Wheezing   A coarse whistling sound produced when airways are partially obstructed

Further Reading

Hinkle, J.L. (2014) *Brunner & Suddarth's Textbook of Medical-surgical Nursing*, 13th edn. Philadelphia: Lippincott.

Nair, M. and Peate, I. (eds) (2013) *Fundamentals of Applied Pathophysiology*, 2nd edn. Oxford: Wiley.

Peate, I. and Nair, M. (2011) (eds) *Fundamentals of Anatomy and Physiology for Student Nurses*. Oxford: Wiley.

Peate, I., Nair, M., Hemming, L. and Wild, K. (2012) *LeMone and Burke's Adult Nursing: Acute and Ongoing Care*. Harlow: Pearson.

Peate, I., Wild, K. and Nair, M. (eds) (2014) *Nursing Practice, Knowledge and Care*. Oxford: Wiley.

Pudner, R. (2010) *Nursing the Surgical Patient*, 3rd edn. Edinburgh: Baillière Tindall.

Index

Page numbers in *italics* refer to tables and figures